ANESTHESIA
A COMPREHENSIVE REVIEW

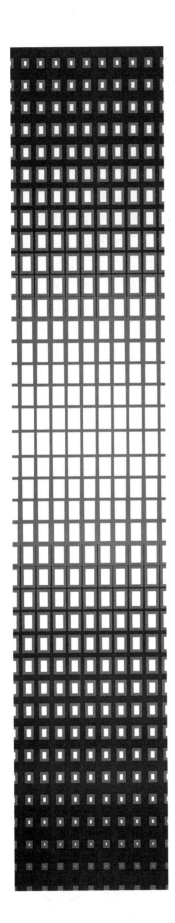

ANESTHESIA
A COMPREHENSIVE REVIEW

Second Edition

Brian A. Hall, M.D.
Assistant Professor of Anesthesiology
Department of Anesthesiology
Mayo Clinic
Rochester, MN

and

Keith A. Jones, M.D.
Assistant Professor of Anesthesiology
Department of Anesthesiology
Mayo Clinic
Rochester, MN

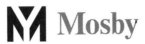 Mosby

St. Louis Baltimore Boston Carlsbad Chicago Naples New York Philadelphia Portland
London Madrid Mexico City Singapore Sydney Tokyo Toronto Wiesbaden

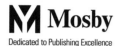
Mosby

Dedicated to Publishing Excellence

A Times Mirror Company

Senior Editor: Laurel Craven
Senior Developmental Editor: Kimberley Cox
Project Manager: Chris Baumle
Production Editor: Anthony Trioli
Design Manager: Nancy McDonald
Manufacturing Manager: William A. Winneberger, Jr.

Second Edition
Copyright © 1997 by Mayo Foundation.

Previous edition copyrighted 1992

Printed in the United States of America
Composition by Clarinda Composition and Prepress Services
Printing and binding by R. R. Donnelley & Sons Company

Mosby–Year Book, Inc.
11830 Westline Industrial Drive
St. Louis, Missouri 63146

Library of Congress Cataloging-in-Publication Data

Hall, Brian A.
    Anesthesia : a comprehensive review / Brian A. Hall and Keith A.
Jones.—2nd ed.
      p.   cm.
    Includes bibliographical references and index.
    ISBN 0-8151-4192-0
    1. Anesthesiology—Examinations, questions, etc.
2. Anesthesiology—Outlines, syllabi, etc.   I. Jones, Keith A.,
M.D. II. Title.
    [DNLM: 1. Anesthesia—examination questions.   WO 218.2 H174a
1997]
RD82.3.H35   1997
617.9'6'076—dc21
DNLM/DLC
for Library of Congress
                   96-45302
                   CIP

98 99 00 01 / 9 8 7 6 5 4 3 2

Contributing Authors

Renee Caswell, M.D.
Instructor in Anesthesiology
Department of Anesthesiology
Mayo Clinic
Rochester, MN

Robert Chantigian, M.D.
Associate Professor of Anesthesiology
Department of Anesthesiology
Mayo Clinic
Rochester, MN

Roger Hofer, M.D.
Assistant Professor of Anesthesiology
Department of Anesthesiology
Mayo Clinic
Rochester, MN

Ronald Kufner, M.D.
Instructor in Anesthesiology
Department of Anesthesiology
Mayo Clinic
Rochester, MN

C. Thomas Wass, M.D.
Instructor in Anesthesiology
Department of Anesthesiology
Mayo Clinic
Rochester, MN

Preface to the Second Edition

The emergence of new techniques and pharmacologic agents as well as a broader understanding of older concepts and ideas add to the ever growing body of knowledge in anesthesiology. The aim of this book is to underscore important principles in the practice of anesthesiology and to question the reader about these.

Many questions from the first edition have been replaced by new problems which relate to material not covered previously. The remaining questions have been re-referenced to the latest editions of major textbooks. New tables have been added to the second edition to summarize, contrast, and review detailed information which does not lend itself to easy retention. Likewise, new figures have been included in both the questions and explanations to visually emphasize major points.

This book is intended for new practitioners of anesthesia preparing for the certifying examination as well as the anesthesia veteran who may be preparing for the re-certification examination or for any individual desiring to test his or her knowledge. This is not a textbook, rather a learning tool which directs the reader to specific sources for additional information about the topic at hand.

Brian A. Hall, M.D.
Keith A. Jones, M.D.

Preface to the First Edition

The acquisition and mastery of knowledge is a lifelong process, the most intense segment of which occurs during residency. From day one the anesthesia resident is confronted with many avenues of learning which include textbook, journals, lectures, refresher courses, colleagues, and of course, his or her own clinical experiences.

Although these sources represent a vast reservoir of information, each of them lacks one essential element; they do not test the participant on the material presented. This book represents a set of questions which was written over the last 4 years for the purpose of teaching our residents specific facts or concepts about anesthesia. Each question is designed to test knowledge of one or more pertinent topics. At the end of each multiple-choice section are located the answers and concise explanations for the material covered in the questions. For the reader desiring additional information, there is a specific reference, usually to an anesthesia textbook, with an exact page location.

With such an abundance of information available in the field of anesthesia, it may be difficult to focus on the clinically relevant material. Our goal is to test knowledge of important principles and not to present trivia or minutia. This book is not intended to replace textbooks, but to augment them.

Brian A. Hall, M.D.
Keith A. Jones, M.D.

Credits

The following figures are reprinted with permission.

Figure with Question 32
van Genderingen HR, Gavenstein N, et al: J Clin Monit 3:198, 1987.

Figure with Question 93-96
Stoelting RK, Miller RD (eds): Basics of Anesthesia, ed 3. New York, Churchill Livingstone, Inc., 1994, p 135.

Figure with Question 102
Bonica JJ (ed): Principles and Practice of Obstetric Analgesia and Anesthesia. Baltimore, Waverly, 1967, p 24.

Figure with Question 524
Stoelting RK, Dierdorf SF (eds): Anesthesia and Co-existing Disease, ed 3. New York, Chruchilll Livingstone, Inc., 1993, p 172.

Figure with Question 574
Avery ME: Lung and Its Disorders in the Newborn, ed 3. Philadelphia, W. B. Saunders, 1974, p 134.

Figure with Question 590
Moore KL (ed): Clinically Oriented Anatomy. Baltimore, Williams & Wilkins, 1980, p 653.

Figure with Question 640
Benedetti TJ: Obstetric hemorrhage. In: Gabbe SG, Niebyl JR, Simpson JL (eds): Obstetrics: Normal and Problem Pregnancies, ed 2. New York, Churchill Livingstone, 1991, p 585.

Figure with Question 750
Miller RD (ed): Anesthesia, ed 3. New York, Churchill Livingstone, 1990, p 1745.

Figure with Question 825
Raj PP: Practical Management of Pain ed 2. St Louis, Mosby–Year Book, 1992, p 785.

Figure with Question 947
Jackson JM, Thomas SJ, Lowenstein E: Anesthetic Management of Patients with Valvular Heart Disease. Seminars in Anesthesia 1:244, 1982.

Figure with Question 961
Morgan GE, Mikhail MS: Clinical Anesthesiology, ed 1. East Norwalk, Appleton & Lange, 1992, p 301.

Figure with Question 962
Spiess BD, Ivankovich AD: Thromboelastography: A Coagulation-Monitoring Technique Applied to Cardiopulmonary Bypass. In: Effective Hemostasis in Cardiac Surgery. Philadelphia, W. B. Saunders Company, 1988, p 165.

Figure with Question 986
Rorie DK: Monitoring During Cardiovascular Surgery. In: Tarhan S: Cardiovascular Anesthesia and Postoperative Care ed. 2. St. Louis, Mosby–Year Book, Inc., 1989, p 69.

Figure with Question 986A
Rorie DK: Monitoring During Cardiovascular Surgery. In: Tarhan S: Cardiovascular Anesthesia and Postoperative Care, ed 2. St. Louis, Mosby–Year Book, Inc., 1980, p 70.

Figure with Question 986B
Rorie DK: Monitoring During Cardiovascular Surgery. In: Tarhan S: Cardiovascular Anesthesia and Postoperative Care, ed 2. St. Louis, Mosby–Year Book, Inc., 1980, p 71.

Acknowledgements

Completion of the second edition would never have occurred were it not for the assistance of many individuals. In addition to the contributing authors, the authors would like to express their gratitude to Drs. Alison Albrecht, Raul Buelvas, Paul Carns, Jonathan Cohen, Philip Leeds, Christine Liu, Douglas Loveless, David Martin, Brian McGlinch, David Ransom, and Lawrence Schroeder for painstakingly re-referencing all of the questions from the first edition which were used in the second edition. The authors would also like to thank Drs. Borislav Banjac, Roxann Barnes, Stephen Foster, Jack Gaspari, James Hough, Todd Kor, David Martin, Angel Martinez, Brian McGlinch, Jeff Mueller, Scott Nelson, Malcolm Sanders, and Lawrence Schroeder for proofreading the chapters. Several other individuals deserve recognition for reviewing and advising us on specific points in the text. These include but are not limited to Drs. Dorothee Bremerich, Brian Donahue, Ronald Faust, Randall Flick, Scott LeBard, Robert Lunn, David Munce, Lee Nauss, Steven Rettke, Edwin Rho, Klaus Torp, Denise Wedel, and Roger White.

We also wish to thank Susan Gay for initiating the second edition project, Laurel Craven for seeing the project through to the end, and Kimberley Cox and Anthony Trioli for managing the technical aspect of the production of the second edition.

We are also indebted to our secretary, Michelle Schendel, for meticulously typing and re-typing hundreds of pages of manuscript.

Brian A. Hall, M.D.
Keith A. Jones, M.D.

Contents

PART I / BASIC SCIENCES

Physics, Biochemistry, and Anesthesia Equipment

DIRECTIONS (Questions 1 through 69): Each of the questions or incomplete statements in this section is followed by answers or by completions of the statement, respectively. Select the ONE BEST answer or completion for each item.

1. A 58-year-old patient has severe shortness of breath and "wheezing." On examination, the patient has inspiratory and expiratory stridor. Further evaluation reveals marked extrinsic compression of the proximal trachea by a tumor. The type of air flow at the point of obstruction within the trachea is

   A. Laminar flow
   B. Orifice flow
   C. Undulant flow
   D. Stenotic flow
   E. None of the above

2. Concerning the patient in question 1, administration of 70% helium in O_2 instead of 100% O_2 will decrease the resistance to air flow through the stenotic region within the trachea because

   A. Helium decreases the viscosity of the gas mixture
   B. Helium decreases the friction coefficient of the gas mixture
   C. Helium decreases the density of the gas mixture
   D. Helium decreases the Reynold's number of the gas mixture
   E. None of the above

3. A 56-year-old patient is brought to the OR for elective replacement of a stenotic aortic valve. An awake 20-gauge arterial catheter is placed into the right radial artery and is then connected to a transducer located at the same level as the patient's left ventricle. The entire system is zeroed at the transducer. Several seconds later the patient raises both arms into the air such that his right wrist is 20 cm above his heart. As he is yawning, the blood pressure on the monitor reads 120/80. What would this patient's true blood pressure be at this time?

   A. 140/100 mm Hg
   B. 135/95 mm Hg
   C. 120/80 mm Hg
   D. 105/65 mm Hg
   E. 100/60 mm Hg

4. To avoid cardiac microshock, total leakage current for catheters or electrodes placed close to the heart must be less than

   A. 1 μamp
   B. 10 μamp
   C. 20 μamp
   D. 50 μamp
   E. 1 mamp

5. The relationship between intra-alveolar pressure, surface tension, and the radius of an alveolus is described by

    A. Graham's law
    B. Beer's law
    C. Newton's law
    D. Laplace's law
    E. Bernoulli's law

6. A size "E" compressed-gas cylinder completely filled with N_2O contains how many liters?

    A. 1,160
    B. 1,470
    C. 1,590
    D. 1,640
    E. 1,750

7. Halothane is administered from a vernitrol vaporizer to a patient in a submarine cabin (pressurized to 1,200 mm Hg). The carrier-gas flow through the vaporizing chamber is 200 mL/min. What diluent fresh gas flow is required to deliver 2% halothane to the patient?

    A. 1,000 mL/min
    B. 2,250 mL/min
    C. 3,500 mL/min
    D. 4,750 mL/min
    E. Cannot be calculated

8. Which of the following valves prevents transfilling between compressed-gas cylinders?

    A. Fail-safe valve
    B. Pop-off valve
    C. Pressure-sensor shutoff valve
    D. Adjustable pressure-limiting valve
    E. Outlet check valve

9. The expression that for a fixed mass of gas at constant temperature, the product of pressure and volume is constant is known as

    A. Graham's law
    B. Bernoulli's law
    C. Boyle's law
    D. Dalton's law
    E. Charles' law

10. The pressure gauge on a size "E" compressed-gas cylinder containing O_2 reads 1,600 psia (pounds per square inch at absolute temperature). How long could O_2 be delivered from this cylinder at a rate of 2 L/min?

    A. 90 min
    B. 140 min
    C. 245 min
    D. 320 min
    E. Cannot be calculated

11. A 25-year-old healthy patient is anesthetized for a femoral hernia repair. Anesthesia is maintained with isoflurane and N_2O 50% in O_2 and the patient's lungs are mechanically ventilated. Suddenly, the "low-arterial-saturation" warning signal on the pulse oximeter alarms. After disconnecting the patient from the anesthesia machine, he is ventilated with an AMBU bag with 100% O_2 without difficulty and the arterial saturation quickly improves. During inspection of your anesthesia equipment, you notice that the bobbin in the O_2 rotameter is not rotating. This most likely indicates

    A. The flow of N_2O through the O_2 rotameter
    B. No flow of O_2 through the O_2 rotameter
    C. A flow of O_2 through the O_2 rotameter that is markedly lower than indicated
    D. A leak in the O_2 rotameter above the bobbin
    E. A leak in the O_2 rotameter below the bobbin

12. The O_2 pressure-sensor-shutoff valve requires what O_2 pressure to remain open and allow N_2O to flow into the N_2O rotameter?

    A. 10 psia
    B. 25 psia
    C. 50 psia
    D. 100 psia
    E. 600 psia

13. A 78-year-old patient is anesthetized for resection of a liver tumor. After induction and tracheal intubation, a 20-gauge arterial line is placed and is connected to a transducer which is located 20 cm below the level of the heart. The system is zeroed at the stopclock located at the wrist while the patient's arm is stretched out on an arm board. How will the arterial line pressure compare with the true blood pressure?

    A. It will be 20 mm Hg higher
    B. It will be 15 mm Hg higher
    C. It will be the same
    D. It will be 15 mm Hg lower
    E. It will be 20 mm Hg lower

14. The second-stage O_2 pressure regulator delivers a constant O_2 pressure to the rotameters of

    A. 4 psia
    B. 8 psia
    C. 16 psia
    D. 32 psia
    E. 64 psia

15. The highest trace concentration of N_2O allowed in the operating room atmosphere by the National Institute for Occupational Safety and Health (NIOSH) is

    A. 1 part per million (ppm)
    B. 5 ppm
    C. 25 ppm
    D. 50 ppm
    E. 100 ppm

16. A Fluotec (halothane) vaporizer will deliver an accurate concentration of an unknown volatile anesthetic if the latter shared which property with halothane?

    A. Molecular weight
    B. Viscosity
    C. Vapor pressure
    D. Blood:gas partition coefficient
    E. Oil:gas partition coefficient

17. The portion of the ventilator on the anesthesia machine which compresses the bellows is driven by

    A. Compressed oxygen
    B. Compressed air
    C. Electricity alone
    D. Electricity and compressed oxygen
    E. Electricity and compressed air

18. Which of the following rotameter flow indicators is read in the middle of the dial?

    A. Bobbin
    B. "H" float
    C. Ball float
    D. Skirted float
    E. Nonrotating float

19. When the pressure gauge on a size "E" compressed-gas cylinder containing N_2O begins to fall from its previous constant pressure of 750 psia, how many liters of gas will remain in the cylinder?

    A. 200
    B. 400
    C. 600
    D. 800
    E. Cannot be calculated

20. A 3-year-old child with severe congenital facial anomalies is anesthetized for extensive facial reconstruction. After inhalation induction with halothane and oral tracheal intubation, a 22-gauge arterial line is placed in the right radial artery. The arterial cannula is then connected to a transducer which is located 10 cm below the patient's heart. After zeroing the arterial line at the transducer, how will the given pressure compare with the true arterial pressure?

    A. It will be 10 mm Hg higher
    B. It will be 7.5 mm Hg higher
    C. It will be the same
    D. It will be 7.5 mm Hg lower
    E. It will be 10 mm Hg lower

21. If the diameter of an intravenous catheter is doubled, flow through the catheter will

    A. Decrease by a factor of 2
    B. Decrease by a factor of 4
    C. Increase by a factor of 8
    D. Increase by a factor of 16
    E. Increase by a factor of 32

22. Of the following statements concerning the safe storage of compressed-gas cylinders, choose the one that is **FALSE**.

    A. Should not be handled with oily hands
    B. Should not be stored near flammable material
    C. Should not be stored in extreme heat or cold
    D. Paper or plastic covers should not be removed from the cylinders before storage
    E. All of the above statements are true

23. For any given concentration of volatile anesthetic, the splitting ratio is dependent on which of the following characteristics of that volatile anesthetic?

    A. Vapor pressure
    B. Barometric pressure
    C. Molecular weight
    D. Specific heat
    E. Minimum alveolar concentration at 1 atmosphere

24. A mechanical ventilator is set to deliver a tidal volume (V_T) of 500 mL at a rate of 10 breaths/min and an inspiratory-to-expiratory (I:E) ratio of 1:2. The fresh-gas flow into the breathing circuit is 6 L/min. In a patient with normal total pulmonary compliance, the actual V_T delivered to the patient would be

    A. 400 mL
    B. 500 mL
    C. 600 mL
    D. 700 mL
    E. 800 mL

25. In reference to question 24, if the ventilator rate is decreased from 10 to 6 breaths/min, the actual V_T delivered to the patient would be

    A. 600 mL
    B. 700 mL
    C. 800 mL
    D. 900 mL
    E. 1,000 mL

26. Vaporizers for which of the following volatile anesthetics could be used interchangeably with accurate delivery of the concentration of anesthetic set on the vaporizer dial?

    A. Halothane, enflurane, and isoflurane
    B. Enflurane, isoflurane
    C. Halothane, enflurane
    D. Halothane, isoflurane
    E. None of the above

27. Which of the following is the basis for the mechanism of air-O_2 dilution systems that utilize the Venturi principle?

    A. Newton's law
    B. Hagen-Poiseuille's law
    C. Henry's law
    D. Graham's law
    E. Bernoulli's law

28. According to NIOSH regulations, the highest concentration of volatile anesthetic contamination allowed in the operating room atmosphere when administered in conjunction with N_2O is

    A. 0.5 ppm
    B. 2 ppm
    C. 5 ppm
    D. 25 ppm
    E. 50 ppm

29. The device on anesthesia machines that most reliably detects delivery of hypoxic gas mixtures is the

    A. Fail-safe valve
    B. O_2 analyzer
    C. Second-stage O_2 pressure regulator
    D. Proportion-limiting control system
    E. Diameter index safety system

30. A ventilator pressure-relief valve stuck in the closed position can result in

    A. Barotrauma
    B. Hypoventilation
    C. Hypoxia
    D. Hyperventilation
    E. A low breathing-circuit pressure

31. 1% enflurane, 70% N_2O and 30% O_2 are administered to a patient for 30 minutes. The expired enflurane concentration measured is 1%. N_2O is shut off and a mixture of 30% O_2, 70 N_2 with 1% enflurane is administered. The expired enflurane concentration measured 10 minutes after the start of this new mixture is 2.3%. The best explanation for this observation is

    A. Intermittent back pressure (pumping effect)
    B. Diffusion hypoxia
    C. Concentration effect
    D. Effect of N_2O solubility in enflurane
    E. Effect of similar mass:charge ratios of N_2O and CO_2

32.

    The mass spectrometer wave form above represents which of the following situations?

    A. Cardiac oscillations
    B. Kinked endotracheal tube
    C. Bronchospasm
    D. Incompetent inspiratory valve
    E. Incompetent expiratory valve

33. Select the **FALSE** statement.

    A. If a Magill forceps is used for a nasotracheal intubation, the right nares is preferable for insertion of the nasotracheal tube
    B. Extension of the neck can convert an endotracheal intubation to an endobronchial intubation
    C. Bucking signifies the return of the coughing reflex
    D. Postintubation pharyngitis is more likely to occur in females
    E. Stenosis becomes symptomatic when the adult tracheal lumen is reduced to less than 5 mm

34. Gas from a N_2O compressed-gas cylinder enters the anesthesia machine through a pressure regulator that reduces the pressure to

    A. 60 psia
    B. 45 psia
    C. 30 psia
    D. 15 psia
    E. 10 psia

35. Which of the following factors is least responsible for killing bacteria in anesthesia machines?

    A. Metallic ions
    B. High O_2 concentration
    C. Anesthetic gases (at clinical concentrations)
    D. Shifts in humidity
    E. Shifts in temperature

36. Which of the following systems prevents attachment of gas-administering equipment to the wrong type of gas line?

    A. Pin-index safety system
    B. Diameter index safety system
    C. Fail-safe system
    D. Proportion-limiting control system
    E. None of the above

37. A volatile anesthetic has a saturated vapor pressure of 360 mm Hg at room temperature. At what flow would this agent be delivered from a bubble-through vaporizer if the carrier-gas flow through the vaporizing chamber is 100 mL/min?

    A. 30 mL/min
    B. 60 mL/min
    C. 90 mL/min
    D. 120 mL/min
    E. 150 mL/min

38. The total saturated vapor pressure in a half-full size "E" compressed-gas cylinder containing 50% O_2 and 50% N_2O by volume (entonox) is 1,100 psia. The partial saturated vapor pressure of N_2O within this cylinder is

    A. 375 psia
    B. 450 psia
    C. 500 psia
    D. 550 psia
    E. Cannot be calculated

39. Which of the following would result in the greatest decrease in the arterial hemoglobin saturation (SpO_2) value measured by the dual wave length pulse oximeter?

    A. Intravenous injection of indigo carmine
    B. Intravenous injection of indocyanine green
    C. Intravenous injection of methylene blue
    D. Presence of elevated bilirubin
    E. Presence of fetal hemoglobin

40. Body plethysmography can be used to measure lung volumes by application of

    A. Boyle's law
    B. Dalton's law
    C. Newton's law
    D. Laplace's law
    E. Bernoulli's law

41. Which of the following combinations would result in delivery of a higher-than-expected concentration of volatile anesthetic to the patient?

    A. Halothane vaporizer filled with enflurane
    B. Halothane vaporizer filled with isoflurane
    C. Isoflurane vaporizer filled with halothane
    D. Isoflurane vaporizer filled with enflurane
    E. Enflurane vaporizer filled with halothane

42. The factors that determine the net flow of fluid across capillary membranes are described in

    A. Fick's law
    B. Graham's law
    C. Fick's principle
    D. Starling's law
    E. Henry's law

43. The most important determinant of resistance to laminar gas flow through a tube is the

    A. Length of the tube
    B. Radius of the tube
    C. Viscosity of the gas
    D. Density of the gas
    E. Mass of the gas

44. All of the following would result in less trace gas pollution of the operating room atmosphere **EXCEPT**

    A. Using a high gas flow in a circular system
    B. Tight mask seal during mask induction
    C. Use of a scavenger system
    D. Periodic maintenance of the anesthesia machine
    E. Allow patient to breath 100% O_2 as long as possible before extubation

45. The greatest source for contamination of the operating room atmosphere is leakage of volatile anesthetics

    A. Around the anesthesia mask
    B. At the vaporizer
    C. At the rotameter
    D. At the CO_2 absorber
    E. At the endotracheal tube

46. Uptake of enflurane from the lungs during the first minute of general anesthesia is 200 mL. How much enflurane would be taken up from the lungs between the 16th and 36th minutes?

    A. 100 mL
    B. 200 mL
    C. 400 mL
    D. 700 mL
    E. 2,000 mL

47. The predominant component of baralyme granules is

    A. Water
    B. Silica
    C. Barium hydroxide
    D. Calcium hydroxide
    E. Potassium hydroxide

48. Select the **FALSE** statement regarding iatrogenic bacterial infections from anesthetic equipment.

    A. Even low concentrations of O_2 are lethal to airborne bacteria
    B. Bacteria that are released from the airway during violent exhalation originate almost exclusively from the anterior oropharynx
    C. Of all the bacterial forms, acid fast bacteria are the most resistant to destruction
    D. Shifts in temperature and humidity are probably the most important factors responsible for bacterial killing
    E. Bacterial filters in the anesthesia breathing system lower the incidence of postoperative pulmonary infections

49. Frost develops on the outside of an N_2O compressed-gas cylinder during general anesthesia. This phenomenon indicates that

    A. The saturated vapor pressure of N_2O within the cylinder is rapidly increasing
    B. The cylinder is almost empty
    C. There is a rapid transfer of heat to the cylinder
    D. The flow of N_2O from the cylinder into the anesthesia machine is rapid
    E. None of the above

50. The **LEAST** reliable site for central temperature monitoring is the

    A. Rectum
    B. Skin on forehead
    C. Distal third of the esophagus
    D. Nasopharynx
    E. Tympanic membrane

51. A balanced anesthetic is administered to an otherwise healthy 38-year-old patient undergoing repair of a right inguinal hernia. During mechanical ventilation, the anesthesiologist notices that the scavenging-reservoir bag is distended during inspiration. The most likely cause of this is

    A. An incompetent pressure-relief valve in the mechanical ventilator
    B. An incompetent pressure-relief valve in the patient breathing circuit
    C. An incompetent inspiratory unidirectional valve in the patient breathing circuit
    D. An incompetent expiratory unidirectional valve in the patient breathing circuit
    E. None of the above; the scavenging-reservoir bag is supposed to distend during inspiration

52. The reason a 40:60 mixture of helium:O_2 is more desirable than a 40:60 mixture of nitrogen:O_2 for a spontaneously breathing patient with tracheal stenosis is

    A. Helium has a lower density than nitrogen
    B. Helium is a smaller molecule than O_2
    C. Absorption atelectasis decreased
    D. Helium has a lower critical velocity for turbulent flow than does O_2
    E. Helium is toxic to most microorganisms

53. The maximum F_IO_2 that can be delivered by a nasal cannula is

    A. 0.25
    B. 0.30
    C. 0.35
    D. 0.40
    E. 0.45

54. Each of the following statements concerning rotameters is true **EXCEPT** which one?

    A. Rotation of the bobbin within the Thorpe tube is important for accurate function
    B. The Thorpe tube increases in diameter from bottom to top
    C Its accuracy is affected by changes in temperature and atmospheric pressure
    D. The rotameter for N_2O and CO_2 are interchangeable
    E. The rotameter for O_2 should be the last in the series

55. Which color of nail polish would have the greatest effect on the accuracy of dual-wavelength pulse oximeters?

    A. Red
    B. Yellow
    C. Blue
    D. Green
    E. White

56. The minimum macroshock current required to elicit ventricular fibrillation is

    A. 1 mamp
    B. 10 mamp
    C. 100 mamp
    D. 500 mamp
    E. 5,000 mamp

57. The line isolation monitor

    A. Prevents microshock
    B. Prevents macroshock
    C. Provides electrical isolation in the operating room
    D. Sounds an alarm when grounding occurs in the operating room
    E. Provides a safe electrical ground

58. Kinking of the transfer tubing from the patient breathing circuit to the closed scavenging-system interface can result in

    A. Barotrauma
    B. Hypoventilation
    C. Hypoxia
    D. Hyperventilation
    E. None of the above

59. At what concentration should the isoflurane vaporizer dial be set to deliver 1 minimum alveolar concentration (MAC) of isoflurane in Denver, Colorado (assume P_B is 630 mm Hg)?

    A. 0.75%
    B. 0.9%
    C. 1.15%
    D. 1.4%
    E. 1.6%

60. Select the **FALSE** statement regarding noninvasive arterial blood-pressure-monitoring devices.

    A. If the width of the blood-pressure cuff is too narrow, the measured blood pressure will be falsely lowered
    B. The width of the blood-pressure cuff should be 40% of the circumference of the patient's arm
    C. If the blood-pressure cuff is too loosely wrapped around the arm, the measured blood pressure will be falsely elevated
    D. Oscillometric blood-pressure measurements are accurate in neonates
    E. Frequent cycling of automated blood pressure-monitoring devices can result in edema distal to the cuff

61. An incompetent ventilator pressure-relief valve can result in

    A. Hypoxia
    B. Barotrauma
    C. A low-circuit-pressure signal
    D. Hypoventilation
    E. Hyperventilation

62. The pressure gauge of a size "E" compressed-gas cylinder containing air shows a pressure of 900 psia. How long could air be delivered from this cylinder at the rate of 10 L/min?

    A. 10 min
    B. 20 min
    C. 30 min
    D. 40 min
    E. 50 min

63. The most frequent cause of mechanical failure of the anesthesia-delivery system to deliver adequate O_2 to the patient is

    A. Attachment of the wrong compressed-gas cylinder to the O_2 yoke
    B. Crossing of pipelines during construction of the operating room
    C. Improperly assembled O_2 rotameter
    D. Fresh-gas line disconnection from the anesthesia machine to the in-line hosing
    E. Disconnection of the O_2 supply system from the patient

64. How many mL of vapor at 37°C are derived from 1 mL of liquid enflurane at 20°C?

    A. 100 mL
    B. 200 mL
    C. 300 mL
    D. 400 mL
    E. 500 mL

65. The expression that the rate of passive diffusion of a gas across a lipid membrane is inversely proportional to the square root of the molecular weight of the gas is known as

    A. Dalton's law
    B. Graham's law
    C. Boyle's law
    D. Nagen-Poiseuille's law
    E. Fick's law

66. The volume of O_2 in a half-full compressed-gas cylinder can be calculated by application of

    A. Boyle's law
    B. Dalton's law
    C. Graham's law
    D. Charles' law
    E. None of the above

67. A 75-year-old patient with COPD is ventilated with a mixture of 50% oxygen with 50% helium. 2% isoflurane is added to this mixture. What effect will helium have on mass spectrometer reading of the isoflurane concentration?

    A. The mass spectrometer will give a slightly increased false value.
    B. The mass spectrometer will give a false value equal to double the isoflurane concentration.
    C. The mass spectrometer will give the correct value.
    D. The mass spectrometer will give a wrong value equal to half the isoflurane concentration.
    E. The mass spectrometer will give an erroneous value slightly less than the correct value of isoflurane.

68. At high altitudes, the flow of a gas through a rotameter will be

    A. Greater than expected
    B. Less than expected
    C. Greater than expected at high flows but less than expected at low flows
    D. Less than expected at high flows but greater than expected at low flows
    E. Greater than expected at high flows but accurate at low flows

69. The volume of N_2O in a half-full compressed-gas cylinder can be calculated by application of

    A. Boyle's Law
    B. Dalton's Law
    C. Graham's Law
    D. Charles' Law
    E. None of the above

DIRECTIONS (Questions 70 through 92): For each of the items in this section, ONE or MORE of the numbered options is correct. Select the answer:

Select A if options *1, 2 and 3* are correct,
Select B if options *1 and 3* are correct,
Select C if options *2 and 4* are correct,
Select D if only option *4* is correct,
Select E if *all* options are correct.

70. During spontaneous breathing through a circle system, the anesthesia bag contracts during inspiration. To flow from the anesthesia bag to the patient, O_2 must pass through which of the following devices?

    1. Common gas outlet
    2. Inspiratory valve
    3. Ventilator bellows
    4. CO_2 absorber

Select A if options *1, 2 and 3* are correct,
Select B if options *1 and 3* are correct,
Select C if options *2 and 4* are correct,
Select D if only option *4* is correct,
Select E if *all* options are correct.

71. Advantages of the Bain anesthesia breathing circuit include

   1. Improved humidification of the fresh-gas inflow as a result of partial rebreathing
   2. Ease of scavenging waste anesthetic gases from the overflow valve
   3. Rewarming of the fresh-gas inflow by the surrounding exhaled gases
   4. Ease of detecting kinking of the inner tube

72. Which of the following alarms would sound if the anesthesia breathing circuit became disconnected from the patient's endotracheal tube?

   1. The high pressure alarm
   2. The continuing pressure alarm
   3. The subatmospheric pressure alarm
   4. The minimum ventilation pressure alarm

73. True statements concerning the arterial pressure waveform generated in the radial artery compared with that generated in the aortic root include which of the following?

   1. The systolic pressure is higher
   2. The pulse pressure is greater
   3. The diastolic pressure is lower
   4. The mean arterial pressure is higher

74. Which of the following mechanical ventilator parameters can influence the tidal volume delivered to patients?

   1. The ventilator rate
   2. The fresh-gas flow
   3. The inspiratory-to-expiratory (I:E) ratio
   4. Positive end-expiratory pressure

75. Mass spectrometry readings of nitrogen are taken in a patient who is intubated and on a ventilator. The inspired nitrogen concentration is 0 and expired nitrogen is 3.2%. Possible explanations for these findings would include:

   1. Nitrogen washout
   2. A leak in the CO_2 absorber
   3. Air embolism
   4. A deflated endotracheal cuff

Select A if options *1, 2 and 3* are correct,
Select B if options *1 and 3* are correct,
Select C if options *2 and 4* are correct,
Select D if only option *4* is correct,
Select E if *all* options are correct.

76. The markings on compressed-gas cylinders designate

    1. The contents of the cylinder
    2. The maximal permissible pressure allowed within the cylinder
    3. Dates of prior transportation of the cylinder
    4. The size of the cylinder

77. Turbulent gas flow through a tube increases

    1. Linearly with the pressure gradient down the tube
    2. Linearly with the density of the gas
    3. To the fourth power of the radius of the tube
    4. Approximately to the square of the radius of the tube

78. Which of the following materials will not ignite during laser surgery of the airway?

    1. Rubber
    2. Silicone
    3. Polyvinylchloride
    4. Metal

79. Prior to administering general anesthesia to a patient, the anesthesiologist checks for leaks in the anes-
    thesia machine by closing the adjustable pressure-limiting (pop-off) valve, occluding the patient end
    of the breathing circuit, and filling the system *via* the O_2 flush valve until the reservoir bag is full and
    there is a pressure within the circuit of approximately 15 to 20 cm H_2O. The anesthesia machine con-
    tains an outlet-check valve at the common gas outlet. The O_2 flow is then slowly decreased until the
    pressure no longer rises. This technique will identify *gross* leaks in which of the following compo-
    nents of the anesthesia machine?

    1. Unidirectional expiratory valve
    2. Unidirectional inspiratory valve
    3. CO_2 absorber
    4. Vaporizer

80. True statements concerning the structure and function of the Bain anesthesia-breathing circuit include
    which of the following?

    1. The fresh-gas inflow is located near the patient
    2. The overflow valve is located near the reservoir bag
    3. The amount of rebreathing depends on the fresh-gas inflow rate
    4. Can be used efficiently during controlled ventilation

Select A if options *1, 2 and 3* are correct,
Select B if options *1 and 3* are correct,
Select C if options *2 and 4* are correct,
Select D if only option *4* is correct,
Select E if *all* options are correct.

81. True statements concerning a closed scavenging-system interface include which of the following?

    1. Failure to connect the system interface to the wall suction will result in barotrauma to the patient
    2. Excessive wall suction will result in hypoventilation of the lungs
    3. The scavenging reservoir bag will distend during inspiration
    4. The scavenging reservoir bag will distend during expiration

82. Baralyme granules are composed of

    1. Calcium hydroxide
    2. Sodium hydroxide
    3. Water
    4. Silica

83. True statements concerning soda lime granules include which of the following?

    1. A specific water content is required for optimal activity
    2. The hardness of the granules is caused by the addition of silica
    3. The reaction of CO_2 with the granules produces heat
    4. The granules consist primarily of sodium and potassium hydroxide

84. Which of the following determine the efficiency of CO_2 neutralization by CO_2 absorption canisters?

    1. Channeling
    2. Tidal volume
    3. Size of the granules
    4. pH of the fluid inside the canister

85. Which of the following factors cause over-damping of direct arterial pressure waveforms?

    1. Long length of tubing
    2. Low viscosity of fluid in tubing
    3. Small radius of tubing
    4. Low compliance of tubing

86. The pin-index safety system prevents

    1. Attachment of gas-administration equipment to the wrong gas line
    2. Delivery of a hypoxic mixture from the rotameters to the patient
    3. Delivery of the wrong gas from the central supply source
    4. Incorrect yoke to compressed-gas cylinder connections

Select A if options *1, 2 and 3* are correct,
Select B if options *1 and 3* are correct,
Select C if options *2 and 4* are correct,
Select D if only option *4* is correct,
Select E if *all* options are correct.

87. The saturated vapor pressure of volatile anesthetics

    1. Is dependent on the temperature of the liquid
    2. Is dependent on the atmospheric pressure above the liquid
    3. Decreases during use of the vaporizer
    4. Increases during use of the vaporizer

88. Which of the following can result in excessive overflow of gas from the scavenging system reservoir bag?

    1. High fresh-gas flow into the patient breathing circuit
    2. A positive-end expiratory pressure (PEEP) valve located in the patient breathing circuit
    3. A scavenging-system interface not connected to the wall suction
    4. Excessive suction applied to the scavenging-system interface

89. Of the following arrangements of rotameters on the anesthesia machine, which is (are) safe (gas flow is from left to right)?

    1. N_2O, air, O_2
    2. O_2, air, N_2O
    3. Air, N_2O, O_2
    4. Air, O_2, N_2O

90. Operation at high altitudes will affect the accurate function of which of the following devices?

    1. Mechanical ventilator
    2. Vaporizer
    3. CO_2 absorber
    4. O_2 rotameter

91. Hazards associated with laser surgery include

    1. Endotracheal tube fire
    2. Atmospheric contamination
    3. Ocular injury
    4. Venous gas embolism

92. Disadvantage(s) of the Bain anesthesia breathing circuit include

    1. Requirement for high fresh-gas inflow rates when used during spontaneous ventilation
    2. Increased resistance to breathing
    3. Unrecognized disconnection or kinking of the inner tube
    4. Inability to scavenge waste anesthetic gases

DIRECTIONS (Questions 93 through 96): This group of questions consists of several numbered statements followed by lettered headings. For each numbered statement, select the ONE lettered heading that is most closely associated with it. Each lettered heading may be selected once, more than once, or not at all.

93. Best for spontaneous ventilation

94. Best for controlled ventilation

95. Bain system

96. Jackson-Rees system

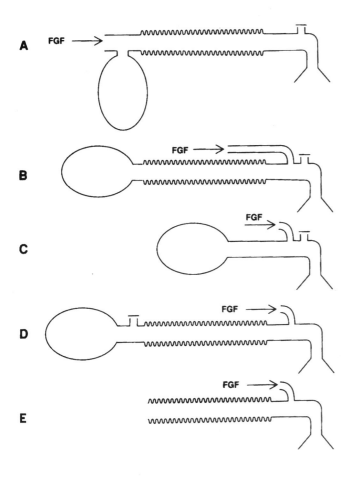

PHYSICS, BIOCHEMISTRY, AND ANESTHESIA EQUIPMENT
ANSWERS, REFERENCES, AND EXPLANATIONS

1. **(B)** Orifice flow occurs when gas flows through a region of severe constriction such as described in this question. Orifice flow is a special case of turbulent gas flow where the diameter of the tube is considerably larger than its length (e.g., in the larynx). Laminar flow occurs when gas flows down parallel-sided tubes at a rate less than critical velocity. When the gas flow exceeds the critical velocity, it becomes turbulent *(Miller: Anesthesia, ed 4, p 191; Ehrenwerth: Anesthesia Equipment: Principles and Applications, pp 224 & 225).*

2. **(C)** During orifice flow, the resistance to gas flow is directly proportional to the density of the gas mixture. Substituting helium for nitrogen will decrease the density of the gas mixture, thereby decreasing the resistance to gas flow (as much as threefold) through the region of constriction *(Miller: Anesthesia, ed 4, p 586; Ehrenwerth: Anesthesia Equipment: Principles and Applications, pp 224 & 225).*

3. **(C)** Modern electrotonic blood pressure monitors are designed to interface with electromechanical transducer systems. These systems do not require extensive technical skill on the part of the anesthesia provider for accurate usage. A static zeroing of the system is built in to most modern electrotonic monitors. Thus, after the zeroing procedure is accomplished, the system is ready for operation. The system should be zeroed with the reference point of the transducer at the approximate level of the aortic root, eliminating the effect of the fluid column of the system on arterial blood pressure readings *(Ehrenwerth: Anesthesia Equipment: Principles and Applications, pp 275-278).*

4. **(B)** Microshock occurs when a small amount of electrical power is delivered directly to the heart. The minimum electrical current required to cause ventricular fibrillation of the human heart is approximately 50 µamp. To provide a margin of safety, 10 µamp is the maximum permissible total leakage current allowed through electrodes or catheters that contact the heart *(Miller: Anesthesia, ed 4, p 2631).*

5. **(D)** The relationship between intra-alveolar pressure, surface tension, and the radius of alveoli is described by Laplace's law for a sphere, which states that the surface tension of the sphere is directly proportional to the radius of the sphere and pressure within the sphere. With regard to pulmonary alveoli, the mathematical expression of Laplace's law is as follows: $T = \frac{1}{2} PR$, where T is the surface tension, P is the intra-alveolar pressure, and R is the radius of the alveolus. In pulmonary alveoli, surface tension is produced by a liquid film lining the alveoli. This occurs because the attractive forces between the molecules of the liquid film are much greater than the attractive forces between the liquid film and gas. Thus, the surface area of the liquid tends to become as small as possible, which could collapse the alveoli *(Miller: Anesthesia, ed 4, pp 585 & 586).*

6. **(C)** The World Health Organization requires that compressed-gas cylinders containing N_2O for medical use be painted blue. Size "E" compressed-gas cylinders completely filled with N_2O contain approximately 1,590 liters of gas *(Stoelting: Basics of Anesthesia, ed 3, pp 127-130).*

7. **(B)** The amount of volatile anesthetic vapor leaving the vaporizing chamber will constitute a fractional volume of the total gas leaving the chamber. This fractional volume is proportional to the saturated vapor pressure of the volatile anesthetic relative to the atmospheric pressure. Therefore, the percent of vapor concentration in the effluent gas from the vaporizing chamber is directly proportional to the ratio of the saturated vapor pressure of the volatile anesthetic and barometric pressure. This relationship is mathematically expressed by the following equation:

$$VCanes\ (\%) = \frac{SVP\ anes}{Pb} \cdot 100,$$

where VC_{anes} is the vapor concentration (%) of the effluent anesthetic gas from the vaporizing chamber, SVP_{anes} is the saturated vapor pressure (mm Hg) of the volatile anesthetic at 22°C, and P_b is the barometric pressure (mm Hg). Under steady state conditions of temperature and pressure, the saturated vapor pressure is the only determinant of the concentration of volatile anesthetic leaving the vaporizing chamber. In this example, 20% of the carrier-gas flow leaving the vaporizing chamber will be halothane vapor (240 mm Hg/1,200 mm Hg x 100 = 20%). Since the carrier gas flow is 200 mL/min, 50 mL of halothane vapor plus the 200 mL of carrier gas will exit the vaporizing chamber (i.e., 250 mL of 20% halothane). The question asks what diluent-gas flow will result in the delivery of 2% halothane to the patient. Simple calculation will reveal that a diluent-gas flow of approximately 2,250 mL/min will be required to mix with the 250 mL of 20% halothane emerging from the vaporizing chamber to produce a delivered concentration of 2% halothane *(Ehrenwerth: Anesthesia Equipment: Principles and Applications, pp 60-63).*

8. **(E)** Check valves permit only unidirectional flow of gases. These valves prevent retrograde flow of gases from the anesthesia machine or the transfer of gas from a compressed-gas cylinder at high pressure into a container at a lower pressure. Thus, these unidirectional valves will allow an empty compressed-gas cylinder to be exchanged for a full one during operation of the anesthesia machine with minimal loss of gas. The adjustable pressure-limiting valve is a synonym for a pop-off valve. A fail-safe valve is a synonym for a pressure-sensor shutoff valve. The purpose of a fail-safe valve is to discontinue the flow of N_2O if the O_2 pressure within the anesthesia machine falls below 25 psia *(Ehrenwerth: Anesthesia Equipment: Principles and Applications, pp 46 & 47; Stoelting: Basics of Anesthesia, ed 3, p 129).*

9. **(C)** Boyle's law states that for a fixed mass of gas at constant temperature, the product of pressure and volume is constant. This concept can be used to estimate the volume of gas remaining in a compressed-gas cylinder by measuring the pressure within the cylinder *(Ehrenwerth: Anesthesia Equipment: Principles and Applications, p 224).*

10. **(C)** United States manufacturers require that all compressed-gas cylinders containing O_2 for medical use be painted green. A compressed-gas cylinder completely filled with O_2 has a pressure of approximately 2,000 psia and contains approximately 625 L of gas. According to Boyle's law (see explanation to question 9) the volume of gas remaining in a closed container can be estimated by measuring the pressure within the container. Therefore, when the pressure gauge on a compressed-gas cylinder containing O_2 shows a pressure of 1,600 psia, the cylinder contains 490 L of O_2. At a gas flow of 2 L/min, O_2 could be delivered from the cylinder for approximately 245 minutes *(Stoelting: Basics of Anesthesia, ed 3, pp 128-130).*

11. **(B)** All of the choices listed in this question can potentially result in inadequate flow of O_2 to the patient; however, given the description of the problem, no flow of O_2 through the O_2 rotameter is the correct choice. In a normally functioning rotameter, gas flows between the rim of the bobbin and the wall of the Thorpe tube, causing the bobbin to rotate. If the bobbin is rotating you can be certain that gas is flowing through the rotameter and that the bobbin is not stuck *(Ehrenwerth: Anesthesia Equipment: Principles and Applications, pp 40-42).*

12. **(B)** Fail-safe valve is a synonym for pressure-sensor shutoff valve. The purpose of the fail-safe valve is to prevent delivery of hypoxic gas mixtures from the anesthesia machine to the patient due to failure of the O_2 supply. When the O_2 pressure within the anesthesia machine decreases below 25 psia, this valve discontinues the flow of N_2O or proportionally decreases the flow of all gases. It is important to realize that this valve will not prevent delivery of hypoxic gas mixtures or pure N_2O when the O_2 rotameter is off but the O_2 pressure within the circuits of the anesthesia machine is maintained by an open O_2 compressed-gas cylinder or central supply source. Under these circumstances, an O_2 analyzer would be needed to detect delivery of a hypoxic gas mixture *(Ehrenwerth: Anesthesia Equipment: Principles and Applications, pp 37 & 38).*

13. **(C)** Also see explanation to question 3. It is important to zero the electromechanical transducer system with the reference point at the approximate level of the heart. This will eliminate the effect of the fluid column of the transducer system on the arterial blood pressure reading of the system. In this question, the system was zeroed at the stopclock which was located at the patient's wrist (approximate level of the ventricle) *(Ehrenwerth: Anesthesia Equipment: Principles and Applications, p 276).*

14. **(C)** O_2 and N_2O enter the anesthesia machine from a central supply source or compressed-gas cylinders at pressures greater than 2,000 psia. First-stage pressure regulators reduce this pressure to approximately 50 psia. Prior to entering the rotameters, second-stage O_2 pressure regulators further reduce the pressure to approximately 16 psia *(Miller: Anesthesia, ed 4, p 187).*

15. **(C)** The National Institute of Occupational Safety and Health (NIOSH) sets guidelines and issues recommendations concerning the control of waste anesthetic gases. NIOSH mandates that the highest trace concentration of N_2O contamination of the operating room atmosphere should be less than 25 ppm *(Ehrenwerth: Anesthesia Equipment: Principles and Applications, pp 114 & 115).*

16. **(C)** Agent-specific vaporizers, such as the Fluotec (halothane) vaporizer, are designed for each volatile anesthetic. However, volatile anesthetics with identical saturated vapor pressures could be used interchangeably with accurate delivery of the volatile anesthetic. See explanation to question 7 *(Ehrenwerth: Anesthesia Equipment: Principles and Applications, pp 60-63; Stoelting: Basics of Anesthesia, ed 3, pp 130-133).*

17. **(A)** The control mechanism of standard anesthesia ventilators, such as the North American Dräger AV-E, utilizes compressed oxygen to compress the ventilator bellows and electrical power for the timing circuits *(Ehrenwerth: Anesthesia Equipment: Principles and Applications, p 155).*

18. **(C)** Five types of rotameter indicators are commonly used to indicate the flow of gases delivered from the anesthesia machine. As with all anesthesia equipment, proper understanding of their function is necessary for safe and proper use. All rotameter flow indicators should be read at the upper rim except ball floats, which should be read in the middle *(Ehrenwerth: Anesthesia Equipment: Principles and Applications, pp 40-43).*

19. **(B)** The pressure gauge on a size "E" compressed-gas cylinder containing N_2O shows 750 psia when it is full and will continue to register 750 psia until approximately three-quarters of the gas has left the cylinder. A full cylinder of N_2O contains 1,600 L. Therefore, when 400 L of gas remain in the cylinder, the pressure within the cylinder will begin to fall *(Stoelting: Basics of Anesthesia, ed 3, pp 128-130).*

20. **(B)** Also see explanations to questions 3 and 13. In this question the reference point was the transducer, which was located 10 cm below the level of the patient's heart. Thus, there is an approximate 10 cm H_2O fluid column from the level of the patient's heart to the transducer. This will cause the pressure reading from the transducer system to read approximately 7.5 mm Hg higher than a true arterial pressure of the patient *(Ehrenwerth: Anesthesia Equipment: Principles and Applications, p 275).*

21. **(D)** Factors that influence the rate of laminar flow of a substance through a tube is described by the Hagen-Poiseuille law of friction. The mathematical expression of the Hagen-Poiseuille law of friction is as follows:

$$\dot{V} = \frac{\Pi r^4 (\Delta P)}{8 L \mu},$$

where $\dot{V}$ is the flow of the substance, r is the radius of the tube, ΔP is the pressure gradient down the tube, L is the length of the tube, and μ is the viscosity of the substance. Note that the rate of laminar flow is proportional to the radius of the tube to the fourth power. If the diameter of an intravenous catheter is doubled, flow would increase by a factor of 2 raised to the fourth power (i.e., a factor of 16) *(Ehrenwerth: Anesthesia Equipment: Principles and Applications, p 225).*

22. **(D)** The safe storage and handling of compressed-gas cylinders is of vital importance. Compressed-gas cylinders should not be stored in extremes of heat or cold, and should be unwrapped when stored or when in use. Flames should not be used to detect the presence of a gas. Oily hands can lead to difficulty in handling of the cylinder, which can result in dropping the cylinder. This can cause damage to or rupture of the cylinder, which can lead to an explosion *(Ehrenwerth: Anesthesia Equipment: Principles and Applications, pp 8-11).*

23. **(A)** Vaporizers can be categorized into variable-bypass and measured-flow vaporizers. Measured-flow vaporizers (non-concentration calibrated vaporizers) include the copper kettle or vernitrol vaporizer. With measured-flow vaporizers, the flow of oxygen is selected on a separate flow meter to pass into the vaporizing chamber from which the anesthetic vapor emerges at its saturated vapor pressure. By contrast, in variable-bypass vaporizers, the total gas flow is split between a variable bypass and the vaporizer chamber containing the anesthetic agent. The ratio of these two flows is called the splitting ratio. The splitting ratio depends on the anesthetic agent, temperature, the chosen vapor concentration set to be delivered to the patient, and the

saturated vapor pressure of the anesthetic *(Ehrenwerth: Anesthesia Equipment: Principles and Applications, p 63).*

24. **(D)**   The contribution of the fresh-gas flow from the anesthesia machine to the patient's V_T should be considered when setting the V_T of a mechanical ventilator. Because the ventilator pressure-relief valve is closed during inspiration, both the gas from the ventilator bellows and the fresh-gas flow will be delivered to the patient breathing circuit. In this question, the fresh-gas flow is 6 L/min or 100 mL/sec (6000 mL/60). Each breath lasts 6 sec (60 sec/10 breaths) with inspiration lasting 2 sec (I:E ratio = 1:2). Under these conditions, the V_T delivered to the patient by the mechanical ventilator will be augmented by approximately 200 mL *(Scheller: J Cardiothoracic Anesth 3:564-567, 1989).*

25. **(C)**   Also see explanation to question 24. The ventilator rate is decreased from 10 breaths/min to 6 breaths/min. Thus, each breath will last 10 sec (60 sec/6 breaths) with inspiration lasting approximately 3.3 sec (I:E ratio = 1:2). Under these conditions, the actual V_T delivered to the patient by the mechanical ventilator will be 830 mL (500 mL + 330 mL) *(Scheller: J Cardiothoracic Anesth 3:564-567, 1989).*

26. **(D)**   Also see explanation to questions 7 and 16. The saturated vapor pressures of halothane and isoflurane are very similar (approximately 240 mm Hg at room temperature) and therefore could be used interchangeably in agent-specific vaporizers *(Ehrenwerth: Anesthesia Equipment: Principles and Applications, pp 60-63; Stoelting: Basics of Anesthesia, ed 3, pp 130-133).*

27. **(E)**   Bernoulli's law states that the total energy of a substance flowing through a tube is equal to the sum of the internal potential energy of the substance, its gravitational potential, and the energy of its motion. The flow of a gas through a tube of varying cross-sectional diameter (e.g., a Venturi tube) is one application of this principle. Since the total energy of the gas remains constant, the velocity of the gas (kinetic energy) within the narrow region or "throat" of the Venturi tube is increased; this increase is matched by a drop in the pressure within this region of the tube (internal potential energy). This drop in pressure is known as the Venturi effect, which is responsible for the function of Venturi masks for measured O_2 delivery. The flow of O_2 through the Venturi apparatus pulls air into the Venturi throat by the force of the negative pressure gradient produced at the throat *(Miller: Anesthesia, ed 4, p 1100).*

28. **(A)**   NIOSH mandates that the highest trace concentration of volatile anesthetic contamination of the operating room atmosphere when administered in conjunction with N_2O is 0.5 ppm *(Ehrenwerth: Anesthesia Equipment: Principles and Applications, pp 114 & 115).*

29. **(B)**   The O_2 analyzer is the last line of defense against inadvertent delivery of hypoxic gas mixtures. It should be located in the inspiratory (not expiratory) limb of the patient breathing circuit to provide maximum safety. Since the O_2 concentration in the fresh-gas supply line may be different from that of the patient breathing circuit, the O_2 analyzer should not be located in the fresh-gas supply line *(Ehrenwerth: Anesthesia Equipment: Principles and Applications, pp 216-220).*

30. **(A)**   The ventilator pressure-relief valve is pressure-controlled *via* pilot tubing that communicates with the ventilator bellows chamber. As pressure within the bellows chamber increases during the inspiratory phase of the ventilator cycle, the pressure is transmitted *via* the pilot tubing to

close the pressure-relief valve, thus making the patient breathing circuit "gas-tight." This valve should open during the expiratory phase of the ventilator cycle to allow the release of excess gas from the patient breathing circuit into the waste-gas scavenging circuit after the bellows has fully expanded. If the ventilator pressure-relief valve were to stick in the closed position, there would be a rapid buildup of pressure within the circle system which would be readily transmitted to the patient. Barotrauma to the patient's lungs would result if this situation were to continue unrecognized *(Eisenkraft: J Clin Anesth 1:452-456, 1989).*

31. **(D)**   Vaporizer output can be affected by the composition of the carrier gas used to vaporize the volatile agent in the vaporizing chamber, especially when nitrous oxide is either initiated or discontinued. This observation can be explained by the solubility of nitrous oxide in the volatile agent. When nitrous oxide and oxygen enter the vaporizing chamber, a portion of the nitrous oxide dissolves in the liquid agent. Thus, the vaporizer output transiently decreases. Conversely, when nitrous oxide is withdrawn as part of the carrier gas, the nitrous oxide dissolved in the volatile agent comes out of solution, thereby transiently increases the vaporizer output *(Ehrenwerth: Anesthesia Equipment: Principles and Applications, pp 68-69).*

32. **(E)**   The capnogram can provide a variety of information, such as verification of the presence of exhaled CO_2 following tracheal intubation, estimation of the difference in P_aCO_2 and P_eCO_2, abnormalities of ventilation, and the presence of hypercapnia or hypocapnia. The four phases of the capnogram include inspiratory baseline, expiratory upstroke, expiratory plateau, and inspiratory downstroke. The shape of the capnogram can be used to recognize and diagnose a variety of potentially adverse circumstances. Under normal conditions, the inspiratory baseline should be 0, indicating that there is no rebreathing of CO_2 with a normal functioning circle breathing system. If the inspiratory baseline is elevated above 0, there is rebreathing of CO_2. If this occurs, the differential diagnosis should include an incompetent expiratory valve, exhausted CO_2 absorbent, or gas channeling through the CO_2 absorbent. However, the inspiratory baseline may or may not be elevated when the inspiratory valve is incompetent (e.g., there may be a slanted inspiratory downstroke). The expiratory upstroke occurs when the fresh gas from the anatomic dead space is quickly replaced by CO_2-rich alveolar gas. Under normal conditions the upstroke should be steep; however, it may become slanted during partial airway obstruction, if a side-stream analyzer is sampling gas too slowly, or if the response time of the capnograph is too slow for the patient's respiratory rate. Partial obstruction may be the result of an obstruction in the breathing system (e.g., by a kinked endotracheal tube) or in the patient's airway (e.g., the presence of chronic obstructive pulmonary disease or acute bronchospasm). The expiratory plateau is normally characterized by a slow but shallow progressive increase in CO_2 concentration. This occurs because of imperfect matching of ventilation and perfusion in all lung units. Partial obstruction of gas flow either in the breathing system or in the patient's airways may cause a prolonged increase in the slope of the expiratory plateau, which may continue rising until the next inspiratory downstroke begins. The inspiratory downstroke is caused by the rapid influx of fresh gas, which washes the CO_2 away from the CO_2 sensing or sampling site. Under normal conditions, the inspiratory downstroke is very steep. Causes of a slanted or blunted inspiratory downstroke include an incompetent inspiratory valve, slow mechanical inspiration, slow gas sampling, and partial CO_2 rebreathing *(Ehrenwerth: Anesthesia Equipment: Principles and Applications, p 240).*

33. **(B)** Complications of tracheal intubation can be divided into those associated with direct laryngoscopy and intubation of the trachea, tracheal tube placement, and extubation of the trachea. The most frequent complication associated with direct laryngoscopy and tracheal intubation is dental trauma. If a tooth is dislodged and not found, radiographs of the chest and abdomen should be taken to determine whether the tooth has passed through the glottic opening into the lungs. Should dental trauma occur, immediate consultation with a dentist is indicated. Other complications of direct laryngoscopy and tracheal intubation include hypertension, tachycardia, cardiac dysrhythmias, and aspiration of gastric contents. The most common complication that occurs while the endotracheal tube is in place is inadvertent endobronchial intubation. Flexion, not extension, of the neck or change from the supine to the head-down position can shift the carina upward, which may convert a midtracheal tube placement into a bronchial intubation. Extension of the neck can cause cephalad displacement of the tube into the pharynx. Lateral rotation of the head can displace the distal end of the endotracheal tube approximately 0.7 cm away from the carina. Complications associated with extubation of the trachea can be immediate or delayed. The two most serious immediate complications associated with extubation of the trachea are laryngospasm and aspiration of gastric contents. Laryngospasm is most likely to occur in patients who are lightly anesthetized at the time of extubation. If laryngospasm occurs, positive pressure mask-bag ventilation with 100% O_2 and forward displacement of the mandible may be sufficient treatment. However, if laryngospasm persists, succinylcholine should be administered intravenously or intramuscularly. Pharyngitis is another frequent complication following extubation of the trachea. This complication occurs most commonly in females, presumably because of the thinner mucosal covering over the posterior vocal cords compared with males. This complication usually does not require treatment and spontaneously resolves in 48 to 72 hours. Delayed complications associated with extubation of the trachea include laryngeal ulcerations, tracheitis, tracheal stenosis, vocal-cord paralysis, and arytenoid cartilage dislocation *(Stoelting: Basics of Anesthesia, ed 3, pp 154-156).*

34. **(B)** Gas leaving a compressed-gas cylinder is directed through a pressure-reducing valve (first-stage pressure regulator), which lowers the pressure within the metal tubing of the anesthesia machine to 45 to 55 psia *(Stoelting: Basics of Anesthesia, ed 3, p 129).*

35. **(C)** There is considerable controversy regarding the role of bacterial contamination of anesthesia machines and equipment in cross-infection between patients. The incidence of postoperative pulmonary infection is not reduced by the use of sterile disposable anesthetic breathing circuits (as compared with the use of reusable circuits that are cleaned with basic hygienic techniques). Furthermore, inclusion of a bacterial filter in the anesthesia-breathing circuit has no effect on the incidence of cross-infection. Clinically relevant concentrations of volatile anesthetics have no bacteriocidal or bacteriostatic effects. Low concentrations of volatile anesthetics, however, may inhibit viral replication. Shifts in humidity and temperature in the anesthesia-breathing and scavenging circuits are the most important factors responsible for killing bacteria. In addition, high O_2 concentration and metallic ions present in the anesthesia machine and other equipment have a significant lethal effect on bacteria. Acid-fast bacilli are the most resistant bacterial form to destruction. Nevertheless, there has been no case documenting transmission of tuberculosis via a contaminated anesthetic machine from one patient to another. When managing patients that can potentially cause cross-infection of other patients (e.g., patients with tuberculosis, pneumonia, or known viral infections, such as acquired immune deficiency syndrome [AIDS]) a disposable anesthetic breathing circuit should be used and nondisposable equipment should be disinfected

with glutaraldehyde (Cidex). Sodium hypochlorite (bleach), which destroys the human immuno-deficiency virus, should be used to disinfect nondisposable equipment, including laryngoscope blades, if patients with AIDS require anesthesia *(Ehrenwerth: Anesthesia Equipment: Principles and Applications, p 100; Stoelting: Basics of Anesthesia, ed 3, pp 141 & 142).*

36. **(B)** The diameter index safety system prevents incorrect connections of medical gas lines. This system consists of two concentric and specific bores in the body of one connection, which correspond to two concentric and specific shoulders on the nipple of the other connection *(Ehrenwerth: Anesthesia Equipment: Principles and Applications, pp 21, 30, & 37).*

37. **(C)** The amount of anesthetic vapor (mL) in effluent gas from a vaporizing chamber can be calculated using the following equation:

$$VO = \frac{CG \cdot SVP_{anes}}{P_b - SVP_{anes}},$$

where VO is the vapor output (mL) of effluent gas from the vaporizer, CG is the carrier gas flow (mL/min) into the vaporizing chamber, SVP_{anes} is the saturated vapor pressure (mm Hg) of the anesthetic gas at room temperature, and P_b is the barometric pressure (mm Hg). In this question,

$$VO = \frac{100 \cdot 360}{760 - 360}$$

$$VO = \frac{36,000}{400}$$

$$VO = 90 \ mL$$

(Ehrenwerth: Anesthesia Equipment: Principles and Applications, p 61).

38. **(D)** Entonox is a commercially available single-cylinder gas mixture that contains 50% O_2 and 50% N_2O by volume. Because the attractive forces between N_2O molecules are not as strong when mixed with O_2, condensation of N_2O does not occur when the ambient temperature is greater than −5.5°C. Therefore, this gas mixture obeys the principles of Dalton's law, which states that the total pressure exerted by a gas mixture is the sum of the individual pressures exerted by the constituents of the gas mixture. The pressure within a size "E" compressed-gas cylinder completely filled with Entonox is 2,200 psia (the partial pressure on N_2O is 1,100 psia). Thus, the partial pressure exerted by N_2O in a half-full cylinder is 550 psia *(Miller: Anesthesia, ed 2, p 81).*

39. **(C)** Pulse oximeters estimate arterial hemoglobin saturation (S_aO_2) by measuring the amount of light transmitted through a pulsatile vascular tissue bed. Pulse oximeters measure the alternating current (AC) component of light absorbance at each of two wavelengths (660 nanometers and 940 nanometers) and then divides this measurement by the corresponding direct current component. Then the ratio (R) of the two absorbance measurements is determined by the following equation:

$$R = \frac{AC_{660}/DC_{660}}{AC_{940}/DC_{940}}$$

Using an empirical calibration curve which relates arterial hemoglobin saturation to R, the actual arterial hemoglobin saturation is calculated. Based on the physical principles outlined above, the sources of error in SpO_2 readings can be easily predicted. Pulse oximeters can function accurately when only two hemoglobin species, oxyhemoglobin and reduced hemoglobin, are present. If any light absorbing species other than oxyhemoglobin and reduced hemoglobin are present, the pulse oximeter measurements will be inaccurate. Fetal hemoglobin has minimal effect on the accuracy of pulse oximetry, because the extinction coefficients for fetal hemoglobin at the two wavelengths used by pulse oximetry are very similar to the corresponding values for adult hemoglobin. In addition to abnormal hemoglobins, any substance present in the blood that absorbs light at either 660 or 940 nanometers, such as intravenous dyes used for diagnostic purposes, will affect the value of R, making accurate measurements of the pulse oximeter impossible. These dyes include methylene blue and indigo carbine. Methylene blue has the greatest effect on S_aO_2 measurements since the extinction coefficient is so similar to that of oxyhemoglobin *(Ehrenwerth: Anesthesia Equipment: Principles and Applications, pp 254 & 255).*

40. **(A)** Boyle's law states that at a constant temperature, the product of pressure and volume is constant. This principle can be applied to the measurement of lung volumes; a change in plethysmograph pressure will reflect a change in the lung volume. This technique is most frequently used to measure the functional residual capacity *(West: Respiratory Physiology, ed 5, p 14).*

41. **(E)** Since halothane and isoflurane have similar saturated vapor pressures, the vaporizers for these volatile anesthetics could be used interchangeably with accurate delivery of the anesthetic concentration set by the vaporizer dial. If an enflurane vaporizer were filled with a volatile anesthetic which has a greater saturated vapor pressure than enflurane (e.g., halothane or isoflurane), a higher-than-expected concentration would be delivered from the vaporizer. If a halothane or isoflurane vaporizer were filled with a volatile anesthetic which had a lower saturated vapor pressure than halothane or isoflurane (e.g., enflurane or methoxyflurane), a lower-than-expected concentration would be delivered from the vaporizer *(Ehrenwerth: Anesthesia Equipment: Principles and Applications, pp 66 & 67).*

42. **(D)** Starling's law of fluid exchange across capillaries states that the net direction of fluid flow is determined by the forces tending to move fluid out of the capillaries relative to the forces tending to move fluid into the capillaries. The total outward force is the sum of the pressures generated by the capillary hydrostatic pressure, negative interstitial free-fluid pressure, and interstitial fluid colloid osmotic pressure. The total inward force is the sum of the pressures generated by the interstitial pressure and plasma colloid osmotic pressure *(West: Respiratory Physiology, ed 5, pp 45, 170).*

43. **(B)** Also see explanation to questions 1 and 21. Laminar flow occurs when a substance flows down a parallel-sided tube at a rate less than critical velocity. Resistance to laminar gas flow through a tube is directly proportional to the viscosity of the gas and length of the tube, and is inversely proportional to the fourth power of the radius of the tube. This is known as the Hagan-Poiseuille Law of Friction. Based on this law, a change in the radius of the tube will have the greatest effect on the resistance to laminar gas flow though a tube *(Ehrenwerth: Anesthesia Equipment: Principles and Applications, pp 224 & 225).*

44. **(A)** Although controversial, chronic exposure to low concentrations of volatile anesthetics may constitute a health hazard to operating room personnel. Therefore, removal of trace concentrations of volatile anesthetic gases from the operating room atmosphere with a scavenging system and steps to reduce and control gas leakage into the environment are required. High-pressure system leakage of volatile anesthetic gases into the operating room atmosphere occurs when gas escapes from compressed-gas cylinders attached to the anesthetic machine (e.g., faulty yokes) or from tubing delivering these gases to the anesthesia machine from a central supply source. The most common cause of low-pressure leakage of anesthetic gases into the operating room atmosphere is the escape of gases from sites located between the flowmeters of the anesthesia machine and the patient, such as a poor mask seal. The use of high gas flows in a circle system will not reduce trace gas contamination of the operating room atmosphere. In fact, this could contribute to the contamination if there is a leak in the circle system *(Stoelting: Basics of Anesthesia, ed 3, p 143)*.

45. **(A)** Some epidemiology studies suggest that chronic exposure to trace concentrations of volatile anesthetic gases constitutes a health hazard to operating room personnel. For this reason, proper and routine use of scavenging systems is recommended in the operating room. It is extremely difficult to keep trace volatile anesthetic gas concentrations within safe limits when they are delivered using a face mask. Although all of the choices in this question can contribute as sources of contamination, leakage around the anesthesia face mask poses the greatest threat *(Ehrenwerth: Anesthesia Equipment: Principles and Applications, pp 128 & 129)*.

46. **(C)** The amount of volatile anesthetic taken up by the patient in the first minute is equal to that amount taken up between the squares of any two consecutive minutes. Accordingly, 200 mL would be taken up between the 16th (4 x 4) and 25th (5 x 5) minute, and another 200 mL would be taken up between the 25th and 36th (6 x 6) minute *(Miller: Anesthesia, ed 4, pp 116)*.

47. **(D)** Baralyme granules are composed primarily of barium hydroxide (20%) and calcium hydroxide (80%). Unlike soda lime, baralyme granules are inherently hard and thus the addition of silica to the granules is not necessary. Furthermore, baralyme granules contain water in the form of barium hydroxide octahydrate salt, and therefore can be used more efficiently in dry climates *(Stoelting: Basics of Anesthesia, ed 3, p 140)*.

48. **(E)** Also see explanation to question 35. There is no evidence that the incidence of postoperative pulmonary infection is altered by the use of sterile disposable anesthesia-breathing systems (compared with the use of reusable systems that are cleaned with basic hygienic techniques) or by the inclusion of a bacterial filter in the anesthesia-breathing system *(Ehrenwerth: Anesthesia Equipment: Principles and Applications, p 100; Stoelting: Basics of Anesthesia, ed 3, pp 141 & 142)*.

49. **(D)** Vaporization of a liquid requires the transfer of heat from the objects in contact with the liquid (e.g., the metal cylinder and surrounding atmosphere). For this reason, at high gas flows, atmospheric water will condensate as frost on the outside of compressed-gas cylinders *(Stoelting: Basics of Anesthesia, ed 3, pp 128-130)*.

50. **(B)** Rectal, esophageal, axillary, nasopharyngeal, and tympanic membrane temperature measurements correlate with central temperature in patients undergoing noncardiac surgery. Skin temperature does not reflect central temperature and does not warn adequately of malignant hyperthermia or excessive hypothermia *(Miller: Anesthesia, ed 4, p 1364)*.

51. **(A)** In a closed scavenging system interface, the reservoir bag should distend during expiration and deflate during inspiration. During the inspiratory phase of mechanical ventilation, the ventilator pressure-relief valve closes, thereby directing the gas inside the ventilator bellows into the patient breathing circuit. If the ventilator pressure-relief valve is incompetent, there will be a direct communication between the patient breathing circuit and scavenging circuit. This would result in delivery of part of the mechanical ventilator V_T directly to the scavenging circuit, causing the reservoir bag to inflate during the inspiratory phase of the ventilator cycle *(Ehrenwerth: Anesthesia Equipment: Principles and Applications, p 128)*.

52. **(A)** Also see explanation to questions 2 and 3. The critical velocity for helium is greater than that for nitrogen. For this reason, there is less work of breathing when helium is substituted for nitrogen *(Miller: Anesthesia, ed 4, p 191; Ehrenwerth: Anesthesia Equipment: Principles and Applications, pp 224 & 225)*.

53. **(E)** The F_1O_2 delivered to patients from low-flow systems (e.g., nasal prongs) is determined by the size of the O_2 reservoir, the O_2 flow, and the patient's breathing pattern. As a rule of thumb, assuming a normal breathing pattern, the F_1O_2 delivered by nasal prongs increases by approximately 0.04 for each L/min increase in O_2 flow up to maximum F_1O_2 of approximately 0.45 (at an O_2 flow of 6 L/min). In general, the larger the patient's V_T or faster the respiratory rate, the lower the F_1O_2 for a given O_2 flow *(Miller: Anesthesia, ed 4, pp 2399 & 2400)*.

54. **(D)** Rotameters consist of a vertically positioned tapered tube which is smallest in diameter at the bottom (Thorpe tube). Gas enters at the bottom of the Thorpe tube elevating a bobbin or float, which comes to rest when gravity on the float is balanced by the fall in pressure across the float. The rate of gas flow through the tube depends on the pressure drop along the length of the tube, the resistance to gas flow through the tube, and the physical properties (density and viscosity) of the gas. Because few gases have the same density and viscosity, rotameters cannot be used interchangeably *(Ehrenwerth: Anesthesia Equipment: Principles and Applications, pp 38-43)*.

55. **(C)** The accurate function of dual-wavelength pulse oximeters is altered by nail polish. Because blue nail polish has a peak absorbance similar to that of adult deoxygenated hemoglobin (near 660 nm), blue nail polish has the greatest effect on the S_pO_2 reading. Nail polish causes an artifactual and fixed decrease in the S_pO_2 reading by these devices *(Miller: Anesthesia, ed 4, p 1264)*.

56. **(C)** The minimum macroshock current required to elicit ventricular fibrillation is 100 mamp *(Brunner: Electricity, Safety, and the Patient, ed 1, pp 22 & 23)*.

57. **(D)** The line isolation monitor alarms when grounding occurs in the operating room or when the maximum current that a short circuit could cause exceeds 2 mamp. Therefore, the line isolation monitor will not prevent microshock or macroshock *(Brunner: Electricity, Safety, and the Patient, ed 1, p 304)*.

58. **(A)** A scavenging system with a closed interface is one in which there is communication with the atmosphere through positive and negative pressure-relief valves. The positive pressure-relief valve will prevent transmission of excessive pressure buildup to the patient breathing circuit, even if there is an obstruction distal to the interface or if the system is not connected to wall suction. However, obstruction of the transfer tubing from the patient breathing circuit to the scavenging circuit is proximal to the interface. This will isolate the patient breathing circuit from the positive pressure-relief valve of the scavenging system interface. Should this occur,

barotrauma to the patient's lungs can result *(Ehrenwerth: Anesthesia Equipment: Principles and Applications, pp 127 & 128).*

59. **(C)** Agent-specific vaporizers (in contrast to measured-flow vaporizers such as the copper kettle vaporizer) will deliver the same partial pressure of volatile anesthetic regardless of atmospheric pressure. Since the partial pressure of the volatile anesthetic in the brain, not the absolute concentration delivered to the patient, is the most important factor in achieving depth of anesthesia, the clinical effect of a given setting on the vaporizer dial will not be affected by atmospheric pressure. In contrast, the concentration of volatile anesthetic (measured as volumes percent) delivered from the vaporizer is influenced by atmospheric pressure. This effect may be calculated using the following equation:

$$Cx = C \cdot \frac{P}{Px},$$

where C_x is the output concentration in volumes percent at atmospheric pressure x, C is the dial setting of the vaporizer in volumes percent, P is the atmospheric pressure for which the vaporizer is calibrated, and P_x is the atmospheric pressure for which C_x is being established *(Ehrenwerth: Anesthesia Equipment: Principles and Applications, pp 69 & 70).*

60. **(A)** Automated noninvasive blood pressure (ANIBP) devices provide consistent and reliable arterial blood pressure measurements. Variations in the cuff pressure resulting from arterial pulsations during cuff deflation are sensed by the device and are used to calculate mean arterial pressure. Then, values for systolic and diastolic pressures are derived from formulae which utilize the rate of change of the arterial pressure pulsations and the mean arterial pressure (oscillometric principle). This methodology provides accurate measurements of arterial blood pressure in neonates, infants, children, and adults. The main advantage of ANIBP devices is that they free the anesthesia provider to perform other duties required for optimal anesthesia care. In addition, these devices provide alarm systems to draw attention to extreme blood pressure values and have the capacity to transfer data to automated trending devices or recorders. The improper use of these devices can lead to erroneous measurements and complications. The width of the blood-pressure cuff should be approximately 40% of the circumference of the patient's arm. If the width of the blood-pressure cuff is too narrow or if the blood-pressure cuff is too loosely wrapped around the arm, the blood-pressure measurement by the device will be falsely elevated. Frequent blood-pressure measurements can result in edema of the extremity distal to the cuff. For this reason, cycling of these devices should not be more frequent than every 1 to 3 minutes. Other complications associated with improper use of ANIBP devices include ulnar nerve paresthesia, superficial thrombophlebitis, and compartment syndrome. Fortunately, these complications are rare occurrences *(Miller: Anesthesia, ed 4, pp 1164 & 1165; Stoelting: Basics of Anesthesia, ed 3, pp 201 & 202).*

61. **(D)** Also see explanation to question 51. If the ventilator pressure-relief valve were to become incompetent, there would be a direct communication between the patient breathing circuit and the scavenging system circuit. This would result in delivery of part of the V_T during the inspiratory phase of the ventilator cycle directly to the scavenging reservoir bag. Therefore, adequate positive pressure ventilation may not be achieved and hypoventilation of the patient's lungs may result *(Ehrenwerth: Anesthesia Equipment: Principles and Applications, p 120).*

62. **(C)** A size "E" compressed-gas cylinder completely filled with air contains 625 L and would show a pressure gauge reading of 1,800 psia. Therefore, a cylinder with a pressure gauge reading of 900 psia would be half-full, containing approximately 310 L of air. A half-full size "E" compressed-gas cylinder containing air could be used for approximately 30 minutes at a flowrate of 10 L/min (see definition of Boyle's law in explanation to question 9) *(Stoelting: Basics of Anesthesia, ed 3, pp 128-130).*

63. **(E)** Failure to oxygenate patients adequately is the leading cause of anesthesia-related morbidity and mortality. All of the choices listed in this question are potential causes of inadequate delivery of O_2 to the patient; however, the most frequent cause is inadvertent disconnection of the O_2 supply system from the patient (e.g., disconnection of the patient breathing circuit from the endotracheal tube) *(Barash: Clinical Anesthesia, ed 2, p 664).*

64. **(B)** One mL of enflurane at 20°C will yield 210 mL of vapor at 37°C. Under the same conditions, isoflurane will yield 206 mL and halothane will yield 240 mL *(Barash: Clinical Anesthesia, ed 2, p 678).*

65. **(B)** The rate of simple diffusion of molecules through a lipid membrane is influenced by factors described in both Graham's law and Fick's law. Graham's law states that the rate of diffusion of a gas through a lipid membrane is directly proportional to the solubility of the gas and is inversely proportional to the square root of the molecular weight of the gas. Fick's law states that the rate of diffusion of a gas through a lipid membrane is directly proportional to the pressure gradient of the gas across the membrane and the area of the membrane, and is inversely proportional to the thickness of the membrane *(West: Respiratory Physiology, ed 4, pp 163 & 164).*

66. **(A)** Boyle's law states that for a fixed mass of gas at constant temperature, the product of pressure and volume is constant. This principle can be used to estimate the volume of gas remaining in compressed-gas cylinders *(Ehrenwerth: Anesthesia Equipment: Principles and Applications, p 224).*

67. **(B)** The mass spectrometer functions by separating the components of a stream of charged particles into a spectrum based on their mass/charge ratio. The amount of each ion at specific mass/charge ratios is then determined and expressed as the fractional composition of the original gas mixture. The charged particles are created and manipulated in a high vacuum to avoid interference by outside air and minimize random collisions among the ions and residual gases. An erroneous reading will be displayed by the mass spectrometer when a gas that is not detected by the collector plate system is present in the gas mixture to be analyzed. Helium, which has a mass charge ratio of 4, is not detected by standard mass spectrometers. Consequently, the standard gases (i.e., halothane, enflurane, isoflurane, oxygen, nitrous oxide, nitrogen, and carbon dioxide) will be summed to 100 percent as if helium were not present. All readings would be approximately twice their real values in the original gas mixture in the presence of 50 percent helium *(Ehrenwerth: Anesthesia Equipment: Principles and Applications, pp 203-205).*

68. **(E)** Gas density decreases with increasing altitude (i.e., the density of a gas is directly proportional to atmospheric pressure). Atmospheric pressure will influence the function of rotameters (see

explanation to question 54) because the accurate function of rotameters is influenced by the physical properties of the gas, such as density and viscosity. The magnitude of this influence, however, depends on the rate of gas flow. At low gas flows, the pattern of gas flow is laminar. Atmospheric pressure will have little effect on the accurate function of rotameters at low gas flows (see explanation to questions 21 and 43) because laminar gas flow is influenced by gas viscosity (which is minimally affected by atmospheric pressure) and not gas density. However, at high gas flows, the gas flow pattern is turbulent, and is influenced by gas density (see explanation to questions 2 and 3). At high altitudes (i.e., low atmospheric pressure), the gas flow through the rotameter will be greater than expected at high flows but accurate at low flows *(Ehrenwerth: Anesthesia Equipment: Principles and Applications, pp 38-43, 224 & 225).*

69. **(E)** The critical temperature (that temperature at which a substance exists as a liquid) for N_2O is far greater than room temperature. Therefore, N_2O exists as a liquid in compressed-gas cylinders and does not obey Boyle's law. Since N_2O does not obey Boyle's law, the volume of N_2O in the compressed-gas cylinder cannot be estimated by measuring the pressure within the cylinder *(Stoelting: Basics of Anesthesia, ed 3, pp 128-130).*

70. **(C)** During spontaneous breathing through a circle system, O_2 would pass through the CO_2 absorber and the inspiratory valve on its way from the anesthesia bag to the patient *(Ehrenwerth: Anesthesia Equipment: Principles and Applications, p 36).*

71. **(A)** The Bain anesthesia-breathing circuit is a coaxial version of a Mapleson D breathing circuit. The fresh-gas inflow enters through a tube located within the corrugated expiratory limb of the circuit and an adjustable pressure-relief valve is located near the reservoir bag. Advantages of this design include improved humidification of the fresh-gas inflow as a result of partial rebreathing, ease of scavenging waste anesthetic gases from the overflow valve, and warming of the fresh-gas inflow by the surrounding exhaled gases. Unfortunately, this design can lead to serious complications. Unrecognized disconnection or kinking of this tube within the expiratory limb of the circuit may lead to hypoxia or rebreathing of exhaled gases. *(Stoelting: Basics of Anesthesia, ed 3, pp 135 & 136).*

72. **(D)** Alarm systems are integrated into anesthesia machines to aid and assist the anesthesia provider in making diagnoses of abnormal functions of the anesthesia machine. The location of the alarm and alarm method varies with the particular model of machine. With regard to ventilator alarm systems, a high pressure alarm occurs whenever the circuit pressure exceeds approximately 65 cm of water. The subatmospheric pressure alarm is triggered when the pressure in the breathing circuit decreases to less than 10 cm of water below atmospheric pressure. The continuing pressure alarm alerts the anesthesia provider that the airway pressure remains above 18 cm of water for more than 10 seconds. A continuing pressure situation can occur with a blocked or closed pop-off valve, a malfunctioning ventilator pressure relief valve, or obstruction of the scavenging system interface. The minimum ventilation pressure or "disconnect" alarm is triggered when the amplitude of the pressure wave during the inspiration cycle does not achieve a preselected minimum value. A disconnection of the patient's endotracheal tube from the anesthesia breathing circuit would trigger this alarm *(Ehrenwerth: Anesthesia Equipment: Principles and Applications, p 157).*

73. **(A)**   The arterial pulse is caused by a wave of vascular distention which results from the combined effects of the forward-propagating pressure wave (caused by the impact of the stroke volume of the heart into a closed system) and its reflectance back toward the heart from various parts of the vasculature. The arterial pulse wave is not due to the passage of blood itself. The characteristics of the arterial pulse wave change as it moves peripherally. In the peripheral vasculature, the arterial pulse wave has a higher systolic pressure, a lower diastolic pressure, a greater pulse pressure (i.e., the difference between the systolic and diastolic pressures), and a lower mean arterial pressure than in the aorta *(Barash: Clinical Anesthesia, ed 2, p 1012).*

74. **(A)**   During the inspiratory phase of the mechanical ventilator cycle, the ventilator pressure-relief valve is closed so that gas from the ventilator bellows and the fresh-gas flow entering the circuit from the anesthesia machine are delivered to the patient. Thus, the fresh-gas flow will influence the actual V_T delivered to the patient. Since the ventilator rate and I:E ratio determine the time during which the ventilator is in the inspiratory phase, these variables will also influence the actual V_T. Accordingly, the magnitude of the effect these variables will have on the actual V_T delivered to the patient is inversely related to the total pulmonary compliance of the patient relative to that of the anesthesia breathing circuit components *(Scheller: J Cardiothorac Anesth 3:564-567, 1989).*

75. **(B)**   Monitoring end-expired and inspired nitrogen by mass spectrometer can be a useful tool during anesthesia. For example, monitoring of end-tidal nitrogen during pre-oxygenation prior to rapid sequence induction of anesthesia will ensure adequate denitrogenation of the patient. Additionally, an increase in end-tidal nitrogen is a sensitive means for detecting air entering the cardiovascular system, such as venous air embolism via open veins during pelvic, thoracic, or intracranial surgery. An equipment fault causing an air leak into the anesthetic breathing system or into the mass spectrometry sampling system would be detected by an increase in inspired nitrogen *(Ehrenwerth: Anesthesia Equipment: Principles and Applications, p 208).*

76. **(C)**   The letters and numbers imprinted near the top of compressed-gas cylinders refer to the Department of Transportation (DOT) specification number, service pressure number, serial numbers of the purchaser, user, or manufacturer of the cylinder, the maximal permissible pressure, and the original and retest dates for pressure tolerance. In addition, the cylinders are designated by a letter indicating the size of the cylinder. The contents of the cylinder are designated by a detachable label and the color of the cylinder (green for O_2, blue for N_2O, gray for CO_2, and yellow for air) *(Ehrenwerth: Anesthesia Equipment: Principles and Applications, pp 3-7).*

77. **(D)**   Also see explanation to questions 1, 2, and 21. The Hagan-Poiseuille Law of Friction does not apply when gas flow through a tube is turbulent. Turbulent gas flow increases approximately with the square of the radius of the tube (instead of the radius raised to the fourth power), the square root of the pressure gradient down the tube, and the reciprocal of gas density (instead of gas viscosity) *(Ehrenwerth: Anesthesia Equipment: Principles and Applications, pp 224 & 225).*

78. **(D)**   Any endotracheal tube not constructed of metal has the potential to ignite in an O_2-enriched environment. Polyvinylchloride (PVC) tubes are ignited most easily. Silicone endotracheal tubes are more difficult to ignite than PVC tubes *(Barash: Clinical Anesthesia, ed 2, p 1117).*

79. **(A)**   The technique described in this question will detect gross leaks in components of the anesthesia machine located "downstream" from the rotameters. These components include gaskets, vaporizers, Thorpe tubes, and the patient breathing circuit. However, in anesthesia machines that have an outlet check valve, the integrity of the low-pressure components of the machine (i.e., vaporizer, rotameter) cannot be assessed using this technique *(Ehrenwerth: Anesthesia Equipment: Principles and Applications, pp 47-54)*.

80. **(E)**   Also see explanation to question 71. The Bain anesthesia-breathing circuit is a coaxial version of a Mapleson D breathing circuit. The fresh-gas inflow is located near the patient and an adjustable pressure-relief valve is located near the reservoir bag. This design allows for efficient use during both spontaneous and controlled ventilation. Fresh-gas flows of 200 to 300 mL/kg/min are necessary to prevent rebreathing of CO_2 when the Bain breathing circuit is used during spontaneous ventilation; fresh-gas flows of 70 mL/kg/min are required when the Bain breathing circuit is used during controlled ventilation *(Stoelting: Basics of Anesthesia, ed 3, pp 135 & 136)*.

81. **(D)**   Also see explanation to question 51. A scavenging system with a closed interface is one in which there is communication with the atmosphere through positive and negative pressure-relief valves. The negative pressure-relief valve prevents the transfer of negative pressure from wall suction to the patient breathing circuit. The scavenging reservoir bag should distend during expiration, not inspiration *(Ehrenwerth: Anesthesia Equipment: Principles and Applications, pp 120-123)*.

82. **(B)**   Also see explanation to question 47. Baralyme granules consist of 80% calcium hydroxide and 20% barium hydroxide, and contain water as the barium hydroxide octohydrate salt *(Barash: Clinical Anesthesia, ed 2, p 657)*.

83. **(A)**   In semiclosed or closed anesthesia breathing circuits, CO_2 is eliminated by chemical neutralization. This process can be accomplished by mixing exhaled gases with soda lime or baralyme. Soda lime granules consist primarily of calcium hydroxide. The hardness of these granules is due to the addition of silica. This hardness decreases the amount of dust, which if present can be carried throughout the breathing circuit to the patient, causing chemical injury to the lungs. The reaction of CO_2 with calcium hydroxide is exothermic and requires a specific water content to assure optimal activity *(Stoelting: Basics of Anesthesia, ed 3, pp 138-140)*.

84. **(E)**   The optimal CO_2 absorptive condition of soda lime or baralyme canisters exists when the patient's V_T is accommodated entirely within the void space of the canister. This optimal condition depends on the size of the granules and the presence or absence of channeling within the canister. Channeling is the passage of exhaled gases through low-resistance pathways within the canister, such that the majority of the granules are bypassed *(Stoelting: Basics of Anesthesia, ed 3, pp 138-141)*.

85. **(B)**   The mechanical characteristics of transducer systems can be understood by the description of two parameters: natural frequency and damping coefficient. The natural frequency of a transducer system is the frequency at which the system will resonate. Any physiologic frequency occurring near the natural frequency of the transducer system is amplified. For this reason, the natural frequency of standard transducer systems used to measure arterial blood pressure is

greater than that which exists in a blood pressure signal (which is approximately 20 Hz). The damping coefficient represents the tendency of the transducer system to extinguish oscillations through viscous and frictional forces. The damping coefficient is dependent on several mechanical characteristics of the transducer system and is mathematically expressed as follows:

$$\oint = \frac{16\mu}{d^3} \sqrt{\frac{3LV\!d}{\Pi\rho}},$$

where $\oint$ is the damping coefficient, μ is the viscosity of the fluid, d is the diameter of the tubing, L is length of the tubing, V_d is the transducer fluid volume displacement, and ρ is the density of the fluid. Thus, high fluid viscosity and low fluid density, small tube diameter, long tube length, and high tube compliance will increase the damping coefficient of the transducer system, and produce damping of the arterial pressure waveform *(Miller: Anesthesia, ed 4, pp 1166-1169)*.

86. **(D)**   The pin-index safety system consists of two pins projecting from the inner surface of the yoke corresponding to holes in the valve casing of the compressed-gas cylinder. This system prevents the incorrect attachment of compressed-gas cylinders to the anesthesia machine *(Ehrenwerth: Anesthesia Equipment: Principles and Applications, p 397)*.

87. **(B)**   The saturated vapor pressure of a liquid within a closed container is that pressure produced by the molecules in the vapor phase when they collide with each other and the walls of the container. This pressure is directly proportional to the temperature of the liquid. As the volatile becomes vaporized in the vaporizer, the temperature falls as this is an endothermic reaction *(Ehrenwerth: Anesthesia Equipment: Principles and Applications, pp 172-174)*.

88. **(B)**   Excessive overflow of gas from the scavenging system reservoir bag into the operating room atmosphere can result from several causes. The most common causes are excessive fresh-gas flow into the patient breathing circuit, kinking or obstruction of the tubing to the wall suction (e.g., by the wheels of the anesthesia machine), and failure to connect the scavenging system interface to wall suction. These malfunctions will not result in excessive pressure buildup within the patient breathing circuit if a positive pressure-relief valve is incorporated into the scavenging system interface and is functioning correctly *(Ehrenwerth: Anesthesia Equipment: Principles and Applications, pp 120-123)*.

89. **(B)**   The last gas added to a gas mixture should always be O_2. This arrangement is the safest since it assures that leaks proximal to the O_2 inflow cannot result in delivery of a hypoxic gas mixture to the patient. With this arrangement (O_2 added last), leaks distal to the O_2 inflow will result in a decreased volume of gas, but the F_1O_2 will not be reduced *(Barash: Clinical Anesthesia, ed 2, p 645)*.

90. **(D)**   Also see explanations to questions 59 and 68. Changes in atmospheric pressure will affect gas density. Because rotameters are calibrated at an atmospheric pressure of 760 mm Hg, use of these devices at an atmospheric pressure other than 760 mm Hg will alter the accuracy of these devices *(Ehrenwerth: Anesthesia Equipment: Principles and Applications, pp 69 & 70)*.

91. **(E)** The term LASER refers to Light Amplification by Stimulated Emission of Radiation. This device is capable of producing very intense beams of light that can be focused to produce controlled coagulation, incision, or vaporization of tissues. The primary advantage of using laser light is that edema and damage to surrounding tissues is minimal, and thus healing is rapid. All of the choices listed in this question are potential disadvantages and hazards associated with laser surgery. In addition to those listed, another potential complication is that the personnel may be struck by a misdirected beam of light, potentially causing burns to the skin and mucous membranes. Additionally, corneal burns are a possibility, emphasizing the need for personnel to wear safety glasses. Because endotracheal tubes not made of metal may be ignited by the laser beam, inhaled concentrations of oxygen are typically maintained at the lowest concentrations acceptable (approximately 40 percent) and nitrous oxide, which can support combustion, is not usually administered *(Stoelting: Basics of Anesthesia, ed 3, p 350).*

92. **(A)** Also see explanations to questions 71 and 80. The Bain anesthesia-breathing circuit has an adjustable pressure-relief valve located near the reservoir bag. This design allows for ease of scavenging waste anesthetic gasses. The other choices are disadvantages of this breathing system *(Stoelting: Basics of Anesthesia, ed 3, pp 135 & 136).*

93. **(A)** 94. **(D)** 95. **(D)** 96. **(E)** There are five different types of Mapleson breathing circuits (designated A through E). These circuits vary in arrangement of the fresh-gas-flow inlet, tubing, mask, reservoir bag, and unidirectional expiratory valve. These systems are lightweight, portable, easy to clean, offer low resistance to breathing, and because of high fresh-gas inflows, prevent rebreathing of exhaled gases. In addition, with these breathing circuits, the concentration of volatile anesthetic gases and O_2 delivered to the patient can be accurately estimated. The reservoir bag enables the anesthesia provider to provide assisted or controlled ventilation of the lungs. The unidirectional expiratory valve functions to direct fresh gas into the patient and exhaled gases out of the circuit. In the Mapleson A breathing circuit, the unidirectional expiratory valve is located near the patient and the fresh-gas-flow inlet is located proximal to the reservoir bag. This arrangement is the most efficient for elimination of CO_2 during spontaneous breathing. However, since the unidirectional expiratory valve must be tightened to permit production of positive airway pressure when the gas reservoir bag is manually compressed, this breathing circuit is less efficient in preventing rebreathing of CO_2 during assisted or controlled ventilation of the lungs. The structure of the Mapleson D breathing circuit is similar to that of the Mapleson A breathing circuit except that the positions of the fresh-gas-flow inlet and the unidirectional expiratory valve are reversed. The placement of the fresh-gas-flow inlet near the patient produces efficient elimination of CO_2, regardless of whether the patient is breathing spontaneously or whether the patient's ventilation is controlled. The Bain anesthesia breathing circuit is a coaxial version of the Mapleson D breathing circuit except that the fresh gas enters through a narrow tube within the corrugated expiratory limb of the circuit (see explanation to question 71, 80, and 92). The Jackson-Rees breathing circuit is a modification of the Mapleson E breathing circuit. In the Jackson-Rees breathing circuit, the adjustable unidirectional expiratory valve is incorporated into the reservoir bag and the fresh-gas-flow inlet is located close to the patient. This arrangement offers the advantage of ease of instituting assisted or controlled ventilation of the lungs, as well as monitoring ventilation by movement of the reservoir bag during spontaneous breathing *(Miller: Anesthesia, ed 4, pp 203-206; Ehrenwerth: Anesthesia Equipment: Principles and Applications, pp 102-108).*

Respiratory Physiology

DIRECTIONS (Questions 97 through 143): Each of the questions or incomplete statements in this section is followed by answers or by completions of the statement, respectively. Select the ONE BEST answer or completion for each item.

97. The normal FEV_1/FVC ratio is

    A. 0.95
    B. 0.80
    C. 0.60
    D. 0.50
    E. 0.40

98. The degree of transpulmonary shunt can be estimated to equal 1% of the cardiac output for each

    A. 10 mm Hg increase in the alveolar-to-arterial difference in O_2 tension $P(A - a)O_2$
    B. 20 mm Hg increase in the $P(A - a)O_2$
    C. 30 mm Hg increase in the $P(A - a)O_2$
    D. 40 mm Hg increase in the $P(A - a)O_2$
    E. 50 mm Hg increase in the $P(A - a)O_2$

99. During the first minute of apnea, the P_aCO_2 will rise

    A. 2 mm Hg/min
    B. 4 mm Hg/min
    C. 6 mm Hg/min
    D. 8 mm Hg/min
    E. 10 mm Hg/min

100. What is the maximum compensatory increase in serum bicarbonate concentration ($[HCO_3^-]$) for every 10 mm Hg increase in P_aCO_2 with chronic respiratory acidosis?

    A. 1 mEq/L
    B. 3 mEq/L
    C. 7 mEq/L
    D. 10 mEq/L
    E. 15 mEq/L

101. O_2 requirement for a 70-kg adult under general anesthesia is

    A. 150 mL/min
    B. 250 mL/min
    C. 350 mL/min
    D. 450 mL/min
    E. 550 mL/min

102. The functional residual capacity is composed of the

    A. Expiratory reserve volume and residual volume
    B. Inspiratory reserve volume and residual volume
    C. Inspiratory capacity and vital capacity
    D. Expiratory capacity and tidal volume
    E. Expiratory reserve volume and tidal volume

103. Which of the following statements correctly defines the relationship between minute ventilation ($\dot{V}_E$), dead space ventilation ($\dot{V}_D$), and P_aCO_2?

    A. If $\dot{V}_E$ is constant and V_D increases, then P_aCO_2 will increase
    B. If $\dot{V}_E$ is constant and V_D increases, then P_aCO_2 will decrease
    C. If V_D is constant and $\dot{V}_E$ increases, then P_aCO_2 will increase
    D. If V_D is constant and $\dot{V}_E$ decreases, then P_aCO_2 will decrease
    E. None of the above

104. A 22-year-old patient who sustained a closed head injury is brought to the operating room from the ICU for placement of a dural bolt. Hemoglobin has been stable at 15 gm/dL. Blood gas analysis immediately prior to induction reveals a P_aO_2 of 120 mm Hg and an arterial saturation of 100%. After induction the P_aO_2 rises to 150 mm Hg and the saturation remains the same. How has the oxygen content of this patient's blood changed?

    A. It has increased by 10%
    B. It has increased by 5%
    C. It has increased by less than 1%
    D. Cannot be determined with P_aCO_2
    E. Cannot be determined without pH

105. Inhalation of CO_2 increases $\dot{V}_E$ by

    A. 0.5 L/min/mm Hg increase in P_aCO_2
    B. 1 to 3 L/min/mm Hg increase in P_aCO_2
    C. 3 to 5 L/min/mm Hg increase in P_aCO_2
    D. 5 to 10 L/min/mm Hg increase in P_aCO_2
    E. 10 to 20 L/min/mm Hg increase in P_aCO_2

106. What is the O_2 content of whole blood if the hemoglobin concentration is 10 mg/dL, the P_aO_2 is 60 mm Hg, and the S_aO_2 is 90%?

    A. 10 mL/dL
    B. 13 mL/dL
    C. 15 mL/dL
    D. 18 mL/dL
    E. 21 mL/dL

107. Each of the following will cause erroneous readings by dual-wavelength pulse oximeters **EXCEPT**

      A. Carboxyhemoglobin
      B. Methylene blue
      C. Fetal hemoglobin
      D. Methemoglobin
      E. Nail polish

108. The mechanism for the compensatory shift of the oxyhemoglobin dissociation curve toward normal in response to chronic (>24 hours) respiratory alkalosis is

      A. Increased renal excretion of HCO_3^-
      B. An influx of potassium into red blood cells
      C. Altered erythrocyte 2,3-diphosphoglycerate (2,3-DPG) metabolism
      D. Decreased sensitivity of the central nervous system to changes in P_aCO_2
      E. None of the above

109. The P_{50} for normal adult hemoglobin is approximately

      A. 15
      B. 25
      C. 35
      D. 45
      E. 50

110. During a normal V_T (500 mL) breath, the transpulmonary pressure increases from 0 to 5 cm H_2O. The product of transpulmonary pressure and V_T is 2,500 cm H_2O-mL. This expression of the pressure-volume relationship during breathing determines what parameter of respiratory mechanics?

      A. Lung compliance
      B. Airway resistance
      C. Pulmonary elastance
      D. Work of breathing
      E. Closing capacity

111. An acute increase in P_aCO_2 of 10 mm Hg will result in an immediate compensatory increase in plasma $[HCO_3^-]$ of

      A. 1 mEq/L
      B. 2 mEq/L
      C. 4 mEq/L
      D. 5 mEq/L
      E. 7 mEq/L

112. The normal vital capacity for a 70-kg man is

    A. 1 L
    B. 2 L
    C. 5 L
    D. 7 L
    E. 9 L

113. The most important mechanism for the transport of CO_2 from peripheral tissues to the lungs is

    A. CO_2 dissolved in plasma
    B. Carbonic acid
    C. Carbaminohemoglobin
    D. HCO_3^-
    E. CO_3^{-2}

114. An increase in P_aCO_2 of 10 mm Hg will result in a decrease in pH of

    A. 0.01 pH units
    B. 0.02 pH units
    C. 0.04 pH units
    D. 0.08 pH units
    E. None of the above

115. A 20-year-old, 80-kg patient with a history of insulin-dependent diabetes mellitus arrives in the emergency room in diabetic ketoacidosis. The arterial blood gases (on room air) are as follows: pH 6.95, P_aCO_2 30 mm Hg, P_aO_2 98 mm Hg, $[HCO_3^-]$ 6 mEq/L. What is the total body deficit of HCO_3^- in this patient?

    A. 500 mEq
    B. 400 mEq
    C. 300 mEq
    D. 200 mEq
    E. 100 mEq

116. A 44-year-old patient is hyperventilated to a P_aCO_2 of 24 mm Hg for 48 hours. What $[HCO_3^-]$ would you expect (normal $[HCO_3^-]$ is 24 mEq/L)?

    A. 10 mEq/L
    B. 12 mEq/L
    C. 14 mEq/L
    D. 16 mEq/L
    E. 18 mEq/L

117. The normal arterial-to-alveolar ratio (a/A) is greater than

    A. 0.10
    B. 0.65
    C. 0.75
    D. 0.50
    E. 0.25

118.   What is the rate of O_2 transported to peripheral tissues in a healthy 70-kg patient with a hemoglobin
        concentration of 10 mg/dL, a P_aO_2 of 60 mm Hg, an S_aO_2 of 90%, and a cardiac output of 5 L/min?

   A.   300 mL/min
   B.   400 mL/min
   C.   500 mL/min
   D.   600 mL/min
   E.   700 mL/min

119. The P_{50} of sickle cell hemoglobin is

   A.   19
   B.   26
   C.   31
   D.   35
   E.   40

120.   The leftward shift of the oxyhemoglobin dissociation curve caused by hypocarbia is known as the

   A.   Fick principle
   B.   Bohr effect
   C.   Haldane effect
   D.   Law of Laplace
   E.   None of the above

121.   Which of the following is the correct mathematical expression of Fick's law of diffusion of a gas
        through a lipid membrane ($\dot{V}$ = rate of diffusion, D = diffusion coefficient of the gas, A = area of the
        membrane, $P_1 - P_2$ = transmembrane partial pressure gradient of the gas, T = thickness of the mem-
        brane)?

   A. $\dot{V} = D \cdot \dfrac{A \cdot T}{P_1 - P_2}$

   B. $\dot{V} = \dfrac{A \cdot T}{D\,(P_1 - P_2)}$

   C. $\dot{V} = D \cdot \dfrac{A(P_1 - P_2)}{T}$

   D. $\dot{V} = D \cdot \dfrac{T\,(P_1 - P_2)}{A}$

   E. $\dot{V}_E = \dfrac{D \cdot T \cdot A}{P_1 - P_2}$

122. Each of the following is decreased in elderly patients compared with their younger counterparts **EXCEPT**

    A. P_aO_2
    B. FEV_1
    C. Ventilatory response to hypercarbia
    D. Vital capacity
    E. Closing volume

123. Calculate the V_D/V_T ratio (physiologic dead-space ventilation) based on the following data: P_aCO_2 45 mm Hg, mixed expired CO_2 tension (P_ECO_2) 30 mm Hg.

    A. 0.1
    B. 0.2
    C. 0.3
    D. 0.4
    E. 0.5

124. The shift of the CO_2-hemoglobin dissociation curve which occurs in response to changes in P_aO_2 is known as the

    A. Fick principle
    B. Bohr effect
    C. Haldane effect
    D. Law of Laplace
    E. Le Chatelier principle

125. Which of the following acid-base disturbances is the least well compensated?

    A. Metabolic alkalosis
    B. Respiratory alkalosis
    C. Increased anion gap metabolic acidosis
    D. Normal anion gap metabolic acidosis
    E. Respiratory acidosis

126. What is the P_aO_2 of air in a patient in Denver, Colorado (assume a barometric pressure of 630 mm Hg, respiratory quotient of 0.8, and P_aCO_2 of 34 mm Hg)?

    A. 40 mm Hg
    B. 50 mm Hg
    C. 60 mm Hg
    D. 70 mm Hg
    E. 80 mm Hg

127. A venous blood sample from which of the following sites would correlate most reliably with P_aO_2 and P_aCO_2?

    A. Jugular vein
    B. Subclavian vein
    C. Antecubital vein
    D. Femoral vein
    E. Vein on posterior surface of a warmed hand

128. Which of the following pulmonary function tests is least dependent on patient effort?

    A. FEV_1
    B. FVC
    C. $FEF_{800-1200}$
    D. FEF_{25-75}
    E. MVV

129. A 33-year-old woman with 20% carboxyhemoglobin is brought to the emergency room for treatment of smoke inhalation. Which of the following is **LEAST** consistent with a diagnosis of carbon monoxide poisoning?

    A. Cyanosis
    B. P_aO_2 105 mm Hg, oxygen saturation 80% on initial room air ABGs
    C. 98% oxygen saturation on dual wave pulse oximeter
    D. Dizziness
    E. Oxyhemoglobin dissociation curve shifted far to the left

130. The $P(A - a)O_2$ of a patient breathing 100% O_2 is 240 mm Hg. The estimated fraction of the cardiac output shunted past the lungs without exposure to ventilated alveoli (i.e., transpulmonary shunt) is

    A. 5%
    B. 12%
    C. 17%
    D. 20%
    E. 34%

131. Each of the following will alter the position or slope of the CO_2-ventilatory response curve **EXCEPT**

    A. Hypoxemia
    B. Fentanyl
    C. N_2O
    D. Volatile anesthetics
    E. Ketamine

132. Which of the following statements concerning the distribution of alveolar ventilation (V_A) in the upright lungs is true?

   A. The distribution of V_A is not affected by body posture
   B. Alveoli at the apex of the lungs (nondependent alveoli) are better ventilated than those at the base
   C. All areas of the lungs are ventilated equally
   D. Alveoli at the base of the lungs (dependent alveoli) are better ventilated than those at the apex
   E. Alveoli at the central regions of the lungs are better ventilated than those at the base or apex

133. In the resting adult, what percent of total body O_2 consumption is due to the work of breathing?

   A. 2%
   B. 5%
   C. 10%
   D. 20%
   E. 50%

134. The anatomic dead space in a 70-kg male is

   A. 50 mL
   B. 150 mL
   C. 250 mL
   D. 500 mL
   E. 700 to 1,000 mL

135. Reynold's number is an important factor in the determination of

   A. O_2 transport
   B. Surface tension
   C. Turbulent vs. laminar flow
   D. Physiologic dead-space ventilation
   E. Functional residual capacity

136. A decrease in P_aCO_2 of 10 mm Hg will result in

   A. A decrease in serum potassium concentration ($[K^+]$) of 0.5 mEq/L
   B. A decrease in $[K^+]$ of 1.0 mEq/L
   C. No change in $[K^+]$ under normal circumstances
   D. An increase in $[K^+]$ of 0.5 mEq/L
   E. An increase in $[K^+]$ of 1.0 mEq/L

137. An increase in [HCO_3^-] of 10 mEq/L will result in an increase in pH of

   A. 0.10 pH units
   B. 0.15 pH units
   C. 0.20 pH units
   D. 0.25 pH units
   E. None of the above

138. A 28-year-old female (70 kg) with ulcerative colitis is undergoing general anesthesia for colon resection and ileostomy. Current medications include sulfasalazine and corticosteroids. Induction of anesthesia and tracheal intubation are uneventful. Anesthesia is maintained with isoflurane, N_2O and 50% O_2, and fentanyl, and the patient is paralyzed with atracurium. The patient's lungs are mechanically ventilated with the following parameters: $\dot{V}_E$ 5,000 mL, respiratory rate 10 breaths/min. How would $\dot{V}_A$ change if the respiratory rate were increased from 10 to 20 breaths/min?

   A. Increase by 500 mL
   B. Increase by 1,000 mL
   C. No change
   D. Decrease by 750 mL
   E. Decrease by 1,500 mL

139. Each of the following will shift the oxyhemoglobin dissociation curve to the right **EXCEPT**

   A. Volatile anesthetics
   B. Decreased P_aO_2
   C. Decreased pH
   D. Increased temperature
   E. Increased red blood cell (RBC) 2,3-DPG content

140. The half-life of carboxyhemoglobin in a patient breathing 100% O_2 is

   A. 5 minutes
   B. 1 hour
   C. 2 hours
   D. 4 hours
   E. 12 hours

141. The most important buffering system in the body is

   A. Hemoglobin
   B. Plasma proteins
   C. Bone
   D. HCO_3^-
   E. Phosphate

142. Which of the following statements concerning the distribution of O_2 and CO_2 in the upright lungs is true?

    A. $P_{A}O_2$ is greater at the apex than at the base
    B. $P_{A}CO_2$ is greater at the apex than at the base
    C. Both $P_{A}O_2$ and $P_{A}CO_2$ are greater at the apex than at the base
    D. Both $P_{A}O_2$ and $P_{A}CO_2$ are greater at the base than at the apex
    E. The $P_{A}CO_2$ is equal throughout the lung

143. Which of the following choices correctly describes the effect a bilateral carotid endarterectomy resulting in denervation of the carotid bodies would have on the control of breathing?

    A. Loss of the ventilatory response to CO_2
    B. Loss of the ventilatory response to hypoxia
    C. Loss of the ventilatory response to hydrogen ions
    D. Loss of the ventilatory response to fever
    E. No change in the control of breathing

DIRECTIONS (Questions 144 through 168): For each of the items in this section, ONE or MORE of the numbered options is correct. Select the answer:

Select A if options *1, 2 and 3* are correct,
Select B if options *1 and 3* are correct,
Select C if options *2 and 4* are correct,
Select D if only option *4* is correct,
Select E if *all* options are correct.

144. Adverse effect(s) of respiratory or metabolic alkalosis include

    1. Decreased plasma ionized calcium concentration ($[Ca^{2+}]$)
    2. Coronary artery vasoconstriction
    3. Bronchial smooth muscle constriction
    4. Increased right-to-left transpulmonary shunting

145. A 22-year-old black male comes to the emergency room diaphoretic and short of breath. The patient is given 100% O_2 by nonrebreathing face mask. Arterial blood gases are as follows: $P_{a}O_2$ 309 mm Hg, $P_{a}CO_2$ 24 mm Hg, pH 7.57, and $S_{a}O_2$ 89%. Causes of these findings could include the presence of

    1. Methemoglobin
    2. Carboxyhemoglobin
    3. Sulfhemoglobin
    4. Sickle cell hemoglobin

Select A if options *1, 2 and 3* are correct,
Select B if options *1 and 3* are correct,
Select C if options *2 and 4* are correct,
Select D if only option *4* is correct,
Select E if *all* options are correct.

146. Adverse effect(s) of respiratory or metabolic acidosis include

   1. Increased incidence of cardiac dysrhythmias
   2. Hypovolemia
   3. Increased serum potassium concentration
   4. Increased pulmonary vascular resistance

147. Which of the following can cause metabolic acidosis?

   1. Chronic renal failure
   2. Pancreatic-duodenal fistula
   3. Excessive diarrhea
   4. Cirrhotic liver disease

148. Which of the following can increase physiologic dead-space ventilation?

   1. PEEP
   2. Venous air embolus
   3. Hypotension
   4. Pregnancy

149. Which of the following can cause a rightward shift of the oxyhemoglobin dissociation curve?

   1. Methemoglobinemia
   2. Carboxyhemoglobinemia
   3. Rapid transfusion of large amounts of citrate-preserved packed erythrocytes
   4. Pregnancy

150. True statements concerning pulmonary vascular resistance (PVR) include which of the following?

   1. PVR increases with increasing lung volume from functional residual capacity
   2. PVR increases with decreasing lung volume from functional residual capacity
   3. PVR decreases with increasing cardiac output
   4. PVR increases with decreasing P_aO_2

151. Factor(s) that determine the diffusing capacity of the lungs for carbon monoxide (DL_{co}) include the

   1. Area of the alveolar membrane
   2. Blood volume of the pulmonary vasculature
   3. Thickness of the alveolar membrane
   4. Red blood cell hemoglobin concentration

Select A if options *1, 2 and 3* are correct,
Select B if options *1 and 3* are correct,
Select C if options *2 and 4* are correct,
Select D if only option *4* is correct,
Select E if *all* options are correct.

152. On arterial blood gas sampling, an oxygen saturation of 95% is noted with a P_aO_2 of 60 mm Hg. Possible explanations for this include

    1. Sepsis
    2. Intracardiac shunt
    3. Cyanide toxicity
    4. Abnormal hemoglobin

153. PVR is increased by which of the following?

    1. Hypocarbia
    2. Vasopressin
    3. Hyperthermia
    4. Metabolic acidosis

154. Which of the following respiratory variables can be measured by simple spirometry?

    1. Vital capacity
    2. Expiratory reserve volume
    3. Inspiratory capacity
    4. Residual volume

155. Pulmonary surfactant is decreased in which of the following situations?

    1. After cardiopulmonary bypass
    2. With pulmonary embolism
    3. Prolonged inhalation of 100% O_2
    4. Administration of corticosteroids to parturients

156. Which of the following will increase the closing capacity?

    1. Smoking
    2. Obesity
    3. Supine position
    4. Aging

157. Compensatory mechanism(s) for metabolic acidosis include which of the following?

    1. Secretion of H^+ and absorption of HCO_3^- by the renal tubules
    2. Increased V_A caused by direct stimulation of the carotid bodies by H^+
    3. Buffering of nonvolatile acids by bone
    4. Buffering of nonvolatile acids by hemoglobin

Select A if options *1, 2 and 3* are correct,
Select B if options *1 and 3* are correct,
Select C if options *2 and 4* are correct,
Select D if only option *4* is correct,
Select E if *all* options are correct.

158. Correct mathematical expression of static lung capacities and volumes include which of the following?

    1. Total lung capacity = vital capacity + residual volume
    2. Functional residual capacity = expiratory reserve volume + residual volume
    3. Inspiratory capacity = inspiratory reserve volume + tidal volume
    4. Closing capacity = residual volume + closing volume

159. Mechanism(s) responsible for the compensatory decrease in [HCO_3^-] in response to respiratory alkalosis include

    1. Production of CO_2 by the bicarbonate buffer system
    2. Generation of lactic acid by glycolysis
    3. Decreased absorption of HCO_3^- by the proximal convoluted renal tubules
    4. Hydration of CO_2

160. The factors that influence the rate of diffusion of molecules through a lipid membrane are described in

    1. Laplace's Law
    2. Graham's Law
    3. Boyle's Law
    4. Fick's Law

161. Effects of carboxyhemoglobin include

    1. A leftward shift of the oxyhemoglobin dissociation curve
    2. Overestimation of S_aO_2 by pulse oximeters
    3. Negative inotropic effect on the heart
    4. Increased incidence of deep vein thrombosis

162. Structures that contribute to physiologic shunt include

    1. Thebesian veins
    2. Bronchial veins
    3. Pleural veins
    4. Nonperfused alveoli

163. Which of the following is associated with a decreased DL_{co}?

    1. Emphysema
    2. Severe anemia
    3. Pulmonary hypertension
    4. Asthma

Select A if options *1, 2 and 3* are correct,
Select B if options *1 and 3* are correct,
Select C if options *2 and 4* are correct,
Select D if only option *4* is correct,
Select E if *all* options are correct.

164. Which of the following can cause the formation of methemoglobinemia?

    1. O-toluidine
    2. Nitroglycerin
    3. Sodium nitroprusside
    4. Phencyclidines

165. The respiratory quotient

    1. Describes the relationship between the rate of CO_2 production and the rate of O_2 utilization
    2. Is not dependent on diet
    3. Is increased when the diet consists predominately of carbohydrates
    4. Is increased when the diet consists predominately of fats

166. The cilia of the respiratory tract

    1. Are not affected by the temperature and humidity of inspired gases
    2. Are inhibited by the presence of a cuffed endotracheal tube
    3. Are part of goblet cells
    4. Are a protective mechanism for removing particles from conducting airways

167. Anatomic dead space is

    1. Dependent on lung size
    2. Approximately 1 mL/kg body weight
    3. Affected by anesthesia equipment
    4. Of less importance in the newborn than in the adult

168. The vital capacity is composed of the

    1. Expiratory reserve volume
    2. Inspiratory reserve volume
    3. Tidal volume
    4. Functional residual capacity

RESPIRATORY PHYSIOLOGY
ANSWERS, REFERENCES, AND EXPLANATIONS

97. **(B)** The forced expiratory volume in one second (FEV_1) is the total volume of air that can be exhaled in the first second. Normal healthy adults can exhale approximately 75% to 80% of their forced vital capacity (FVC) in the first second. Therefore, the normal FEV_1/FVC ratio is ≥ 0.80. In the presence of obstructive airway disease, the FEV_1/FVC ratio is < 0.80. This ratio can be used to determine the severity of obstructive airway disease and to monitor the efficacy of bronchodilator therapy *(Miller: Anesthesia, ed 4, p 884)*.

98. **(B)** The fraction of the cardiac output shunted through the lungs without exposure to ventilated alveoli (i.e., transpulmonary shunt) can be estimated using the general rule that for every increase in the alveolar-to-arterial difference in O_2 tension $P(A - a)O_2$ of 20 mm Hg, there is a shunt fraction of approximately 1% of the cardiac output (i.e., $Q_s/Q_t = P(A - a)O_2/20$, where Q_s/Q_t is the shunt fraction) *(Stoelting: Basics of Anesthesia, ed 3, p 227)*.

99. **(C)** During apnea, the P_aCO_2 will increase approximately 6 mm Hg during the first minute and then 3 to 4 mm Hg each minute thereafter *(Miller: Anesthesia, ed 4, p 1717)*.

100. **(B)** The kidneys respond to chronic respiratory acidosis by conserving bicarbonate (HCO_3^-) and secreting hydrogen (H^+). In respiratory acidosis, there is an immediate hydration of CO_2 in plasma to produce HCO_3^-. This acute process produces approximately 1 mEq/L of HCO_3^- for every 10 mm Hg increase in P_aCO_2. Hydration of CO_2 in the proximal and distal renal tubules stimulates the secretion of H^+ into the urine. This compensatory response requires 12 to 48 hours. The compensatory response to chronic respiratory acidosis is rarely complete such that the pH does not fully return to 7.4. The maximum compensatory increase in serum bicarbonate concentration ($[HCO_3^-]$) in response to chronic respiratory acidosis is 3 mEq/L for each 10 mm Hg increase in P_aCO_2 *(Stoelting: Basics of Anesthesia, ed 3, p 222)*.

101. **(B)** The O_2 requirement for an adult under general anesthesia is 3 to 4 mL/kg/min. The O_2 requirement for a newborn under general anesthesia is 7 to 9 mL/kg/min. Alveolar ventilation (V_A) in neonates is double that of adults to help meet their increased O_2 requirements. This increase in V_A is achieved primarily by an increase in respiratory rate as tidal volume (V_T) is similar to that of adults. Although CO_2 production is also increased in neonates, the elevated V_A maintains the P_aCO_2 near 38 to 40 mm Hg *(Barash: Clinical Anesthesia, ed 2, p 1313)*.

102. **(A)**

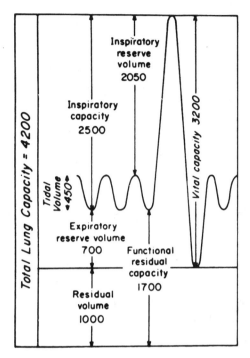

A comprehensive understanding of respiratory physiology is important for understanding the effects of both regional and general anesthesia on respiratory mechanics and pulmonary gas exchange. The volume of gas remaining in the lungs after a normal expiration is called the functional residual capacity. The volume of gas remaining in the lungs after a maximal expiration is called the residual volume. The difference between these two volumes is called the expiratory reserve volume. Therefore, the functional residual capacity is composed of the expiratory reserve volume and residual volume *(Stoelting: Pharmacology and Physiology, ed 2, pp 723 & 724).*

103. **(A)**   The volume of gas in the conducting airways of the lungs (and not available for gas exchange) is called the anatomic dead space. The volume of gas in ventilated alveoli that are unperfused (and also not available for gas exchange) is called the functional dead space. The anatomic dead space together with the functional dead space is called the *physiologic dead space*. Physiologic dead-space ventilation can be calculated by the Bohr dead-space equation which is mathematically expressed as follows:

$$V_D/V_T = \frac{P_aCO_2 - P_ECO_2}{P_aCO_2},$$

where V_D/V_T is the ratio of physiologic dead-space ventilation (V_D) to V_T, and the subscripts a and E represent arterial and mixed expired, respectively. Of the choices given, only the first is correct. A large increase in physiologic dead-space ventilation will result in an increase in P_aCO_2 *(West: Respiratory Physiology, ed 5, pp 2 & 19).*

104. **(C)**   The oxygen content of blood can be calculated with the following formula:

$$O_2 \text{ content} = (1.39 \times \text{hemoglobin} \times \text{arterial saturation}) + 0.003 \times PaO_2$$

first oxygen content $= (1.39 \times 15 \times 1.0) + .003 \times 120 = 21.21 \text{ ml/dL}$

second oxygen content $= (1.39 \times 15 \times 1.0) + .003 \times 150 = 21.30 \text{ ml/dL}$

The difference in the oxygen content is 0.09 ml/dL. This represents a change of 0.42% *(Stoelting: Basics of Anesthesia, ed 3, p 229)*.

105. **(B)**   The degree of ventilatory depression caused by volatile anesthetics can be assessed by measuring resting P_aCO_2, the ventilatory response to hypercarbia and the ventilatory response to hypoxemia. Of these techniques, the resting P_aCO_2 is the most frequently used index. However, measuring the effects of increased P_aCO_2 on ventilation is the most sensitive method of quantifying the effects of drugs on ventilation. In awake, unanesthetized humans, inhalation of CO_2 increases minute ventilation ($\dot{V}_E$) by approximately 1 to 3 L/min/mm Hg increase in P_aCO_2. Using this technique, halothane, isoflurane, enflurane, and N_2O cause a dose-dependent depression of the ventilation *(Stoelting: Basics of Anesthesia, ed 3, p 49)*.

106. **(B)**   The amount of O_2 in blood (O_2 content) is the sum of the amount of O_2 dissolved in plasma and the amount of O_2 combined with hemoglobin. The amount of O_2 dissolved in plasma is directly proportional to the product of the blood:gas solubility coefficient of O_2 (0.003) and P_aO_2. The amount of O_2 bound to hemoglobin is directly related to the fraction of hemoglobin that is saturated. One gram of hemoglobin can bind 1.39 mL of O_2. The mathematical expression of O_2 content is as follows:

$$O_2 \text{ content} = 1.39 \cdot [Hgb] \cdot S_aO_2 = 0.003\,(P_aO_2),$$

where [Hgb] is the hemoglobin concentration (mg/dL), S_aO_2 is the fraction of hemoglobin saturated with O_2, and 0.003 (P_aO_2) is the amount of O_2 dissolved in plasma. The O_2 content of blood in this patient is approximately 13 mL/dL *(Miller: Anesthesia, ed 4, pp 596)*.

107. **(C)**   The presence of hemoglobin species other than oxyhemoglobin can cause erroneous readings by dual-wavelength pulse oximeters. Hemoglobin species, such as carboxyhemoglobin and methemoglobin, dyes such as methylene blue and indocyanine green, and nail polish will cause erroneous readings. Since the absorption spectrum of fetal hemoglobin is similar to that of adult oxyhemoglobin, fetal hemoglobin does not significantly affect the accuracy of these types of pulse oximeters. High levels of bilirubin have no significant effect on the accuracy of dual-wavelength pulse oximeters, but may cause falsely low readings by nonpulsatile oximeters *(Miller: Anesthesia, ed 4, pp 1263-1265)*.

108. **(C)**   The compensatory shift of the oxyhemoglobin dissociation curve toward normal in response to chronic acid-base abnormalities is a result of altered erythrocyte 2,3-diphosphoglycerate (2,3-DPG) metabolism *(Miller: Anesthesia, ed 2, p 1135)*.

109. **(B)** P_{50} is the P_aO_2 required to produce 50% saturation of hemoglobin. The P_{50} for adult hemoglobin is 26 mm Hg *(Stoelting: Anesthesia and Co-existing Disease, ed 3, p 394).*

110. **(D)** The work of breathing is defined as the product of transpulmonary pressure and V_T. The work of breathing is related to two factors: the work required to overcome the elastic forces of the lungs and the work required to overcome airflow or frictional resistances of the airways. Volatile anesthetics cause a marked increase in the elastic component of the work of breathing *(Miller: Anesthesia, ed 4, pp 588 & 589).*

111. **(A)** Also see explanation to question 100. A prolonged increase in P_aCO_2 of 10 mm Hg will result in a maximum compensatory increase in $[HCO_3^-]$ of 3 mEq/L. An acute increase in P_aCO_2 of 10 mm Hg results in an immediate compensatory increase in $[HCO_3^-]$ of 1 mEq/L. This immediate compensatory increase in $[HCO_3^-]$ is caused by the hydration of CO_2 in plasma to produce HCO_3^-. An acute decrease in P_aCO_2 of 10 mm Hg will cause an immediate compensatory decrease in $[HCO_3^-]$ of 2 mEq/L, and a chronic decrease in P_aCO_2 of 10 mm Hg will cause a maximum compensatory decrease in $[HCO_3^-]$ of 5 mEq/L *(Stoelting: Basics of Anesthesia, ed 3, pp 221 & 222).*

112. **(C)** The volume of gas exhaled during a maximum expiration is the vital capacity. In a normal healthy adult, the vital capacity is 60–70 mL/kg. In a 70-kg patient, the vital capacity is approximately 5 L *(Stoelting: Pharmacology & Physiology in Anesthetic Practice, ed 2, p 724).*

113. **(D)** CO_2 is transported from the peripheral tissues to the lungs, primarily in the form of HCO_3^-; there it is eliminated from the body. The conversion of CO_2 to HCO_3^- occurs within erythrocytes and is catalyzed by the enzyme carbonic anhydrase. HCO_3^- then diffuses out of the cell in exchange for a chloride ion (Cl^-) to maintain electrical neutrality. This exchange of HCO_3^- for Cl^- is called the chloride shift. CO_2 is also transported, dissolved in blood, and bound to proteins as carbamino compounds. Carbamino compounds are formed by the combination of CO_2 with terminal amine groups on blood proteins, primarily hemoglobin. This reaction occurs very rapidly without enzymatic catalysts. Approximately 60% of CO_2 is transported from peripheral tissues to the lungs in the form of HCO_3^-, 30% in the form of carbaminohemoglobin, and 10% dissolved in plasma *(Miller: Anesthesia, ed 4, p 599; West: Respiratory Physiology, ed 5, pp 76-79).*

114. **(D)** Respiratory acidosis is present when the P_aCO_2 exceeds 44 mm Hg. Respiratory acidosis is caused by decreased elimination of CO_2 by the lungs (i.e., hypoventilation) or increased metabolic production of CO_2. An acute increase in P_aCO_2 of 10 mm Hg will result in a decrease in pH of approximately 0.08 pH units. The acidosis of arterial blood will stimulate ventilation *via* the carotid bodies and the acidosis of cerebrospinal fluid will stimulate ventilation *via* the medullary chemoreceptors located in the fourth cerebral ventricle. Volatile anesthetics greatly attenuate the carotid body-mediated and aortic body-mediated ventilatory responses to arterial acidosis, but have little effect on the medullary chemoreceptor-mediated ventilatory response to cerebrospinal fluid acidosis *(West: Respiratory Physiology, ed 5, pp 122 & 123; Stoelting: Basics of Anesthesia, ed 3, p 49).*

115. **(C)** Metabolic acidosis occurs when the pH is less than 7.36 and $[HCO_3^-]$ is below 24 mEq/L. A decrease in $[HCO_3^-]$ is caused by decreased elimination of H^+ by the renal tubules (e.g., renal tubule acidosis) or increased metabolic production of H^+ relative to HCO_3^- (e.g., lactic acidosis, ketoacidosis, or uremia). Total body deficit in HCO_3^- can be estimated using the following formula:

Total Body Deficit (mEq) = Total Body Weight (kg) •
Deviation of HCO_3^- From 24 mEq/L •
Extracellular Fluid Volume as a Fraction of Body Mass (L)

The total body deficit in HCO_3^- in this patient is: 80 • (24 − 6) • 0.2 = 288 mEq *(Stoelting: Basics of Anesthesia, ed 3, p 225).*

116. **(D)** Respiratory alkalosis is present when the P_aCO_2 is less than 36 mm Hg. There are three compensatory mechanisms responsible for attenuating the increase in pH that accompanies respiratory alkalosis. First, there is an immediate shift in the equilibrium of the HCO_3^- buffer system, which results in the production of CO_2. Second, alkalosis stimulates the activity of phosphofructokinase, which increases glycolysis and the production of pyruvate and lactic acid. Third, there is a decrease in reabsorption of HCO_3^- by the proximal and distal renal tubules. These three compensatory mechanisms result in a maximum decrease in $[HCO_3^-]$ of approximately 5 mEq/L for every 10 mm Hg decrease in P_aCO_2 below 40 mm Hg *(Stoelting: Basics of Anesthesia, ed 3, pp 222 & 223).*

117. **(C)** Arterial hypoxemia is defined as a decrease in P_aO_2 below 60 mm Hg. Arterial hypoxemia can be caused by low P_AO_2, hypoventilation, or shunt. Shunt can be caused by a right-to-left transpulmonary or intracardiac shunt, or mismatching of ventilation to perfusion. Diffusion limitation to the passage of O_2 from the alveoli to blood has not been documented as a cause of arterial hypoxemia in humans. The degree of shunt can be estimated by calculating the $P(A - a)O_2$ or arterial-to-alveolar (a/A) ratio. It is easier to use the a/A ratio to calculate shunt fraction because the normal range for the $P(A - a)O_2$ changes with the PO_2 of inspired gas. The normal a/A ratio should be greater than 0.75 *(Stoelting: Basics of Anesthesia, ed 3, p 229).*

118. **(D)** Also see explanation to question 106. The amount of O_2 transported from the lungs to peripheral tissues is determined by the O_2 content (see equation in explanation for question 106) and the cardiac output. The mathematical expression of O_2 transport is as follows:

$$O_2 \text{ transport} = CO \cdot O_2 \text{ content,}$$

where CO is the cardiac output (mL/min). In this patient, O_2 transport is approximately 600 mL/min *(Miller: Anesthesia, ed 4, pp 594-597).*

119. **(C)** Also see explanation to question 109. A P_{50} less than 26 mm Hg defines a leftward shift of the oxyhemoglobin dissociation curve. This means that at any given P_aO_2, hemoglobin has a higher affinity for O_2. A P_{50} greater than 26 mm Hg describes a rightward shift of the oxyhemoglobin dissociation curve. This means that at any given P_aO_2, hemoglobin has a lower affinity for O_2. Conditions that cause a rightward shift of the oxyhemoglobin dissociation curve are metabolic

and respiratory acidosis, hyperthermia, increased erythrocyte 2,3-DPG content, pregnancy, and abnormal hemoglobins, such as sickle cell hemoglobin or thalassemia. Alkalosis, hypothermia, fetal hemoglobin, abnormal hemoglobin species, such as carboxyhemoglobin, methemoglobin, and sulfhemoglobin, and decreased erythrocyte 2,3-DPG content will cause a leftward shift of the oxyhemoglobin dissociation curve *(Stoelting: Anesthesia and Co-existing Disease, ed 3, p 401; Stoelting: Pharmacology and Physiology in Anesthetic Practice, ed 2, pp 737 & 738).*

120. **(B)** The effects of P_aCO_2 and pH on the position of the oxyhemoglobin dissociation curve is known as the Bohr effect. Hypercarbia and acidosis shift the curve to the right, and hypocarbia and alkalosis shift the curve to the left. The Bohr effect is attributed primarily to the action of CO_2 and pH on erythrocyte 2,3-DPG metabolism *(Miller: Anesthesia, ed 4, pp 597 & 600).*

121. **(C)** The rate that a gas diffuses through a lipid membrane is directly proportional to the area of the membrane, the transmembrane partial pressure gradient of the gas, and the diffusion coefficient of the gas, and is inversely proportional to the thickness of the membrane. The diffusion coefficient of the gas is directly proportional to the square root of gas solubility and is inversely proportional to the square root of the molecular weight of the gas. This is known as Fick's law of diffusion *(West: Respiratory Physiology, ed 5, pp 21 & 22).*

122. **(E)** Aging is associated with reduced ventilatory volumes and capacities, and decreased efficiency of pulmonary gas exchange. These changes are caused by progressive stiffening of cartilage and replacement of elastic tissue in the intercostal and intervertebral areas, which decreases compliance of the thoracic cage. In addition, progressive kyphosis or scoliosis produces upward and anterior rotation of the ribs and sternum, which further restricts chest wall expansion during inspiration. With aging, the functional residual capacity, residual volume, and closing volume are increased, while the vital capacity, total lung capacity, maximum breathing capacity, FEV_1, and ventilatory response to hypercarbia and hypoxemia are reduced. In addition, age-related changes in lung parenchyma, alveolar surface area, and diminished pulmonary capillary bed density cause ventilation/perfusion mismatch, which decreases resting P_aO_2 *(Stoelting: Anesthesia and Co-existing Disease, ed 3, p 632).*

123. **(C)** Physiologic dead-space ventilation can be estimated using the Bohr equation (described in the explanation to question 103).

$$V_D/V_T = \frac{45 \; mm \; Hg - 30 \; mm \; Hg}{45 \; mm \; Hg} = \frac{15 \; mm \; Hg}{45 \; mm \; Hg} = 0.33$$

(Stoelting: Basics of Anesthesia, ed 3, p 231).

124. **(C)** The shift of the CO_2-hemoglobin dissociation curve which occurs in response to changes in P_aO_2 is known as the Haldane effect. Because of this effect, deoxygenated hemoglobin (in peripheral tissues) has a greater affinity for CO_2 than does oxygenated hemoglobin *(Miller: Anesthesia, ed 4, p 600).*

125. **(A)** The degree to which a person can hypoventilate to compensate for metabolic alkalosis is limited and hence, this is the least well compensated acid-based disturbance. Respiratory compen-

sation for metabolic alkalosis is rarely more than 75% complete. Hypoventilation to a $P_aCO_2 >$ 55 mm Hg is the maximum respiratory compensation for metabolic alkalosis. A $P_aCO_2 > 55$ mm Hg most likely reflects concomitant respiratory acidosis *(Stoelting: Basics of Anesthesia, ed 3, p 226).*

126. **(E)** P_AO_2 can be estimated using the alveolar gas equation which is as follows:

$$P_AO_2 = (P_B - 47)\, F_IO_2 - \frac{P_aCO_2}{R},$$

where P_B is the barometric pressure (mm Hg), F_IO_2 is the fraction of inspired O_2, P_aCO_2 is the arterial CO_2 tension (mm Hg), and R is the respiratory quotient *(West: Respiratory Physiology, ed 5, p 69).*

127. **(E)** When arterial sampling is not possible, "arterialized" venous blood can be used to determine arterial blood gas tensions. Because blood in the veins on the back of the hands have very little O_2 extracted, the O_2 content in this blood best approximates the O_2 content in a sample of blood obtained from an artery *(Stoelting: Basics of Anesthesia, ed 4, p 226).*

128. **(D)** Also see explanation to question 97. Pulmonary function tests can be divided into those that assess ventilatory capacity and into those that assess pulmonary gas exchange. The simplest test to assess ventilatory capacity is the FEV_1/FVC ratio. Other tests to assess ventilatory capacity include the maximum mid-expiratory flow (FEF_{25-75}), maximum voluntary ventilation (MVV), and flow-volume curves. The most significant disadvantage of these tests is that they are dependent on patient effort. However, since the FEF_{25-75} is obtained from the mid-expiratory portion of the flow-volume loop, it is least dependent on patient effort *(Barash: Clinical Anesthesia, ed 2, p 936).*

129. **(A)** Carbon monoxide binds to hemoglobin with an affinity 200 to 250 times that of oxygen. This stabilizes the oxygen hemoglobin complex and hinders release of oxygen to the tissues, i.e. a leftward shift of the oxyhemoglobin dissociation curve. The diagnosis is suggested when there is a low oxygen hemoglobin saturation in the face of a normal P_aO_2. The two-wave pulse oximeter cannot distinguish oxyhemoglobin from carboxyhemoglobin so that a normal oxyhemoglobin saturation would be observed in the presence of high concentrations of carboxyhemoglobin. Carbon monoxide poisoning is not associated with cyanosis *(Rogers: Principles and Practice of Anesthesiology, p 578; Stoelting: Anesthesia and Co-existing Disease, ed 3, p 536; Miller: Anesthesia, ed 4, pp 2431-2432).*

130. **(B)** Also see explanation to question 98.

$$Q_S/Q_t = \frac{A - aDO_2}{20},$$

where Q_S is the cardiac output that is shunted past the lungs without exposure to ventilated alveoli, Q_t is the total cardiac output, and A-aDO_2 is the alveolar-to-arterial difference in O_2 tension. Thus,

$$Q_S/Q_t = \frac{240}{20} = 12\%$$

(Stoelting: Basics of Anesthesia, ed 3, p 227).

131. **(E)** Also see explanation to question 105. Measuring the ventilatory response to increased P_aCO_2 is a sensitive method for quantifying the effects of drugs on ventilation. In general, all volatile anesthetics (including N_2O), narcotics, benzodiazepines, and barbiturates depress the ventilatory response to increased P_aCO_2 in a dose-dependent manner. The magnitude of ventilatory depression by volatile anesthetics is greater in patients with chronic obstructive pulmonary disease (COPD) than in healthy patients. Thus, it is recommended that arterial blood gases are monitored during recovery from general anesthesia in patients with COPD. Ketamine causes minimal respiratory depression. Typically, respiratory rate is decreased only 2 to 3 breaths/min and the ventilatory response to changes in P_aCO_2 is maintained during ketamine anesthesia *(Miller: Anesthesia, ed 4, pp 139 & 140; West: Respiratory Physiology, ed 4, p 126; Stoelting: Pharmacology and Physiology in Anesthetic Practice, ed 2, p 139).*

132. **(D)** The orientation of the lungs relative to gravity has a profound effect on efficiency of pulmonary gas exchange. Because alveoli in dependent regions of the lungs expand more per unit change in transpulmonary pressure (i.e., are more compliant) than alveoli in nondependent regions of the lungs, V_A increases from the top to the bottom of the lungs. Because pulmonary blood flow increases more from the top to the bottom of the lungs than does V_A, the ventilation/perfusion ratio is high in nondependent regions of the lungs and is low in dependent regions of the lungs. Therefore, in the upright lungs, the P_AO_2 and pH are greater at the apex, while the P_ACO_2 is greater at the base *(West: Respiratory Physiology, ed 5, pp 19 & 20, 38-41, 61-66).*

133. **(A)** Also see explanation to question 110. The work required to overcome the elastic recoil of the lungs and thorax, along with airflow or frictional resistances of the airways, contributes to the work of breathing. When the respiratory rate or airway resistance is high, or pulmonary or chest wall compliance is reduced, a large amount of energy is spent overcoming the work of breathing. In the healthy, resting adult, only 1% to 2% of total O_2 consumption is used for the work of breathing *(Stoelting: Pharmacology and Physiology in Anesthetic Practice, ed 2, p 721).*

134. **(B)** Also see explanation to question 103. The conducting airways (trachea, right and left mainstem bronchi, and lobar and segmental bronchi) do not contain alveoli and therefore do not take part in pulmonary gas exchange. These structures constitute the anatomic dead space. In the adult, the anatomic dead space is approximately 1 mL/lb or 2 mL/kg. The anatomic dead space increases during inspiration because of the traction exerted on the conducting airways by the surrounding lung parenchyma. In addition, the anatomic dead space depends on the size and posture of the subject *(Stoelting: Pharmacology and Physiology in Anesthetic Practice, ed 2, p 725).*

135. **(C)** Also see explanations to questions 1, 2, and 3. Reynold's number is a calculated value that represents the overall ratio of inertial forces to viscous forces during flow. Reynold's number is directly proportional to the density of the substance, the flow velocity of the substance, and the radius of the container through which the substance is flowing, and is inversely proportional to

the viscosity of the substance. In general, flow through a long, straight, smooth-walled container becomes turbulent when the Reynold's number is greater than 2,300 *(Miller: Anesthesia, ed 4, p 1101; West: Respiratory Physiology, ed 5, pp 103-105).*

136. **(A)** Cardiac dysrhythmias are a common complication associated with acid-base abnormalities. The etiology of these dysrhythmias is related partly to the effects of pH on myocardial potassium homeostasis. As a general rule, there is an inverse relationship between $[K^+]$ and pH. For every 0.08 unit change in pH, there is a reciprocal change in $[K^+]$ of approximately 0.5 mEq/L *(Stoelting: Pharmacology and Physiology in Anesthetic Practice, ed 2, p 274).*

137. **(B)** There are several guidelines that can be used in the initial interpretation of arterial blood gases that will permit rapid recognition of the type of acid-base disturbance. These guidelines are as follows: 1) a 1 mm Hg change in P_aCO_2 above or below 40 mm Hg results in a 0.008 unit change in the pH in the opposite direction; 2) the P_aCO_2 will decrease by about 1 mm Hg for every 1 mEq/L reduction in $[HCO_3^-]$ below 24 mEq/L; 3) a change in $[HCO_3^-]$ of 10 mEq/L from 24 mEq/L will result in a change in pH of approximately 0.15 pH units in the same direction *(Stoelting: Pharmacology and Physiology in Anesthetic Practice, ed 2, pp 219-226).*

138. **(E)** Also see explanation to questions 103 and 134. A patient with a V_D of 150 mL and a V_A of 350 mL (assuming a normal V_T of 500 mL) will have a V_D minute ventilation ($\dot{V}_D$) of 1,500 mL and a V_A minute ventilation ($\dot{V}_A$) of 3,500 mL (a $\dot{V}_E$ of 5,000 mL) at a respiratory rate of 10 breaths/min. If the respiratory rate is doubled but $\dot{V}_E$ remains unchanged, then the $\dot{V}_D$ would double to 3,000 mL, an increase in $\dot{V}_D$ of 1,500 mL and decrease in $\dot{V}_A$ of 1,500 mL *(Stoelting: Pharmacology and Physiology in Anesthetic Practice, ed 2, p 725).*

139. **(B)** Also see explanation to questions 108 and 109. In addition to the items listed in this question, other factors that shift the oxyhemoglobin dissociation curve to the right include pregnancy and all abnormal hemoglobin S such as hemoglobin S (sickle cell hemoglobin). For reasons unknown, volatile anesthetics increase the P_{50} of adult hemoglobin by 2 to 3.5 mm Hg. A rightward shift of the oxyhemoglobin dissociation curve will decrease the transfer of O_2 from alveoli to hemoglobin and improve release of O_2 from hemoglobin to peripheral tissues *(Stoelting: Pharmacology and Physiology in Anesthetic Practice, ed 2, p 738).*

140. **(B)** The most frequent immediate cause of death from fires is carbon monoxide toxicity. Carbon monoxide is a colorless, odorless gas that exerts its adverse effects by decreasing O_2 delivery to peripheral tissues. This is accomplished by two mechanisms. First, because the affinity of carbon monoxide for the O_2 binding sites on hemoglobin is 240 times that of O_2, O_2 is readily displaced from hemoglobin. Thus, O_2 content is reduced. Second, carbon monoxide causes a leftward shift of the oxyhemoglobin dissociation curve, which increases the affinity of hemoglobin for O_2 at peripheral tissues. Treatment of carbon monoxide toxicity is administration of 100% O_2. Breathing 100% O_2 decreases the half-time of carboxyhemoglobin from 250 minutes to approximately 50 minutes *(Stoelting: Anesthesia and Co-existing Disease, ed 3, p 536).*

141. **(D)** Buffer systems represent the first line of defense against adverse changes in pH. The HCO_3^- buffer system is the most important system and represents >50% of the total buffering capacity of the body. Other important buffer systems include hemoglobin, which is responsible for

approximately 35% of the buffering capacity of blood, phosphates, plasma proteins, and bone *(Miller: Anesthesia, ed 4, pp 1386 & 1387; Stoelting: Basics of Anesthesia, ed 3, p 217).*

142. **(A)**   Also see explanation to question 132. The ventilation/perfusion ratio is greater at the apex of the lungs than at the base of the lungs. Thus, dependent regions of the lungs are hypoxic and hypercarbic compared to the nondependent regions *(West: Respiratory Physiology, ed 5, pp 61-66).*

143. **(B)**   Breathing is controlled by the respiratory center which is a widely dispersed group of neurons located in the medulla and pons. Breathing is regulated in response to a variety of physiologic factors which include P_aCO_2, P_aO_2, hydrogen ion concentration and temperature. Peripheral chemoreceptors which respond to pH, P_aCO_2, and P_aO_2 are located in the aorta (aortic bodies) and at the bifurcation of the common carotid artery (carotid bodies). Denervation or removal of the latter results in a 30% decrease in the ventilatory response to CO_2 and elimination of the ventilatory response to hypoxemia *(Stoelting: Pharmacology and Physiology in Anesthetic Practice, ed 2, pp 727-728).*

144. **(E)**   Maintenance of acid-base equilibrium is necessary to ensure optimal function of enzymes and of the cardiovascular, pulmonary, and neurologic systems. In addition, the acid-base status has direct influence on S_aO_2 and the distribution of electrolytes within the intracellular and extra-cellular fluid spaces. Adverse physiologic effects of alkalosis include coronary artery vasoconstriction, increased cardiac dysrhythmias and airway resistance, decreased cerebral blood flow, central nervous system excitation, decreased $[K^+]$ and ionized calcium concentrations ($[Ca^{2+}]$), and a leftward shift of the oxyhemoglobin dissociation curve, which decreases availability of O_2 to tissues *(Stoelting: Basics of Anesthesia, ed 3, p 219).*

145. **(A)**   Abnormal hemoglobin species, such as methemoglobin, sulfhemoglobin, and carboxyhemoglobin, bind O_2 more avidly than does normal hemoglobin which greatly reduces the O_2 carrying capacity of blood. The presence of these abnormal hemoglobin species is suggested by a low S_aO_2 in the presence of a normal P_aO_2. The diagnosis of these abnormal hemoglobin species is confirmed by direct measurement in plasma *(Stoelting: Anesthesia and Co-existing Disease, ed 3, pp 401-403).*

146. **(E)**   Adverse physiologic effects of respiratory or metabolic acidosis include central nervous system depression, cardiovascular system depression (which is a result of the direct depressant effects of the acidosis on the vasomotor center, arteriolar smooth muscle, and myocardial contractility), increased incidence of cardiac dysrhythmias, hypovolemia (which is a result of decreased pre-capillary and increased postcapillary sphincter tone), pulmonary hypertension, and hyperkalemia. Depression of the cardiovascular system is partially offset by increased secretion of catecholamines and elevated $[Ca^{2+}]$ until severe acidosis occurs *(Stoelting: Basics of Anesthesia, ed 3, p 219).*

147. **(E)**   The causes of metabolic acidosis can be grouped into those associated with an increased anion gap and those associated with a normal anion gap. The anion gap is defined by the following equation:

$$Anion\ gap = [Na^+] - ([Cl^-] + [HCO_3^-])$$

The anion gap is composed of unmeasured anions, such as sulfates, phosphates, plasma proteins, and organic acids. A normal anion gap is approximately 5 to 12 mEq/L. Causes of normal anion gap metabolic acidosis include pancreatic-duodenal fistula, ureteral-enteric fistula, renal tubule acidosis, hyperchloremia (e.g., hyperalimentation), excessive diarrhea, and drugs that produce a HCO_3^- diuresis, such as acetazolamide. Causes of increased anion gap metabolic acidosis include excessive lactate production (e.g., shock), cirrhosis of the liver, uremia (e.g., renal failure), diabetic ketoacidosis, and ingestion of excessive amounts of salicylates, methanol, ethylene glycol, oral hypoglycemic agents (e.g., phenformin), and ethanol *(Stoelting: Basics of Anesthesia, ed 3, p 224)*.

148. **(A)** Also see explanation to questions 103 and 134. Physiologic dead-space ventilation is the ventilation of areas of the lungs that are poorly perfused. Except for pregnancy, all of the choices will increase physiologic dead-space ventilation *(Miller: Anesthesia, ed 4, pp 585, 611, & 612; Shnider: Anesthesia for Obstetrics, ed 3, p 3)*.

149. **(D)** See explanation to questions 108, 109, and 139 *(Miller: Anesthesia, ed 4, p 597; Stoelting: Anesthesia & Co-existing Disease, ed 3, p 394; Stoelting: Pharmacology and Physiology in Anesthetic Practice, ed 2, p 737)*.

150. **(E)** Changes in pulmonary vascular resistance (PVR) may have significant effects on pulmonary gas exchange. Many factors including vasoactive peptides and hormones, cardiac output, and mechanical forces, interact in a complex manner to determine PVR. Lung volume has a significant effect on PVR. In the normal lung, PVR increases with an increase or decrease in lung volume from functional residual capacity. The effect of lung volume on PVR is related to the direct effects of tissue expansion and collapse on the caliber of the extra-alveolar vessels and alveolar capillaries. At low lung volumes, PVR is elevated because the extra-alveolar vessels are compressed. At high lung volumes, PVR is elevated because the alveolar capillaries are compressed. Cardiac output also has a significant effect on PVR. PVR is directly proportional to the mean pulmonary perfusion pressure and is inversely proportional to cardiac output. As cardiac output increases, PVR decreases. The mechanisms responsible for this inverse relationship between cardiac output and PVR are the processes of recruitment and distention of pulmonary vessels. Recruitment of previously closed capillaries in nondependent regions of the lungs is the predominant mechanism for the fall in PVR as cardiac output and pulmonary artery pressure increase from low levels. However, distention of pulmonary vessels is the predominant mechanism for the fall in PVR at relatively high cardiac outputs and pulmonary vascular pressures *(Miller: Anesthesia, ed 4, pp 582 & 584; West: Respiratory Physiology, ed 5, pp 35-38)*.

151. **(E)** The diffusing capacity of the lungs is determined by several processes: 1) diffusion of a gas through the alveolar walls (see explanation to question 121 for discussion of Fick's law of diffusion) and 2) the rate of reaction of the gas with hemoglobin. The mathematical expression of the diffusing capacity of the lungs is as follows:

$$D_L = D_M + (\ominus \cdot V_C),$$

where D_L is the diffusing capacity of the lungs, D_M is the diffusing capacity of the alveolar membrane, $\ominus$ is the rate (in mL/min) a gas can combine with 1 mL of blood/mm Hg partial pressure of the gas in the blood, and V_C is the volume of blood in the pulmonary capillaries.

Thus, D_L is determined by the area and thickness of the alveolar membrane, the blood:gas solubility and molecular weight of the gas, the transmembrane partial pressure difference of the gas, pulmonary blood volume, and hemoglobin concentration *(West: Respiratory Physiology, ed 5, pp 21-30).*

152. **(D)** Normal adult hemoglobin has a P_{50} equal to 27 mm Hg meaning it will be 50% saturated in a PO_2 of 27 mm Hg. The same hemoglobin would be 90% saturated if the PO_2 were 60 mm Hg. If hemoglobin binds oxygen more tightly, i.e. if the P_{50} is less than 27 mm Hg, a leftward shift of the oxyhemoglobin dissociation curve has occurred. There are a number of causes for a leftward shift such as hypothermia, metabolic or respiratory alkalosis, decreased red cell 2,3-DPG, carboxyhemoglobin, methemoglobin, fetal hemoglobin, or other abnormal hemoglobin. Likewise, if the P_{50} for hemoglobin is greater than 27 mm Hg, a rightward shift is said to have taken place. Most of these are the opposite of the factors causing a left shift and include hyperthermia, respiratory or metabolic acidosis, increased red cell 2,3-DPG, pregnancy, inhalational anesthetics, and abnormal hemoglobin. Sepsis, shunting, and cyanide toxicity, unless they cause an acidosis, do not affect the P_{50} of hemoglobin and if they were to cause an acidosis, a rightward not leftward shift in the oxyhemoglobin dissociation curve would result. The three items do not share one common feature. They can produce an elevated mixed venous oxygen saturation *(Miller: Anesthesia, ed 4, pp 596-597).*

153. **(C)** Also see explanation to question 150. Factors that increase pulmonary vascular resistance include acidosis, hypoxia, hypercarbia, sympathetic stimulation, atelectasis, and high hematocrit. Hypocarbia causes alkalosis which decreases pulmonary vascular resistance *(Barash: Clinical Anesthesia, ed 2, p 1015).*

154. **(A)** Also see explanation to question 102. Static lung volumes can be divided into those that can be measured by simple spirometry and into those that cannot. The functional residual capacity and residual volume cannot be measured by simple spirometry. However, these two variables can be measured using gas dilution techniques or body plethysmography *(West: Respiratory Physiology, ed 5, p 12).*

155. **(A)** Also see explanation to question 5. Pulmonary surfactant is lipophilic material that is composed primarily of dipalmitoyl phosphatidyl choline. This substance is produced by type 2 alveolar cells from fatty acids that are extracted from the blood, which are themselves synthesized by the lungs. This process is efficient with very rapid turnover. If blood flow to a region of the lungs is markedly reduced or abolished (e.g., pulmonary embolism or cardiopulmonary bypass) or the type 2 alveolar cells are destroyed (e.g., O_2 toxicity or gastric acid aspiration), surfactant will be depleted causing atelectasis. Administration of corticosteroids during pregnancy has been demonstrated to increase the production of pulmonary surfactant in the fetus *(West: Respiratory Physiology, ed 5, pp 47, 94-98; Stoelting: Pharmacology and Physiology in Anesthetic Practice, ed 2, pp 722 & 723).*

156. **(E)** The closing capacity is the product of residual volume and the volume remaining in the lung when airway closure occurs (i.e., closing volume). Measurement of the closing capacity is a sensitive test of early small airway diseases, such as emphysema, asthma, bronchitis, and pulmonary interstitial edema. Smoking tobacco, obesity, aging, and the supine position increase the closing capacity *(Miller: Anesthesia, ed 4, pp 590-593).*

157. **(E)** The compensatory mechanisms for metabolic acidosis can be divided into two groups: acute compensatory responses and chronic compensatory responses. The acute compensatory responses include increased V_A, which is caused primarily by stimulation of the carotid bodies by H^+, and the buffering of H^+ by HCO_3^-, hemoglobin, phosphates, and proteins. The chronic compensatory responses include secretion of H^+ and the reabsorption of HCO_3^- by the proximal and distal renal tubules, and the buffering of H^+ by bone *(Stoelting: Basics of Anesthesia, ed 3, pp 217 & 224)*.

158. **(E)** Also see explanation to questions 102 and 156. The maximum volume of gas that can be inhaled is called the inspiratory capacity. The volume of gas that can be inhaled from the end of a normal inspiration is called the inspiratory reserve volume. Thus, the inspiratory capacity is composed of the V_T and inspiratory reserve volume *(Miller: Anesthesia, ed 4, pp 589 & 590; West: Respiratory Physiology, ed 5, pp 12-14)*.

159. **(A)** Also see explanation to question 116. There are three compensatory mechanisms for respiratory alkalosis. First, HCO_3^- is oxidized to produce water and CO_2. Second, the alkalosis stimulates the activity of phosphofructokinase, which increases glycolysis and lactic acid production. Finally, reabsorption of HCO_3^- by the proximal convoluted renal tubules is reduced. Hydration of CO_2 in erythrocytes increases $[HCO_3^-]$, which will exacerbate the alkalosis *(Stoelting: Basics of Anesthesia, ed 3, p 223)*.

160. **(C)** Also see explanation to question 151. The rate of simple diffusion of molecules through a lipid membrane is influenced by factors described in both Graham's law and Fick's law. Graham's law states that rate of diffusion of a gas through a lipid membrane is directly proportional to the solubility of the gas and is inversely proportional to the square root of the molecular weight of the gas. Fick's law states that the rate of diffusion of a gas through a lipid membrane is directly proportional to the pressure gradient of the gas across the membrane and the area of the membrane, and is inversely proportional to the thickness of the membrane *(West: Respiratory Physiology, ed 5, pp 169 & 170; Barash: Clinical Anesthesia, ed 2, pp 162-164)*.

161. **(A)** Patients who smoke cigarettes have a higher incidence of postoperative pulmonary complications than those who do not smoke cigarettes. It is thought that part of the morbidity associated with cigarette smoking is associated with the adverse effects of carbon monoxide on the O_2-carrying capacity of hemoglobin. Carbon monoxide combines with hemoglobin to produce carboxyhemoglobin causing a leftward shift of the oxyhemoglobin dissociation curve, which increases the affinity of hemoglobin for O_2 (see explanation to question 140). In addition, carbon monoxide has a negative inotropic effect on myocardial contractility. Although the effects of carbon monoxide on the cardiovascular system are short-lived and readily reversible with cessation of smoking, short-term abstinence from cigarettes prior to elective surgery has not been shown to decrease the incidence of postoperative pulmonary complications. Carboxyhemoglobin will cause dual-wavelength pulse oximeters to display falsely elevated arterial O_2 saturations (see explanation to question 107). There is no evidence that carboxyhemoglobin associated with cigarette smoking will increase the incidence of deep vein thrombosis in the postoperative period *(Miller: Anesthesia, ed 4, p 1263; Stoelting: Anesthesia and Co-existing Disease, ed 3, p 140)*.

162. **(A)** Physiologic shunt is that portion of the cardiac output that perfuses areas of the lungs that are not ventilated. In the normal patient, physiologic shunt accounts for approximately 5% to 10% of the cardiac output. There are several anatomic sources for physiologic shunt. These include bronchial vessels, which supply blood and O_2 to the main conducting airways of the lungs, the Thebesian veins, which drain blood from the coronary vessels that supply the myocardium, and pleural veins, which drain blood that has supplied O_2 to the pleura. Alveoli that are poorly perfused but are adequately ventilated contribute to physiologic dead space ventilation *(West: Respiratory Physiology, ed 5, pp 55-57)*.

163. **(A)** Also see explanation to question 151. The DL_{co} is determined in part by the volume of blood (hemoglobin concentration) within the pulmonary capillaries. Thus, diseases associated with a reduction in pulmonary blood volume, such as anemia, emphysema, dehydration, and pulmonary hypertension, will result in a decrease in DL_{co}. Although the mechanism is not known, acute asthma is associated with an increase in DL_{co} *(West: Respiratory Physiology, ed 5, pp 28 & 29; Miller: Anesthesia, ed 2, p 1375)*.

164. **(A)** Methemoglobin is oxidized adult hemoglobin (i.e., the iron is oxidized from the ferrous to the ferric form). Because methemoglobin is not able to bind O_2, it causes cyanosis despite an adequate P_aO_2. Causes of methemoglobinemia include congenital absence of methemoglobin reductase, the enzyme that reduces methemoglobin to normal hemoglobin, and nitrate-containing compounds. O-toluidine, a metabolite of the local anesthetic prilocaine, oxidizes adult hemoglobin to methemoglobin. Sodium nitroprusside and nitroglycerin are metabolized within erythrocytes by a nonenzymatic reaction which requires the oxidation of oxyhemoglobin to methemoglobin *(Miller: Anesthesia, ed 4, p 515; Barash: Clinical Anesthesia, ed 2, p 529; Stoelting: Anesthesia and Co-existing Disease, ed 3, p 403)*.

165. **(B)** The respiratory quotient is the ratio of the rate of CO_2 production to the rate of O_2 consumption. Metabolic substrate is an important determinant of the rate of CO_2 production and thus affects the respiratory quotient *(Miller: Anesthesia, ed 4, pp 2521 & 2522)*.

166. **(C)** The cilia of the respiratory tract extend from the columnar cells lining the conducting airways. They propel a double layer of mucus up to the epiglottis, an important mechanism for removing small particles from the conducting airways. The rhythmic motion of cilia is altered by changes in gas temperature and humidity *(Miller: Anesthesia, ed 4, pp 133 & 134)*.

167. **(B)** Also see explanation to question 103. Anatomic dead space consists of the conducting airways that contain no alveoli and therefore take no part in gas exchange. Anatomic dead space is approximately 1 mL/lb of body weight *(Miller: Anesthesia, ed 4, p 594; West: Respiratory Physiology, ed 5, pp 2 & 19)*.

168. **(A)** Also see explanation to questions 102 and 156. The vital capacity is the volume of gas that can be exhaled during a maximal expiration. It is composed of the inspiratory and expiratory reserve volumes, and the V_T *(Miller: Anesthesia, ed 4, p 590)*.

Pharmacology and Pharmacokinetics of Intravenous Drugs

DIRECTIONS (Questions 169 through 241): Each of the questions or incomplete statements in this section is followed by answers or by completions of the statement, respectively. Select the ONE BEST answer or completion for each item.

169. Which of the following muscle relaxants is eliminated almost exclusively *via* the kidneys?

    A. Pancuronium
    B. Gallamine
    C. d-Tubocurarine
    D. Metocurine
    E. Doxacurium

170. Special considerations for patients with porphyria cutanea tarda would include which of the following

    A. Avoidance of regional techniques because of neurotoxicity
    B. Avoidance of sodium pentothal
    C. Need for higher doses of nondepolarizing neuromuscular blocking drugs
    D. Special attention to skin pressure
    E. Need for reduced doses of renally metabolized drugs

171. The reason for the shorter duration of action of propofol compared to thiopental is that propofol

    A. Is cleared by the kidneys more rapidly
    B. Has a smaller volume of distribution
    C. Has greater hepatic extraction
    D. Is more lipid soluble
    E. Is less protein bound

172. A 78-year-old patient with Parkinson's disease undergoes a cataract operation under general anesthesia. In the recovery room, the patient has two episodes of emesis and complains of severe nausea. Which of the following antiemetics would be the best choice for treatment of nausea in this patient?

    A. Droperidol
    B. Promethazine
    C. Ondansetron
    D. Thiethylparazine
    E. Metoclopramide

173. Which of the following diseases is associated with increased resistance to neuromuscular blockade with succinylcholine?

    A. Myasthenia gravis
    B. Myasthenic syndrome
    C. Huntington's chorea
    D. Polymyositis
    E. Muscular dystrophy

174. At what dose does dopamine increase renal blood flow?

    A. 1-3 μg/kg/min
    B. 3-10 μg/kg/min
    C. 10-20 μg/kg/min
    D. 20-50 μg/kg/min
    E. Greater than 50 μg/kg/min

175. A 63-year-old male with hypertension is brought to the operating room for a thoracotomy. He has no allergies and has been taking reserpine for 12 years. Following induction his blood pressure decreases from 150/80 mm Hg to 85/50 mm Hg. Which of the following vasopressor agents would be **LEAST** efficacious in treating hypotension in this patient?

    A. Phenylephrine
    B. Ephedrine
    C. Methoxamine
    D. Epinephrine
    E. Norepinephrine

176. A 22-year-old, 70-kg patient is brought to the operating room for resection of an anterior pituitary prolactin-secreting tumor. Anesthesia is maintained with isoflurane, N_2O 50% in O_2, and fentanyl. The surgeon wants to inject lidocaine with epinephrine into the nasal mucosa to minimize bleeding. What is the maximum amount of 1% lidocaine with 1:100,000 epinephrine that can be administered safely to this patient?

    A. 55 mL
    B. 45 mL
    C. 35 mL
    D. 25 mL
    E. 15 mL

177. Patients receiving antihypertensive therapy with propranolol are at increased risk for each of the following **EXCEPT**

    A. Blunted response to hypoglycemia
    B. Bronchoconstriction
    C. Rebound tachycardia after discontinuation
    D. Orthostatic hypotension
    E. Atrioventricular heart block

178. Atropine causes each of the following **EXCEPT**

    A. Decreased gastric acid secretion
    B. Inhibition of salivary secretion
    C. Tachycardia
    D. Mydriasis
    E. Increased lower esophageal sphincter tone

179. Which of the following drugs is capable of crossing the blood-brain barrier?

    A. Neostigmine
    B. Pyridostigmine
    C. Edrophonium
    D. Physostigmine
    E. All of the above

180. Patients treated with which of the following antihypertensive agents may develop paradoxical hypertension if propranolol is administered?

    A. Clonidine
    B. Minoxidil
    C. α-Methyldopa
    D. Hydralazine
    E. Reserpine

181. Which of the following opioid-receptor agonists has anticholinergic properties?

    A. Morphine
    B. Fentanyl
    C. Sufentanyl
    D. Meperidine
    E. Oxymorphone

182. If thiopental is accidently injected into an artery, treatment should include immediate dilution with

    A. Norepinephrine
    B. Lidocaine
    C. Propranolol
    D. Physostigmine
    E. Naloxone

183. Which of the following vasopressor agents increase systemic blood pressure directly by binding to adrenergic receptors and indirectly by stimulating the release of norepinephrine from sympathetic nerve fibers?

    A. Dobutamine
    B. Ephedrine
    C. Epinephrine
    D. Phenylephrine
    E. Methoxamine

184. Which of the following narcotics causes the greatest decreases in myocardial contractility when administered alone?

    A. Morphine
    B. Meperidine
    C. Sufentanyl
    D. Alfentanil
    E. Fentanyl

185. Select the **FALSE** statement about ketamine

    A. May cause purposeful skeletal muscle movements
    B. Visceral pain is better controlled than somatic pain
    C. May increase blood pressure and cardiac output
    D. Inhibits norepinephrine re-uptake into postganglionic sympathetic nerve fibers
    E. Is metabolized by the liver

186. Which of the following anesthetics is most likely to cause myocardial depression?

    A. Morphine
    B. Thiopental
    C. Etomidate
    D. Ketamine
    E. Diazepam

187. Which of the following drugs should be administered with caution if at all to patients receiving echothiopate?

    A. Atropine
    B. Succinylcholine
    C. Ketamine
    D. Pancuronium
    E. Neostigmine

188. What percent of neuromuscular blockade is achieved if 2 out of 4 thumb twitches in the train-of-four stimulation of the ulnar nerve can be elicited?

    A. 25
    B. 50
    C. 75
    D. 80
    E. 90

189. Which of the following muscle relaxants does not cause histamine release?

    A. Metocurine
    B. Gallamine
    C. d-Tubocurarine
    D. Atracurium
    E. Mivacurium

190. Elimination of which of the following muscle relaxants depends **LEAST** on renal function?

   A. Metocurine
   B. Pancuronium
   C. Vecuronium
   D. d-Tubocurarine
   E. Gallamine

191. The incidence of unpleasant dreams associated with emergence from Ketamine anesthesia can be reduced by administration of

   A. Atropine
   B. Scopolamine
   C. Physostigmine
   D. Diazepam
   E. Glycopyrrolate

192. Which of the following premedications is associated with extrapyramidal side-effects?

   A. Metoclopramide
   B. Cimetidine
   C. Scopolamine
   D. Glycopyrrolate
   E. Flurazepam

193. Succinylcholine, when administered to normal patients, will increase serum $[K^+]$ by approximately

   A. 0.1 mEq/L
   B. 0.5 mEq/L
   C. 1.0 mEq/L
   D. 1.5 mEq/L
   E. 2.0 mEq/L

194. Each of the following drugs can potentiate nondepolarizing neuromuscular blockade **EXCEPT**

   A. Calcium
   B. Lithium
   C. Magnesium
   D. Polymyxin B
   E. Procainamide

195. Discontinuation of which of the following medications is recommended prior to elective surgery?

   A. Reserpine
   B. Monoamine oxidase inhibitors
   C. Propranolol
   D. Tricyclic antidepressants
   E. None of the above

196. Laudanosine is a metabolite of

    A. Atracurium
    B. D-tubocurarine
    C. Vecuronium
    D. Pancuronium
    E. Metocurine

197. Pretreatment with a nondepolarizing muscle relaxant is **LEAST** effective in attenuating which of the following side-effects of succinylcholine?

    A. Increased intragastric pressure
    B. Increased intraocular pressure
    C. Hyperkalemia
    D. Myalgias
    E. Bradycardia

198. Which of the following does **NOT** increase neuromuscular blockade?

    A. Clindamycin
    B. Lincomycin
    C. Streptomycin
    D. Erythromycin
    E. Gentamycin

199. Time of onset from most rapid to least rapid

    A. Edrophonium, pyridostigmine, neostigmine
    B. Edrophonium, neostigmine, pyridostigmine
    C. Neostigmine, edrophonium, pyridostigmine
    D. Neostigmine, pyridostigmine, edrophonium
    E. Pyridostigmine, neostigmine, edrophonium

200. The pH of commercially available thiopental is

    A. 4.4
    B. 5.2
    C. 7.4
    D. 8.5
    E. 10.4

201. In which of the following situations is succinylcholine most likely to cause severe hyperkalemia?

    A. 24 hours following a right hemisphere stroke
    B. 10 days following a severe burn injury
    C. 24 hours following a mid-thoracic spinal cord transection
    D. 3 days with an abdominal infection
    E. Chronic renal failure

202. The most common minor side effect reported after flumazenil administration in anesthesia is

    A. Nausea and/or vomiting
    B. Dizziness
    C. Tremors
    D. Hypertension
    E. Pain on injection

203. The most appropriate combination of drugs in terms of onset and duration of action for reversal of nondepolarizing neuromuscular blockade is

    A. Edrophonium and glycopyrrolate
    B. Edrophonium and atropine
    C. Neostigmine and atropine
    D. Pyridostigmine and atropine
    E. None of the above

204. A 37-year-old male with a history of acute intermittent porphyria is scheduled for knee arthroscopy under general anesthesia. Which of the following drugs is contraindicated in this patient?

    A. Pyridostigmine
    B. Droperidol
    C. Propofol
    D. Succinylcholine
    E. Etomidate

205. The combination of dantrolene and verapamil administered intravenously places the patient at increased risk for

    A. Hypotension
    B. Profound bradycardia
    C. Hepatotoxicity
    D. Profound muscular weakness
    E. Increased PT and PTT

206. Severe hypertension can occur when naloxone is administered to patients taking

    A. Clonidine
    B. Nifedipine
    C. Reserpine
    D. Guanethidine
    E. Hydralazine

207. The most important reason for the more rapid onset and shorter duration of action of fentanyl compared with morphine is the difference in

    A. Volume of distribution
    B. Hepatic clearance
    C. Renal clearance
    D. Lipid solubility
    E. Protein binding

208. The term "azeotrope" refers to

    A. A mixture of two volatile anesthetics
    B. A mixture of a volatile anesthetic plus N_2O
    C. A mixture of volatile anesthetic plus N_2
    D. Radioactively labeled N_2O
    E. Radioactively labeled N_2

209. All the following agents inhibit CSF production **EXCEPT**

    A. Digoxin
    B. Steroids
    C. Acetazolamide
    D. Hypothermia
    E. Enflurane

210. The unique advantage of rocuronium over other muscle relaxants is its

    A. Short duration of action
    B. Metabolism by pseudocholinesterase
    C. Onset of action
    D. Lack of need for reversal
    E. Lack of potentiation with aminoglycoside antibiotics

211. Which of the following statements concerning the effect of hypokalemia on nondepolarizing neuro-muscular blockade is correct?

    A. The dose requirement for pancuronium is increased, but the dose requirement for neostigmine is reduced
    B. The dose requirements for both pancuronium and neostigmine are increased
    C. The dose requirements for both pancuronium and neostigmine are reduced
    D. The dose requirement for pancuronium is reduced, but the dose requirement for neostigmine is increased
    E. The dose requirement for pancuronium is reduced, but the dose requirement for neostigmine is unchanged

212. Which of the following neuromuscular blocking drugs cause the greatest release of histamine when administered intravenously?

    A. Succinylcholine
    B. d-Tubocurarine
    C. Metocurine
    D. Atracurium
    E. Mivacurium

213. A 58-year-old female is brought to the emergency room with the following symptoms: miosis, abdominal cramping, salivation, loss of bowel and bladder control, bradycardia, ataxia, and skeletal muscle weakness. The most likely diagnosis is

    A. Central anticholinergic syndrome
    B. Malignant neuroleptic syndrome
    C. Anticholinesterase poisoning
    D. Digitalis overdose
    E. Thorazine overdose

214. Flumazenil

    A. Is contraindicated in narcotic addicts
    B. Partially antagonizes thiopental
    C. Has weak anticonvulsant activity
    D. Has an elimination half-life similar to that of midazolam
    E. Is not effective in antagonizing the muscle relaxing properties of benzodiazepines

215. What percent of neuromuscular receptors could potentially be blocked and still allow patients to carry out a 5 second head lift?

    A. 0
    B. 5
    C. 15
    D. 33
    E. 66

216. Methohexital has a shorter elimination half-time than thiopental because methohexital

    A. Is more lipid soluble
    B. Is more ionized in blood
    C. Has greater protein binding
    D. Has greater hepatic extraction
    E. None of the above

217. Which of the following drugs can prevent tachydysrhythmias in patients with Wolff-Parkinson-White syndrome?

    A. Droperidol
    B. Pancuronium
    C. Ketamine
    D. Gallamine
    E. Meperidine

218. The half-life of pseudocholinesterase is

    A. 3 minutes
    B. 1 hour
    C. 12 hours
    D. 1 week
    E. 2 weeks

219. A 9-year-old girl undergoes a tonsillectomy under general anesthesia. A 30 mg intramuscular dose of ketorolac is administered after the patient is induced and intubated. Four mg of IV morphine are administered at the same time. The operation is carried out uneventfully. The patient is extubated and taken to the recovery room and one hour later is resting quietly and complains of no pain. The effects of ketorolac on transmission of painful stimuli are exerted at which part in the afferent sensory pathway?

   A. At the level of sensory receptors
   B. At the dorsal route ganglia
   C. At spinal thalamic tract
   D. At the thalamus
   E. At the sensory cortex

220. The anti-inflammatory power of 50 mg of prednisone (Deltasone) can be achieved by which of the following?

   A. 100 mg cortisol (Solu-Cortef)
   B. 50 mg methylprednisone (Solu-Medrol)
   C. 8 mg dexamethasone (Decadron)
   D. 4 mg betamethasone (Celestone)
   E. 20 mg prednisolone (Delta-Cortef)

221. The plasma clearance of which of the following nondepolarizing muscle relaxants is not altered by aging?

   A. Atracurium
   B. Vecuronium
   C. d-Tubocurarine
   D. Pancuronium
   E. Metocurine

222. Side effects associated with cyclosporine therapy include each of the following **EXCEPT**

   A. Nephrotoxicity
   B. Pulmonary toxicity
   C. Hypertension
   D. Limb paresthesias
   E. Seizures

223. What is the predominant mechanism for succinylcholine-induced tachycardia?

   A. Histamine release from mast cells
   B. Stimulation of nicotinic receptors at autonomic ganglia
   C. Blockade of nicotinic receptors at autonomic ganglia
   D. Direct vagolytic effect at postjunctional muscarinic receptors
   E. Direct sympathomimetic effect at postjunctional muscarinic receptors

224. Bradycardia observed after administration of succinylcholine to children is attributable to which mechanism

   A. Nicotinic stimulation at the autonomic ganglia
   B. Nicotinic blockade at the autonomic ganglia
   C. Muscarinic stimulation at the sinus node
   D. Muscarinic blockade at the sinus node
   E. Stimulation of the vagus nerve centrally

225. A 72-year-old retired farmer with essential hypertension takes 100 mg of guanethidine daily. Which of the following most accurately describes this patient's blood pressure response to direct- and indirect-acting sympathomimetic agents?

   A. Normal response to indirect-acting agents; exaggerated response to direct-acting agents
   B. Reduced response to indirect-acting agents; exaggerated response to direct-acting agents
   C. Exaggerated response to both direct- and indirect-acting agents
   D. Reduced response to both direct- and indirect-acting agents
   E. Normal response to both direct- and indirect-acting agents

226. Succinylcholine is contraindicated for routine tracheal intubation in children because of an increased incidence of which of the following side effects?

   A. Hyperkalemia
   B. Malignant hyperthermia
   C. Masseter spasm
   D. Bradycardia
   E. Severe myalgias

227. From **MOST** to **LEAST** rapid select the correct temporal sequence of neuromuscular blockade in the adductor of the thumb, the orbicularis oculi, and the diaphragm after administration of an intubating dose of vecuronium to an otherwise healthy patient

   A. Diaphragm, orbicularis oculi, thumb
   B. Orbicularis oculi, diaphragm, thumb
   C. Orbicularis oculi, thumb, diaphragm
   D. Thumb, orbicularis oculi, diaphragm
   E. Orbicularis oculi same as diaphragm, thumb

228. Select the true statement regarding interaction of nondepolarizing neuromuscular blocking drugs when durations of action are dissimilar

   A. If a long-acting drug is administered after a short-acting drug, the duration of the long-acting drug will be longer than normal
   B. If a long-acting drug is administered after a short-acting drug, the duration of the long-acting drug will be about the same as expected
   C. If a short-acting drug is administered after a long-acting drug, the duration of the short-acting drug will be about the same as expected
   D. If a long-acting drug is administered after a short-acting drug, the duration of action of the long-acting drug will be shorter than expected
   E. If a short-acting drug is administered after a long-acting drug, the duration of action of this short-acting drug will be shorter than expected

229. Select the correct statement regarding the effects of volatile anesthetics on nondepolarizing neuromuscular blocking drugs vs the effect of volatile anesthetics on neuromuscular blocking drug antagonists, i.e. anticholinesterase

 A. Volatile anesthetics potentiate neuromuscular blockade, but retard reversal agents
 B. Volatile anesthetics potentiate both neuromuscular blocking drugs and reversal agents
 C. Volatile anesthetics retard both neuromuscular blocking drugs and reversal agents
 D. Volatile anesthetics retard neuromuscular blocking drugs, but potentiate reversal agents
 E. Volatile anesthetics potentiate neuromuscular blocking drugs, but have no effect on reversal agents

230. A 57-year-old woman with severe aortic stenosis is scheduled for aortic valve replacement. A nitrous narcotic anesthetic is planned with nondepolarizing neuromuscular blockade. Which of the following muscle relaxants would be most appropriate for this patient

 A. Pancuronium
 B. d-Tubocurarine
 C. Rocuronium
 D. Pipecuronium
 E. Mivacurium

231. Which of the following benzylisoquinolinium nondepolarizing neuromuscular blocking drugs is unique among this class of drugs in that it does not cause release of histamine?

 A. d-Tubocurarine
 B. Metocurine
 C. Doxacurium
 D. Atracurium
 E. Mivacurium

232. The most common reason for patients to rate anesthesia with etomidate as unsatisfactory is

 A. Postoperative nausea and vomiting
 B. Pain on injection
 C. Recall of intubation
 D. Myoclonus
 E. Postoperative hiccups

233. Which of the following muscle relaxants inhibits the re-uptake of norepinephrine by the adrenergic nerves?

 A. Pancuronium
 B. Pipecuronium
 C. Rocuronium
 D. Doxacurium
 E. Mivacurium

234. The most common side effect of dantrolene as used in the treatment of malignant hyperthermia is

   A. Nausea and vomiting
   B. Muscle weakness
   C. Confusion and disorientation
   D. Hepatitis
   E. Diarrhea

235. Arrange in order from most to least the incidence of myoclonus for the following agents

   A. Etomidate, propofol, thiopental
   B. Etomidate, thiopental, propofol
   C. Propofol, etomidate, thiopental
   D. Thiopental, etomidate, propofol
   E. Thiopental, propofol, etomidate

236. A 37-year-old man is brought to the OR for reattachment of the right index finger after a traumatic amputation. The patient has been in treatment for alcohol and drug abuse and takes naltrexone and disulfiram. Which of the following would be the best technique for management of this patient's post-operative pain?

   A. Continue naltrexone with round-the-clock low dose methadone
   B. Continue naltrexone with small doses of morphine q4h
   C. Continue naltrexone with small doses of nalbuphine q4h prn
   D. Discontinue naltrexone and treat pain with morphine prn
   E. Discontinue naltrexone and treat pain with acetaminophen prn

237. Which of the following muscle relaxants is most suitable for rapid intubation in a patient in whom succinylcholine is contraindicated?

   A. Mivacurium
   B. Rocuronium
   C. Doxacurium
   D. Pipecuronium
   E. Vecuronium

238. The effects of an intubation dose of vecuronium are terminated by

   A. Pseudocholinesterase
   B. Non-specific plasma cholinesterases
   C. The kidneys
   D. The liver
   E. Diffusion from the neuromuscular junction back into the plasma

239. Respiratory depression produced by which of the following analgesics is not readily reversed by administration of naloxone?

   A. Propoxyphene
   B. Methadone
   C. Hydromorphone
   D. Buprenorphine
   E. Opium

240. Which of the following intravenous anesthetic agents is associated with the highest incidence of nausea and vomiting?

   A. Thiopental
   B. Etomidate
   C. Ketamine
   D. Propofol
   E. Midazolam

241. If naloxone is administered to a patient who is receiving ketorolac for postoperative pain, the most likely result would be

   A. Bradycardia
   B. Hypotension
   C. Pain
   D. Somnolence
   E. None of the above

DIRECTIONS (Questions 242 through 282): For each of the items in this section, ONE or MORE of the numbered options is correct. Select the answer:

Select A if options *1, 2 and 3* are correct,
Select B if options *1 and 3* are correct,
Select C if options *2 and 4* are correct,
Select D if only option *4* is correct,
Select E if *all* options are correct.

242. Vasodilators which produce strong effects on the pulmonary arterial tree with minimal or no effect on the systemic circulation include

   1. Sodium nitroprusside
   2. Prostaglandin E_1
   3. Phentolamine
   4. Nitric oxide

Select A if options *1, 2 and 3* are correct,
Select B if options *1 and 3* are correct,
Select C if options *2 and 4* are correct,
Select D if only option *4* is correct,
Select E if *all* options are correct.

243. Characteristics of phase I depolarizing neuromuscular blockade include

    1. Antagonism with neostigmine
    2. Fade in the train-of-four response
    3. Post-tetanic potentiation
    4. Sustained response to a tetanic stimulus

244. Methohexital differs from thiopental in which way(s)

    1. Its elimination half-time is shorter
    2. It activates epileptic foci
    3. Its clearance is faster
    4. Its volume of distribution is smaller

245. Which of the following nondepolarizing muscle relaxants can also block cardiac muscarinic receptors?

    1. d-Tubocurarine
    2. Gallamine
    3. Metocurine
    4. Pancuronium

246. Moricizine (Ethmozine)

    1. Is a type I antiarrhythmic
    2. Is indicated for the treatment of life-threatening ventricular arrhythmias
    3. Blocks sodium channels
    4. Has minimal negative inotropic effects

247. Three hundred mg of intravenous cimetidine are administered to a 78-year-old woman with a history of reactive airways disease 30 minutes prior to induction of anesthesia for an exploratory laparotomy. Possible side effects associated with this drug include:

    1. Bradycardia
    2. Bronchospasm
    3. Delayed awakening
    4. Increased metabolism of diazepam

248. Metabolism of midazolam is inhibited by

    1. Cimetidine
    2. Famotidine
    3. Rantidine
    4. Erythromycin

Select A if options *1, 2 and 3* are correct,
Select B if options *1 and 3* are correct,
Select C if options *2 and 4* are correct,
Select D if only option *4* is correct,
Select E if *all* options are correct.

249. Metoclopramide

    1. May cause extrapyramidal side-effects
    2. Relaxes the lower esophageal sphincter
    3. Facilitates gastric emptying
    4. Reliably raises gastric fluid pH

250. Alfentanil is unique among morphine, meperidine, fentanyl, and sufentanil in that

    1. It undergoes no hepatic metabolism
    2. Continuous intravenous infusions do not produce clinically significant cumulative effects
    3. It has the most rapid clearance
    4. It has the most rapid onset

251. Which of the following medications is effective in the management of acute exacerbations of bronchial asthma?

    1. Corticosteroids
    2. Aminophylline
    3. ß-adrenergic receptor agonists
    4. Cromolyn

252. Clonidine

    1. Reduces the MAC of isoflurane
    2. Reduces the requirement for sufentanil during cardiopulmonary bypass
    3. Decreases extremes in arterial blood pressure during anesthesia
    4. Prevents muscle rigidity seen with narcotics

253. The duration of action of which of the following drugs is prolonged in patients with end-stage cirrhotic liver disease?

    1. Diazepam
    2. Vecuronium
    3. Lidocaine
    4. Procaine

254. The following drug(s) lower(s) the activity of pseudocholinesterase in the plasma

    1. Neostigmine
    2. Echothiophate
    3. Pyridostigmine
    4. Edrophonium

Select A if options *1, 2 and 3* are correct,
Select B if options *1 and 3* are correct,
Select C if options *2 and 4* are correct,
Select D if only option *4* is correct,
Select E if *all* options are correct.

255. Which of the following statements concerning nondepolarizing muscle relaxants is correct?

1. The volume of distribution of d-tubocurarine is less in children than in adults
2. The duration of action of d-tubocurarine is longer in infants than in adults
3. Adults are more sensitive to d-tubocurarine than are infants
4. The initial dose (based on body weight) is the same for infants and adults

256. A 79-year-old male patient is brought to the operating room for elective repair of an inguinal hernia. The patient has a history of awareness during general anesthesia. The patient is preoxygenated prior to induction of general anesthesia, 5 mg of midazolam and 250 mcg of fentanyl are administered. One minute later the patient loses consciousness and chest wall stiffness develops to the extent that positive-pressure ventilation is very difficult. Appropriate therapy for reversal of chest wall stiffness at this point could include

1. Flumazenil
2. Naloxone
3. Sodium pentothal
4. Succinylcholine

257. Thiopental causes hypotension by

1. Reducing cardiac venous return
2. Reducing sympathetic tone
3. Reducing myocardial contractility
4. Histamine release

258. Propofol

1. Possesses significant antiemetic activity at low doses
2. Induces bronchodilation in patients with chronic obstructive pulmonary disease
3. May be used to treat pruritus induced by spinal opiates
4. Does not potentiate neuromuscular blockade produced by vecuronium

259. Treatment of neuroleptic malignant syndrome after administration of droperidol may be carried out with administration of

1. Diphenhydramine
2. Bromocriptine
3. Benztropine
4. Dantrolene

Select A if options *1, 2 and 3* are correct,
Select B if options *1 and 3* are correct,
Select C if options *2 and 4* are correct,
Select D if only option *4* is correct,
Select E if *all* options are correct.

260. Which of the following nondepolarizing neuromuscular blocking drugs inhibit(s) the action of pseudocholinesterase?

    1. Pancuronium
    2. Atracurium
    3. Vecuronium
    4. d-Tubocurarine

261. Cyanide toxicity may be treated with

    1. Sodium nitrate
    2. Hydroxocobalamin
    3. Sodium thiosulfate
    4. Methylene blue

262. The dibucaine number is abnormal in patients

    1. Chronically exposed to malathion
    2. Treated with echothiophate for glaucoma
    3. With metastatic breast cancer treated with cyclophosphamide
    4. Genetically homozygous for atypical pseudocholinesterase

263. The duration of action of which of the following premedications is prolonged in patients with cirrhotic liver disease?

    1. Oxazepam (Serax)
    2. Midazolam (Versed)
    3. Lorazepam (Ativan)
    4. Diazepam (Valium)

264. Bradycardia associated with administration of a second dose of succinylcholine to adults may be prevented by administration of which of the following?

    1. Atropine
    2. Thiopental
    3. Trimethaphan
    4. Gallamine

265. Which of the following anesthetics cause respiratory depression by decreasing tidal volume?

    1. Thiopental
    2. Morphine
    3. Isoflurane
    4. Fentanyl

Select A if options *1, 2 and 3* are correct,
Select B if options *1 and 3* are correct,
Select C if options *2 and 4* are correct,
Select D if only option *4* is correct,
Select E if *all* options are correct.

266. Oral barbiturates are useful for premedicating patients prior to surgery because they

1.   Cause sedation
2.   Have minimal circulatory side-effects
3.   Cause minimal respiratory depression
4.   Provide intense analgesia

267. Advantages of steroidal compounds (e.g., pancuronium, pipecuronium, vecuronium, and rocuronium) over benzylisoquinolinium compounds include

1.   Lack of histamine release
2.   Lack of vagolytic effect
3.   High potency
4.   Lack of renal elimination

268. Treatment for accidental intra-arterial injection of thiopental could include

1.   Stellate ganglion block
2.   Heparin administration
3.   Intra-arterial injection of lidocaine
4.   Intra-arterial injection of papaverine

269. Which of the following intravenous drugs can produce analgesia in subanesthetic doses?

1.   Diazepam
2.   Etomidate
3.   Thiopental
4.   Ketamine

270. Important drug interactions involving phenothiazines include

1.   Potentiation of the depressant effects of narcotics
2.   Lowering of the seizure threshold
3.   Interference with the antihypertensive effects of guanethidine
4.   Potentiation of neuromuscular blockade

271. Amrinone

1.   Is a positive inotrope
2.   Is antagonized by esmolol
3.   Is a vasodilator
4.   Has weak antidysrhythmic properties

Select A if options *1, 2 and 3* are correct,
Select B if options *1 and 3* are correct,
Select C if options *2 and 4* are correct,
Select D if only option *4* is correct,
Select E if *all* options are correct.

272. True statements concerning tricyclic antidepressants in patients receiving general anesthesia include

    1. They should be discontinued two weeks prior to elective operations
    2. They may increase the requirement for volatile anesthetics
    3. Meperidine may produce hyperpyrexia in patients taking tricyclic antidepressants
    4. The response to ephedrine may be exaggerated

273. Drugs useful in the treatment of organophosphate overdose include

    1. Atropine
    2. Pralidoxime
    3. Diazepam
    4. Edrophonium

274. Which of the following intravenous medications would be suitable for the treatment of hypertension and tachycardia in a 68-year-old patient with a reactive airway?

    1. Esmolol
    2. Labetalol
    3. Atenolol
    4. Propranolol

275. The following drug(s) is (are) metabolized by pseudocholinesterase

    1. Trimethaphan
    2. Mivacurium
    3. Procaine
    4. Lidocaine

276. Which of the following agents may cause phlebitis and thrombosis when administered intravenously?

    1. Propofol
    2. Diazepam
    3. Etomidate
    4. Thiopental

277. Which of the following statements concerning the pharmacology of thiopental is (are) correct?

    1. Rapid awakening after induction of anesthesia with thiopental reflects avid hepatic extraction
    2. An induction dose of thiopental will significantly blunt laryngeal reflexes
    3. Thiopental is useful for cerebral protection following cardiac arrest
    4. Can cause hypotension

Select A if options *1, 2 and 3* are correct,
Select B if options *1 and 3* are correct,
Select C if options *2 and 4* are correct,
Select D if only option *4* is correct,
Select E if *all* options are correct.

278. A 59-year-old patient with Parkinson's disease is brought to the recovery room after an emergency appendectomy under general anesthesia. Upon arrival he complains of nausea. Which of the following antiemetic agents is appropriate for treatment of nausea in this patient?

    1. Droperidol
    2. Metoclopramide
    3. Promethazine
    4. Diphenhydramine

279. Bradycardia secondary to excess ß-adrenergic receptor blockade can be treated with

    1. Glucagon
    2. Calcium
    3. Atropine
    4. Dobutamine

280. Side effects of short term administration of dantrolene include

    1. Nausea and vomiting
    2. Phlebitis
    3. Muscle weakness
    4. Hepatotoxicity

281. Which of the following muscle relaxants should be used with caution in patients with impaired renal function?

    1. Pancuronium
    2. Doxacurium
    3. Pipecuronium
    4. Mivacurium

282. Systemic side-effect(s) of etomidate when administered to healthy normovolemic patients include

    1. Myoclonic movements
    2. Suppression of adrenocortical function
    3. Pain on injection
    4. Hypotension

DIRECTIONS (Questions 283 through 320): Each group of questions consist of several numbered statements followed by lettered headings. For each numbered statement, select the ONE lettered heading that is most closely associated with it. Each lettered heading may be selected once, more than once, or not at all.

283. Adrenal suppression

284. Thrombosis, phlebitis, specific antagonist available

285. Pain on injection, severe hypotension in elderly

286. Increased intracranial pressure

287. May precipitate a crisis in patients with acute intermittent porphyria

   A. Thiopental
   B. Diazepam
   C. Etomidate
   D. Propofol
   E. Ketamine

288. Alters MAC

289. Is associated with pericardial effusion and cardiac tamponade

290. With high doses may cause a Lupus-like syndrome

291. Produces α-adrenergic receptor and ß-adrenergic receptor blockade

292. May result in severe rebound hypertension when abruptly discontinued

   A. Guanethidine
   B. Hydralazine
   C. Minoxidil
   D. Labetalol
   E. Clonidine

293. Does not increase cardiac output or heart rate

294. Has the most significant effect on metabolism; possesses $ß_1$ and $ß_2$ properties

295. May lower systemic vascular resistance, increases heart rate

296. Increases cardiac output without increasing heart rate or systemic vascular resistance

297. May decrease mean arterial pressure; may increase heart rate

    A. Dopamine
    B. Norepinephrine
    C. Epinephrine
    D. Isoproterenol
    E. Dobutamine

298. Spinal anesthesia, sedation, miosis

299. Supraspinal analgesia

300. Hypertonia and dysphoria

301. Physical dependence

    A. μ_1 (mu$_1$)
    B. μ_2 (mu$_2$)
    C. σ (sigma)
    D. δ (delta)
    E. κ (kappa)

302. Reversed with neostigmine

303. Post tetanic facilitation

304. Sustained response to tetanic stimulus

305. Prolonged by neostigmine

    A. True of nondepolarizing blockade only
    B. True of phase I depolarizing blockade only
    C. True of phase II depolarizing blockade only
    D. True of nondepolarizing and phase II depolarizing blockade
    E. True of phase I and phase II depolarizing blockade

306. Hypernatremia

307. Hyperkalemia

308. Hyperthyroidism

309. Ethanol

310. Lidocaine

311. Lithium

312. Tricyclic antidepressants

313. Duration of anesthesia

314. Pregnancy

315. P_aO_2 35 mm Hg

    A.   No change in MAC
    B.   Increases MAC
    C.   Decreases MAC
    D.   Chronic administration decreases MAC; acute administration increases MAC
    E.   Acute administration decreases MAC; chronic administration increases MAC

316. Least effective antisialagogue

317. Produces best sedation

318. Increases gastric fluid pH

319. Does not produce central anticholinergic syndrome

320. May produce mydriasis and cycloplegia when given intravenously

    A.   Atropine
    B.   Glycopyrrolate
    C.   Scopolamine
    D.   Atropine and Scopolamine
    E.   None of the above

PHARMACOLOGY AND PHARMACOKINETICS OF INTRAVENOUS DRUGS
ANSWERS, REFERENCES, AND EXPLANATIONS

169. **(B)**   All of the muscle relaxants listed are dependent upon the kidneys for elimination to some extent. However, elimination of gallamine depends almost exclusively on renal function. The following table summarizes the routes for elimination of these nondepolarizing muscle relaxants *(Stoelting: Basics of Anesthesia, ed 3, p 91).*

Summary of Elimination of Nondepolarizing Muscle Relaxants

	Percent Dependence on:		
	Renal Excretion	Biliary Excretion	Hepatic Degradation
d-Tubocurarine	45	10-40	Insignificant
Metocurine	43	<2	Insignificant
Gallamine	95	0	Insignificant
Pancuronium	80	5-10	40%
Pipecuronium	70	20	10%
Doxacurium	70	30	Insignificant

*From Stoelting RK, Miller RD (eds): Basics of Anesthesia, ed 3. New York, Churchill Livingstone, 1994, p 91. Used with permission.

170. **(D)**   Porphyria cutanea tarda is a disease that is caused by an enzymatic defect in the liver. Signs and symptoms of this disease most often appear as photosensitivity in males older than 35 years of age. The patient's skin is often very friable and because of this special attention is required to avoid excessive pressure on the skin that could occur during mask ventilation or endotracheal tube taping. In addition, drugs that are capable of precipitating attacks of other forms of porphyria do not provoke an attack of this disease *(Stoelting: Anesthesia and Co-existing Disease, ed 3, p 377).*

171. **(C)**   Propofol is rapidly metabolized in the liver by conjugation to glucuronide and sulfate (water soluble compounds) which are excreted by the kidneys. Only 1% is excreted unchanged in the urine. The plasma clearance of propofol is greater than total hepatic blood flow, which implies that in addition to liver metabolism, propofol is metabolized by some other source, possibly the lungs *(Miller: Anesthesia, ed 4, pp 269 & 270).*

172. **(C)**   Parkinson's disease (paralysis agitans) is an adult-onset degenerative disease of the central nervous system involving the extrapyramidal system. This disease is characterized by the loss of dopaminergic fibers normally present in the basal ganglia leading to depletion of dopamine, which is presumed to be a neurotransmitter. Dopamine acts by inhibiting the rate of firing of neurons that control the extrapyramidal motor system. Depletion of dopamine results in diminished inhibition of the extrapyramidal motor system and an unopposed action of acetylcholine. The treatment for this disease is to increase the concentration of dopamine in the basal ganglia

or decrease the neuronal effects of acetylcholine. The drugs most often used to achieve these goals are levodopa, anticholinergics, and antihistamines. The selection of drugs to be administered in the preoperative medication and for the production of anesthesia must consider the ability of phenothiazine and butyrophenones to antagonize the effects of dopamine in the basal ganglia. Because droperidol, promethazine, thiethylperazine, and metoclopramide are all dopamine antagonists, odansetron would be the best choice for treatment of nausea in this patient *(Stoelting: Anesthesia and Co-Existing Disease, ed 3, pp 209-211)*.

173. **(A)** Patients with neuromuscular disease frequently have abnormal responses to depolarizing muscle relaxants. Patients with myasthenia gravis tend to be resistant to succinylcholine, whereas patients with myasthenic syndrome (e.g., caused by oat cell carcinoma of the lungs) tend to be sensitive to succinylcholine. In addition, patients with Von Recklinghausen's disease or neurofibromatosis are resistant to succinylcholine, and patients with collagen disorders, such as systemic lupus erythematosus, polymyositis, and polyarteritis nodosa, are sensitive to succinylcholine *(Barash: Clinical Anesthesia, ed 2, p 495)*.

174. **(A)** The pharmacologic effects of dopamine is dose-related. Dopamine can stimulate dopaminergic, β- and α-adrenergic receptors. However, it is the unique ability of this catecholamine to stimulate dopaminergic receptors and redistribute blood flow to the kidneys. These effects on renal blood flow are evident when the dose of dopamine is <3 µg/kg/min. When the dose of dopamine is 3-10 µg/kg/min, β-adrenergic stimulation is seen. This is characterized by increased myocardial contractility without marked changes in heart rate and blood pressure. When the dose of dopamine is between 10 and 20 µg/kg/min, both β- and α-adrenergic effects are seen (i.e., increased cardiac output and systemic vascular resistance). α-adrenergic effects of dopamine predominate at doses at doses >20 µg/kg/min and therefore cardiac output may be reduced *(Stoelting: Basics of Anesthesia, ed 3, p 37)*.

175. **(B)** Reserpine is a sympatholytic agent that depletes catecholamine stores at postganglionic sympathetic nerve terminals. Side-effects of reserpine include sedation and reduced anesthetic requirement, mental depression, bradycardia, abdominal cramps, diarrhea, and increased gastric fluid pH. Patients treated chronically with reserpine demonstrate an increased sensitivity to catecholamines and direct-acting sympathomimetic agents. In contrast, the vasopressor response to indirect-acting sympathomimetic agents, such as ephedrine, is reduced in patients taking reserpine *(Stoelting: Pharmacology and Physiology in Anesthetic Practice, ed 2, p 316)*.

176. **(B)** Volatile anesthetics reduce the concentration of circulating epinephrine required to elicit atrial and ventricular dysrhythmias. This effect is greatest with halothane, less with enflurane, and least with isoflurane. The maximum safe dose of epinephrine when given in association with isoflurane is 6.7 µg/kg. The concentration of epinephrine in the lidocaine solution described in this question is 10 µg/mL. Thus, the maximum amount of this lidocaine solution that can be administered safely to a patient weighing 70 kg is approximately 45 mL *(Stoelting: Basics of Anesthesia, ed 3, p 55)*.

177. **(D)** β-adrenergic receptor antagonists are useful in the treatment of essential hypertension and angina pectoris. β-antagonists may also be effective in decreasing the incidence of postmyocardial infarction mortality and myocardial reinfarction. Side effects associated with the use of these drugs include excessive myocardial depression, bronchoconstriction, atrial ventricular

heart block, excessive sympathetic nervous system activity associated with abrupt discontinuation, accentuated increases in plasma concentrations of potassium associated with infusion of potassium chloride, and blunting of the warning signs and symptoms of hypoglycemia. An important advantage of β-adrenergic receptor antagonists used in treating hypertension is the lack of orthostatic hypotension *(Stoelting: Basics of Anesthesia, ed 3, pp 43 & 44).*

178. **(E)** Atropine is an anticholinergic drug which competes with acetylcholine for muscarinic receptors. It is a tertiary compound and rapidly crosses lipid membranes such as the blood-brain barrier and placenta. Pharmacologic effects of atropine include drying of airway secretions including the inhibition of salivation, sedation and amnesia, central nervous system toxicity (central anticholinergic syndrome) manifesting as delirium or prolonged somnolence after anesthesia, mydriasis and cycloplegia, increased body temperature, tachycardia, and relaxation of the lower esophageal sphincter. The following table compares the effects of various anticholinergics.

Comparative Effects of Anticholinergics Administered Intramuscularly as Pharmacologic Premedication

	Atropine	Scopolamine	Glycopyrrolate
Antisialagogue effect	+	+++	++
Sedative and amnesic effects	+	+++	0
Increased gastric fluid pH	0	0	±
Central nervous system toxicity	+	++	0
Relaxation of lower esophageal sphincter	++	++	++
Mydriasis and cycloplegia	+	+++	0

*From Stoelting RK, Miller RD (eds): Basics of Anesthesia, ed 3. New York, Churchill Livingstone, 1994, p 119. Used with permission.

179. **(D)** Neostigmine, pyridostigmine, edrophonium, and physostigmine all inhibit the enzyme normally responsible for the rapid hydrolysis of acetylcholine, acetylcholinesterase. Neostigmine, pyridostigmine, and edrophonium are all quaternary ammonium compounds. Physostigmine, a tertiary amine, is unique because it is the only anticholinesterase that crosses the blood-brain barrier. This property makes physostigmine an effective treatment for central anticholinergic syndrome *(Stoelting: Basics of Anesthesia, ed 3, p 44).*

180. **(C)** α-Methyldopa is taken up by postganglionic sympathetic nerve fibers where it is metabolized to α-methylnorepinephrine. α-Methylnorepinephrine possesses potent α-adrenergic and ß-adrenergic properties. If propranolol is administered to patients taking α-methyldopa, the ß₂-adrenergic effects of α-methylnorepinephrine are blocked leaving unopposed the vasoconstricting properties of this metabolite. This may result in a paradoxical hypertensive response *(Stoelting: Pharmacology and Physiology in Anesthetic Practice, ed 2, p 313).*

181. **(D)** Opioid-receptor agonists have become an integral part of anesthetic practice. Indeed, high doses of opioid-receptor agonists, such as morphine, fentanyl, and sufentanil, have been used as the sole anesthetic agent in critically ill patients. Unfortunately, these agents are associated with a number of undesirable side-effects including histamine release, bradycardia, hypotension, central nervous system depression, hypoventilation, miosis, skeletal muscle rigidity, spasm of bil-

iary smooth muscle, reduced gastric emptying and intestinal peristalsis, urinary retention, nausea and vomiting, and reduced lower esophageal sphincter tone. Meperidine is a prototype synthetic opioid-receptor agonist derived from phenylpiperidine. It is structurally similar to atropine and therefore, possesses mild anticholinergic properties. In contrast to other opioid-receptor agonists, meperidine rarely causes bradycardia but may increase heart rate *(Stoelting: Pharmacology and Physiology in Anesthetic Practice, ed 2, p 83).*

182. **(B)** Intra-arterial injection of thiopental may result in excruciating pain and intense vasoconstriction, which may cause ischemia to the structures supplied by the artery. Treatment of this complication should include immediate dilution with saline or administration of a drug which will produce vasodilatation (e.g., lidocaine or phentolamine) *(Stoelting: Pharmacology & Physiology in Anesthetic Practice, ed 2, p 114).*

183. **(B)** Indirect-acting sympathomimetic agents increase arterial blood pressure primarily by stimulating the release of norepinephrine from postganglionic sympathetic nerve fibers. Ephedrine, mephenteramine, and metaraminol are all sympathomimetic agents that have some direct-acting properties as well. The following table summarizes the sympathomimetic agents and their effects on the adrenergic receptors *(Stoelting: Basics of Anesthesia, ed 3, pp 39 & 40).*

Classification and Therapeutic Doses of Sympathomimetics

Sympathomimetic	Alpha-1	Alpha-2	Beta-1	Beta-2	Action	Intravenous Dose for an Adult (mg)
Ephedrine	++	?	++	+	I (some D)	10-25
Phenylephrine	+++	?	±	0	D	0.05-0.2
Metaraminol	+++	?	++	0	I (some D)	1.5-5
Mephentermine	+	?	++	+	I	10-25
Methoxamine	+++	?	0	0	D	5-10

*From Stoelting RK, Miller RD (eds): Basics of Anesthesia, ed 3. New York, Churchill Livingstone, 1994, p 39. Used with permission.

184. **(B)** The physiologic effects of meperidine on the cardiovascular system are different from most other opioid-receptor agonists. In contrast to morphine and analogues of meperidine, such as fentanyl, sufentanil, and alfentanil, meperidine reduces myocardial contractility in isolated cardiac muscle preparations and in intact animals. In one study on isolated cat papillary muscle, equianalgesic doses of meperidine reduced contractility 20 times greater than morphine. In clinical studies with humans, morphine-N_2O anesthesia produced far less cardiovascular depression than meperidine-N_2O *(Miller: Anesthesia, ed 4, p 306; Stoelting: Pharmacology and Physiology in Anesthetic Practice, ed 2, p 85).*

185. **(B)** Ketamine is a derivative of phencyclidine used to produce "dissociative anesthesia." This type of anesthesia is characterized by dissociation between the thalamus and limbic system on the electroencephalogram, which resembles a cataleptic state where the patient is noncommunica-

tive, although may appear awake. Ketamine produces varying degrees of hypertonus and skeletal muscle movements, amnesia, and intense analgesia. Although the analgesia produced by ketamine is intense, there is evidence that analgesia is greater for somatic than for visceral pain. Ketamine increases systemic and pulmonary artery blood pressures, heart rate, cardiac output, cardiac work, and myocardial O_2 requirement. The mechanisms for these cardiovascular effects include direct stimulation of the central nervous system, leading to increased sympathetic nervous system outflow and possibly, inhibition of re-uptake of norepinephrine back into postganglionic sympathetic nerve fibers. Ketamine is metabolized almost exclusively in the liver by cytochrome P-450 enzymes to norketamine, which is 1/5 to 1/3 as potent as ketamine *(Stoelting: Pharmacology and Physiology in Anesthetic Practice, ed 2, p 134-141)*.

186. **(B)**   Of the drugs listed in this question, thiopental is the anesthetic most likely to cause myocardial depression *(Thomas: Manual of Cardiac Anesthesia, ed 2, pp 304-311)*.

187. **(B)**   Echothiophate is an organophosphate that irreversibly inhibits acetylcholinesterase by forming a phosphorylate complex of the enzyme. Spontaneous regeneration of acetylcholinesterase either requires several hours or does not occur, thus requiring synthesis of the new enzyme. It is because of this interaction with anticholinesterase that succinylcholine should be administered with caution, if at all, to patients receiving echothiophate *(Stoelting: Pharmacology and Physiology in Anesthetic Practice, ed 2, p 229)*.

188. **(D)**   There is a correlation between the number of receptors occupied by a nondepolarizing muscle relaxant and the number of thumb twitches that can be elicited by train-of-four stimulation of the ulnar nerve. One thumb twitch corresponds to 90% receptor blockade, two thumb twitches corresponds to 80% receptor blockade, three twitches corresponds to 75% receptor blockade, and four thumb twitches corresponds to <75% receptor blockade. Note that the presence of four twitches does not mean that neuromuscular function has completely recovered, in fact a significant number of receptors may still be occupied by the muscle relaxant *(Barash: Clinical Anesthesia, ed 2, p 497)*.

189. **(B)**   Muscle relaxants may exert cardiovascular effects through (1) drug-induced histamine release, (2) effects at cardiac postganglionic muscarinic receptors, or (3) effects on nicotinic receptors at autonomic ganglia. The following table summarizes the mechanisms for the cardiovascular effects of muscle relaxants *(Stoelting: Basics of Anesthesia, ed 3, pp 89 & 93, Table 7-3)*.

Autonomic Nervous System and Histamine Releasing Effects of Muscle Relaxants

Drug[a]	Nicotinic Receptors at Autonomic Ganglia	Cardiac Postganglionic Muscarinic Receptors	Histamine Release
Succinylcholine	Modest stimulation	Modest stimulation	Minimal
d-Tubocurarine	Moderate blockade[b]	None	Marked
Metocurine	Modest blockade[b]	None	Modest[b]
Gallamine	None	Moderate blockade	None
Pancuronium	None	Modest blockade	None
Pipecuronium	None	None	None
Doxacurium	None	None	None
Atracurium	None	None	Minimal[b]
Vecuronium	None	None	None
Mivacurium	None	None	Minimal[b]
Rocuronium	None	None (?)	None

[a]ED_{95} dose equivalent
[b]Occurs only with doses estimated to be two or three times the ED_{95}.
*(From Stoelting RK, Miller RD (eds): Basics of Anesthesia, ed 3. New York, Churchill Livingstone, 1994, p 89. Used with permission.)

190. **(C)** Vecuronium is an analog of pancuronium that lacks vagolytic effects or substantial dependence on renal function for its clearance from the plasma. Up to 60% of an injected dose of vecuronium is excreted predominantly in the bile after deacetylation in the liver. Compared to other nondepolarizing muscle relaxants, vecuronium is unique in its dependence on hepatic metabolism and excretion for elimination from the body *(Stoelting: Basics of Anesthesia, ed 3, p 93)*.

191. **(D)** Administration of ketamine may be associated with visual, auditory, and proprioceptive hallucinations. This unpleasant side-effect of ketamine occurs on emergence and may progress to delirium. The incidence of emergence delirium from ketamine is cited in the literature as 50 to 30 percent. Emergence delirium is less frequent after repeated administrations of ketamine. The most effective prevention of emergence delirium is the administration of benzodiazepines about 5 minutes before induction of anesthesia with ketamine *(Stoelting: Pharmacology and Physiology in Anesthetic Practice, ed 2, pp 140-141)*.

192. **(A)** Metoclopramide is a dopamine antagonist that is structurally similar to procainamide. This drug stimulates gastric and upper intestinal tract motility, and increases lower esophageal sphincter tone. Side-effects associated with metoclopramide include mild sedation, dysphoria, agitation, dry mouth, glossal or periorbital edema, and in rare instances, extrapyramidal reactions *(Stoelting: Pharmacology and Physiology in Anesthetic Practice, ed 2, pp 459-461)*.

193. **(B)** Succinylcholine is a depolarizing muscle relaxant that mimics the action of acetylcholine producing depolarization of the postjunctional membrane. Skeletal muscle paralysis occurs because a depolarized postjunctional membrane cannot respond to a subsequent release of acetylcholine. Hence the designation depolarizing neuromuscular blockade. The sustained depolarization produced by succinylcholine is initially manifested by transient generalized skeletal muscle contractions known as fasciculations. Sustained opening of ion channels pro-

duced by succinylcholine is associated with leakage of potassium from the interior of cells sufficient to increase plasma concentrations of potassium by about 0.5 mEq/L *(Stoelting: Basics of Anesthesia, ed 3, p 87).*

194. **(A)** There are a number of physiologic variables and drugs that enhance nondepolarization neuromuscular blockade. These include antibiotics (e.g., streptomycin, polymyxin B, lincomycin, and clindamycin), magnesium, which reduces the release of acetylcholine from prejunctional neurons, local anesthetics (e.g., lidocaine, mepivacaine, and bupivacaine), antidysrhythmic agents (e.g., quinidine and calcium channel blockers), antihypertensive agents (e.g., hexamethonium and trimethaphan), antiepileptic medications (e.g., phenytoin), antipsychotic medications (e.g., lithium), diuretics (e.g., furosemide), and dantrolene, a drug used for the treatment of malignant hyperthermia. Calcium does not enhance neuromuscular blockade and in fact, may actually antagonize nondepolarizing neuromuscular blockade *(Miller: Anesthesia, ed 4, pp 464 & 465).*

195. **(E)** Monoamine oxidase is the principle intraneuronal enzyme responsible for the metabolism of amine neurotransmitters, such as dopamine, norepinephrine, epinephrine, and serotonin. Thus, monoamine oxidase inhibitors result in accumulation of these amines in the cytoplasm of sympathetic nerve terminals. For this reason, the vasopressor action of indirect-acting sympathomimetic agents, such as ephedrine, can be markedly exaggerated. There are numerous case reports of hyperpyrexia following the administration of meperidine to patients receiving monoamine oxidase inhibitors. In addition, cardiovascular instability, ventilatory depression, muscle rigidity, seizures, and in severe cases, coma and death may occur if meperidine or other narcotics are administered to patients treated with monoamine oxidase inhibitors. For these reasons, it was previously recommended that this class of drugs be withheld 2-3 weeks prior to elective surgery. More recently it has become acceptable to use these drugs up to the time of surgery, since their discontinuance could place the patient at risk for suicide *(Stoelting: Pharmacology and Physiology in Anesthetic Practice, ed 2, p 380).*

196. **(A)** Atracurium is metabolized in blood by the process of Hofmann elimination and by ester hydrolysis. Hofmann elimination is a nonenzymatic, pH- and temperature-dependent phenomenon. Ester hydrolysis of atracurium occurs *via* plasma cholinesterases different from pseudocholinesterase, the enzymes that metabolize succinylcholine. Therefore, in contrast to succinylcholine, patients with atypical pseudocholinesterase will not experience prolonged paralysis after administration of atracurium. The principle metabolite of atracurium is laudanosine. Elimination of laudanosine is almost totally dependent on liver function. Laudanosine readily crosses the blood-brain barrier and in high concentrations, may act as a central nervous system stimulant *(Miller: Anesthesia, ed 4, p 439).*

197. **(C)** Succinylcholine is associated with numerous potential adverse side effects. These side effects may be serious and may limit or contraindicate its use in certain patients. Intravenous administration of subparalyzing doses of nondepolarizing muscle relaxants (pretreatment) 1-3 minutes before succinylcholine will attenuate the occurrence of the following side effects of succinylcholine: myalgia, cardiac dysrhythmias, and elevations in intragastric, intraocular, and intracranial pressures. However, hyperkalemia will not be attenuated by pretreatment with a nondepolarizing muscle relaxant *(Stoelting: Basics of Anesthesia, ed 3, pp 88-90).*

198. **(D)** Streptomycin is one of the most potent of the aminoglycosides in depressing neuromuscular function. The aminoglycosides, including streptomycin and gentamicin, augment both depolarizing and nondepolarizing muscle blockade. Clindamycin and lincomycin have pre- and postjunctional effects and the blockade produced by these antibiotics cannot be reversed with calcium or anticholinesterases. The only drug in this question which does not increase neuromuscular blockade is erythromycin *(Barash: Clinical Anesthesia, ed 2, p 494).*

199. **(B)** Edrophonium, neostigmine, and pyridostigmine are all anticholinesterase drugs. Edrophonium, having a more rapid onset, may reflect a presynaptic (acetylcholine release) rather than postsynaptic (acetylcholinesterase inhibition) action, whereas the postsynaptic action is predominant for neostigmine and pyridostigmine. See the following table for speed of onset, duration of action, and principal site of action *(Stoelting: Pharmacology and Physiology in Anesthetic Practice, ed 2, pp 228-230).*

Comparative Characteristics of Anticholinesterase Drugs Administered to Antagonize Nondepolarizing Neuromuscular Blockade

	Speed of Onset	Duration (min)	Principal Site of Action
Edrophonium ($0.5 \text{ mg} \cdot \text{kg}^{-1}$)	Rapid	60	Presynaptic
Neostigmine ($0.043 \text{ mg} \cdot \text{kg}^{-1}$)	Intermediate	60	Postsynaptic
Pyridostigmine ($0.35 \text{ mg} \cdot \text{kg}^{-1}$)	Delayed	90	Postsynaptic

*From Stoelting RK (ed): Pharmacology and Physiology in Anesthetic Practice, ed 2. Philadelphia, JB Lippincott, 1991, p 228. Used with permission.

200. **(E)** Thiopental is a short-acting thiobarbiturate most commonly used intraoperatively to induce general anesthesia. Thiopental is prepared commercially for clinical use in a 2.5% sodium salt solution. The high alkaline pH of thiopental solutions (pH 10.5) makes this drug incompatible for mixture with opioid-receptor agonists, catecholamines, and nondepolarizing neuromuscular blocking agents, which are acidic solutions. The alkaline pH of thiopental solutions is also responsible for its bacteriostatic properties *(Stoelting: Pharmacology and Physiology in Anesthetic Practice, ed 2, p 102).*

201. **(B)** Hyperkalemia sufficient to cause cardiac arrest may follow administration of succinylcholine to patients with (1) denervation injury as caused by spinal cord injury leading to skeletal muscle atrophy, (2) skeletal muscle injury resulting from third-degree burns, (3) upper motor neuron injury such as stroke, and (4) trauma. The risk of hyperkalemia increases with time and usually peaks 7 to 10 days after the initial injury. All factors considered, it may be prudent to avoid administration of succinylcholine to any patient more than 24 hours after major trauma as listed above. This vulnerability to hyperkalemia may reflect proliferation of extrajunctional receptors and thus providing more sites for potassium to leak outward across the cell membrane during depolarization. The proliferation of extrajunctional receptors are not proven to occur after burn injury *(Stoelting: Basics of Anesthesia, ed 3, p 89).*

202. **(A)** Flumazenil is a specific benzodiazepine antagonist. After an i.v. injection, the onset of its effect is rapid with peak levels occurring in the cerebral cortex and cerebellum within 5 to 8 minutes. Rapid redistribution coupled with a high liver extraction rate produce a relatively short duration of action. Antagonist activity has been shown for all benzodiazepine effects modulated through the CNS benzodiazepine receptor, including sedative, amnestic, muscle relaxant, and anticonvulsant effects. The most common minor side effect reported after administration in anesthesia is nausea and/or vomiting occurring in about 10 percent of patients. Nausea occurs more often when flumazenil is given to patients after general anesthesia than after constant sedation. However, the overall incidence of vomiting alone after general anesthesia is not different with flumazenil than with placebo *(Rogers: Principles and Practice of Anesthesiology, pp 1098-1100)*.

203. **(B)** Combining atropine with edrophonium is logical because the prompt onset of its anticholinergic effects more closely parallels the onset of muscarinic effects produced by edrophonium *(Stoelting: Basics of Anesthesia, ed 3, p 99)*.

204. **(E)** Acute intermittent porphyria is the most serious form of hepatic porphyria. This disease is an inborn error of porphyrin metabolism. This disease affects both the central and peripheral nervous systems. Exacerbation of acute intermittent porphyria can be caused by starvation, dehydration, sepsis, female hormones including pregnancy, and barbiturates. See the following table for the list of safe and unsafe drugs in patients with acute intermittent porphyria *(Stoelting: Anesthesia and Co-existing Disease, ed 3, pp 375-377)*.

Safe and Unsafe Drugs for Administration to a Patient With Acute Intermittent Porphyria

Safe Drugs	Unsafe Drugs
Anticholinergics	Barbiturates
Anticholinesterases	Ethyl alcohol
Depolarizing and nondepolarizing muscle relaxants	Etomidate
Droperidol	Phenytoin
Opioids	Pentazocine
Nitrous oxide	Corticosteroids
Volatile anesthetics	Imipramine
Propofol	Tolbutamide
Benzodiazepines (?)	Benzodiazepines (?)
Ketamine (?)	Ketamine (?)

*From Stoelting RK, Dierdorf SF (eds): Anesthesia and Co-Existing Disease, ed 3. New York, Churchill Livingstone, Inc., 1993, p 377. Used with permission.

205. **(A)** Both verapamil and dantrolene have the ability to inhibit intracellular calcium flux and excitation-contraction coupling. This combination would suggest that this might be useful in the treatment of malignant hyperthermia. In laboratory animals and in case reports, the administration of dantrolene in the presence of verapamil has resulted in hyperkalemia and cardiovascular collapse *(Stoelting: Pharmacology and Physiology in Anesthetic Practice, ed 2, p 360)*.

206. **(A)** Clonidine is a central-acting, α_2-adrenergic receptor agonist. It is thought that stimulation of central nervous system α_2-adrenergic receptors reduces sympathetic nervous system outflow to peripheral tissues, which manifests as a reduction in arterial blood pressure, heart rate, and cardiac output. The most serious side-effect of clonidine is severe rebound hypertension following abrupt discontinuation of the drug. The severity of the rebound hypertension can be exacerbated when ß-adrenergic receptor antagonists and tricyclic antidepressants are administered to these patients. In addition, there have been several reports that naloxone can reverse the antihypertensive effects of clonidine, causing severe hypertension *(Stoelting: Pharmacology and Physiology in Anesthetic Practice, ed 2, p 315)*.

207. **(D)** Fentanyl has a larger volume of distribution, slower plasma clearance, and longer elimination half-life than morphine. However, the duration of action of fentanyl (when given in small doses) is much shorter than morphine because fentanyl is rapidly redistributed from the brain to inactive tissue sites. In larger doses, these tissue sites become saturated, and the pharmacologic action of fentanyl become considerably prolonged *(Stoelting: Pharmacology and Physiology in Anesthetic Practice, ed 2, pp 76, 85, & 86)*.

208. **(A)** An azeotrope is a mixture of two vapors that evaporates to provide a gas mixture from the agents present in the same ratio that occurs in a solution. This type of anesthesia was briefly popular after the introduction of halothane. The idea was to mix it with diethylether and to reap the advantages of two agents having counteracting side effects. However, presently the subject of azeotropes commonly arises when the wrong anesthetic is used to fill a half empty vaporizer *(Miller: Anesthesia, ed 2, pp 83 & 84)*.

209. **(E)** The rate of CSF formation is reduced by acetazolamide, cardiac glycosides, corticosteroids, and hypothermia. Unfortunately, the clinical effect of reducing CSF secretion by these methods is transient; therefore, their use in long-term management of intracranial hypertension has not been substantiated. Interestingly, enflurane has been shown to increase the rate of CSF formation and decrease the rate of CSF resorption. Although the time course of this effect on CSF dynamics is slow, this observation may have relevance when enflurane is administered for prolonged closed cranium procedures in patients with reduced intracranial compliance *(Miller: Anesthesia, ed 4, pp 709, 710, & 1916)*.

210. **(C)** Rocuronium is a relatively new aminosteroid nondepolarizing muscle relaxant. When compared to its cousin, vecuronium, rocuronium has a similar duration of action and pharmacokinetic behavior and also is devoid of cardiovascular effects. However, in some clinical studies it has been shown to have a more rapid onset. However, no studies have been done comparing rocuronium with equipotent doses of succinylcholine *(Barash: Clinical Anesthesia, ed 2, p 493)*.

211. **(D)**   Hypokalemia, as may occur during chronic diuretic therapy, reduces dose requirements for non-depolarizing muscle relaxants and increases the dose of acetylcholinesterase inhibitors required to adequately reverse nondepolarizing neuromuscular blockade *(Stoelting: Pharmacology and Physiology in Anesthetic Practice, ed 2, p 198).*

212. **(B)**   d-Tubocurarine, metocurine, atracurium, and mivacurium all produce decreases in arterial blood pressure principally as a result of the release of histamine. Histamine release evoked by these muscle relaxants is dose-related, occurring with 1 time ED_{95} of d-tubocurarine, 2 times ED_{95} of metocurine, and 3 times ED_{95} of atracurium or mivacurium *(Stoelting: Basics of Anesthesia, ed 3, pp 89-94).*

213. **(C)**   The symptoms described in this patient are consistent with anticholinesterase drug overdose. The treatment of anticholinesterase drug overdose is with atropine and occasionally, the acetylcholinesterase reactivator, pralidoxime. Atropine antagonizes the muscarinic effects of acetylcholine, such as miosis, excess salivation, bronchoconstriction, bradycardia, abdominal cramps, and loss of bladder and/or rectal control, but has no impact on the nicotinic effects at the skeletal muscle neuromuscular junction and autonomic ganglia. The nicotinic effects can be antagonized by intravenous administration of pralidoxime *(Stoelting: Pharmacology and Physiology in Anesthetic Practice, ed 2, p 238).*

214. **(C)**   Flumazenil, a benzodiazepine antagonist, is a drug with a high affinity for the benzodiazepine receptor but with no CNS effects. Flumazenil has clear competitive antagonist activity whether given before, with, or after a benzodiazepine. It can antagonize all the therapeutic benzodiazepines and some of the other drugs that are active at the CNS benzodiazepine receptors. Flumazenil has no antagonistic effect on substances that do not act at the central benzodiazepine receptor (e.g. barbiturates, opiates, alcohol). In addition to its predominantly antagonistic properties, flumazenil may have weak generalized central arousal or anxiogenic activity. It also does have weak anticonvulsant activity as well *(Rogers: Principles and Practice of Anesthesiology, pp 1098-1100).*

215. **(D)**   The most definitive and sensitive indicator of recovery of neuromuscular function following nondepolarizing neuromuscular blockade is the ability of a patient to sustain a head lift for 5 seconds in the supine position. It is estimated that this maneuver can be successfully performed when one-third or fewer of the receptors at the neuromuscular junction are occupied by the muscle relaxant. The major disadvantage of this technique is the need for patient cooperation *(Stoelting: Basics of Anesthesia, ed 3, p 99).*

216. **(D)**   This table summarizes the pharmacokinetics of thiopental and methohexital. Note that the distribution half-times of thiopental and methohexital are very similar. In contrast, methohexital is cleared from plasma approximately 3 times faster than thiopental. The shorter elimination half-time of methohexital compared with that of thiopental reflects the greater hepatic clearance of methohexital *(Stoelting: Pharmacology and Physiology in Anesthetic Practice, ed 2, pp 106 & 107).*

Comparative Pharmacokinetics of Thiopental and Methohexital

	Thiopental	Methohexital
α phase distribution half-time (min)	8.5	5.6
ß phase distribution half-time (min)	62.7	58.3
Elimination half-time (hours)	11.6	3.9
Plasma clearance (mL/kg/min)	3.4	10.9

*From Hudson RJ, Stonski DK, Burch PG (eds): Pharmacokinetics of Methohexital and Thiopental in Surgical Patients. Anesthesiology 1983;59:215. Used with permission.

217. **(A)** In addition to its antidopaminergic properties, droperidol has antidysrhythmic properties which can protect against epinephrine-induced dysrhythmias. The mechanism for this antidysrhythmic effect is not known. However, there is evidence that droperidol may block α-adrenergic receptors in the myocardium, which stabilizes the muscle cell membranes, and blocks α-adrenergic receptors in vascular smooth muscle, which reduces arterial blood pressure. Large doses of droperidol (e.g., 0.2-0.6 mg/kg) can reduce impulse transmission *via* the accessory pathways responsible for the tachydysrhythmias that occur in patients with Wolff-Parkinson-White syndrome. The other drugs listed in this question may exacerbate cardiac impulse transmission along these accessory pathways, because of their anticholinergic properties (pancuronium, gallamine, and meperidine) and sympathomimetic properties (ketamine). Therefore, these drugs should be avoided if possible in patients with Wolff-Parkinson-White syndrome *(Stoelting: Anesthesia and Co-existing Disease, ed 3, p 74; Stoelting: Pharmacology and Physiology in Anesthetic Practice, ed 2, p 371).*

218. **(C)** Pseudocholinesterase is an enzyme found in plasma and most other tissues (except erythrocytes). It is produced in the liver and has a half-life of approximately 8-16 hours. Therefore, pseudocholinesterase levels may be reduced in patients with advanced liver disease, resulting in prolongation of neuromuscular blockade with succinylcholine *(Barash: Clinical Anesthesia, ed 2, p 603).*

219. **(A)** Ketorolac is a non-steroidal antiinflammatory drug which inhibits the enzyme cyclooxygenase which is necessary for prostaglandin synthesis. Prostaglandins are mediators of pain and inflammation and act at the site of injury. Inhibition of cyclooxygenase is therefore a peripheral effect *(Stoelting: Basics of Anesthesia, ed 3, p 445).*

220. **(C)** The actions of corticosteroids are classified according to the potencies of these compounds specifically: 1) reabsorption of sodium ions in exchange for potassium ions (corticoid mineral effect) or 2) production of an anti-inflammatory response (glucocorticoid effect). The following table lists the anti-inflammatory potency and the sodium retaining potency of the various endogenous and synthetic corticosteroids. From the table, it is seen that 50 mg of prednisone is equivalent to 8 mg of dexamethasone *(Stoelting: Pharmacology and Physiology in Anesthetic Practice, ed 2, pp 423).*

Comparative Pharmacology of Endogenous and Synthetic Corticosteroids

	Anti-inflammatory Potency	Sodium Retaining Potency	Equivalent Dose (mg)
Cortisol (Solu-Cortef)	1	1	20
Cortisone (Cortone)	0.8	0.8	25
Prednisolone (Delta-Cortef)	4	0.8	5
Prednisone	4	0.8	5
Methylprednisolone (Solu-Medrol)	5	05	4
Betamethasone (Celestone)	25	0	0.75
Dexamethasone (Decardron)	25	0	0.75
Triamcinolone (Kenalog)	5	0	4
Fludrocortisone (Florinef)	10	125	—

*From Stoelting RK (ed): Pharmacology and Physiology in Anesthetic Practice, ed 2. Philadelphia, JB Lippincott, 1991, p 423. Used with permission.

221. **(A)** Nondepolarizing muscle relaxants, with the exception of atracurium, are highly dependent on urinary excretion, and to a lesser extent, liver metabolism and direct biliary excretion for elimination. Nondepolarizing muscle relaxants are eliminated slowly and have a prolonged duration of action in elderly patients with reduced renal and hepatic function. The duration of action, plasma clearance, and elimination of atracurium, however, is not altered by age *(Barash: Clinical Anesthesia, ed 2, p 1377).*

222. **(B)** Cyclosporin is a drug that selectively inhibits helper T-lymphocyte-mediated immune responses while not affecting the lymphocytes. Use of this drug is important in immunosuppressant therapy and in combination with corticosteroids and has greatly increased the success of organ transplantation. Serious side effects may accompany the administration of cyclosporin. Nephrotoxicity is the most important adverse effect involving 25 to 38 percent of the patients taking it. Other side effects include hypertension, limb paresthesia, headaches, confusion, somnolence, seizures, elevation of liver enzymes, allergic reactions, gum hyperplasia, hirsutism, and hyperglycemia. There appears to be no pulmonary toxicity associated with cyclosporin therapy *(Stoelting: Pharmacology and Physiology in Anesthetic Practice, ed 2, p 426).*

223. **(B)** Succinylcholine consists of two acetylcholine molecules linked by methyl groups. Succinylcholine may exert cardiovascular effects by 1) inducing histamine release from mast cells, 2) stimulating autonomic ganglia, which increases neurotransmission at both the sympathetic and parasympathetic nervous systems, and 3) directly stimulating postjunctional cardiac muscarinic receptors. The effect of succinylcholine on heart rate is mediated primarily by its ability to augment neurotransmission at sympathetic and parasympathetic ganglia, which is greater for the nondominant autonomic nervous system. Therefore, children, who have high sympathetic nervous system tone, are likely to develop bradycardia after succinylcholine is administered. In contrast, adults, who have greater parasympathetic nervous system tone, are more likely to develop tachycardia when succinylcholine is administered. Cardiac bradydysrhythmias are more likely to occur when a second intravenous dose of succinylcholine is administered 4-5 minutes after the first dose *(Barash: Clinical Anesthesia, ed 2, p 484).*

224. **(C)** Succinylcholine, a depolarizing muscle relaxant, stimulates all cholinergic autonomic receptors including the nicotinic receptors in both sympathetic and sympathetic ganglia and muscarinic receptors in the sinus node of the heart. It is this muscarinic effect that causes the bradycardia that can be seen after the administration of succinylcholine in children *(Miller: Anesthesia, ed 4, p 425)*.

225. **(B)** Guanethidine is a peripheral sympatholytic agent most frequently used in the treatment of essential hypertension that is resistant to the less potent antihypertensive drugs. Guanethidine may also be used for the treatment of reflex sympathetic dystrophy. Guanethidine produces its antihypertensive effect by displacing norepinephrine from storage sites within sympathetic nerve fibers. With chronic administration of guanethidine, a denervation hypersensitivity phenomenon occurs, which may result in a hypertensive crisis if direct-acting sympathomimetic agents are administered. Conversely, the vasopressor response to indirect-acting sympathomimetic agents, such as ephedrine or mephentermine, is attenuated, because norepinephrine stores within sympathetic nerve fibers are depleted *(Stoelting: Pharmacology and Physiology in Anesthetic Practice, ed 2, pp 319 & 645)*.

226. **(A)** Hyperkalemia, malignant hyperthermia, masseter spasm, bradycardia, and myalgias are all side effects that can be seen after administration of succinylcholine. In recent years there have been several case reports of intractable cardiac arrest in apparently healthy children after the administration of succinylcholine. In many of these cases, hyperkalemia, rhabdomyolysis, and acidosis have been documented. It is for this reason, hyperkalemia, that succinylcholine is contraindicated for routine tracheal intubation in children *(Miller: Anesthesia, ed 4, p 426)*.

227. **(E)** Recent investigations have shown that the evolution of both depolarizing and non-depolarizing block proceeds more rapidly in the central muscles of the airway (i.e., the larynx, the jaw, and the diagram) than in the more peripheral abductor of the thumb. The neuromuscular block develops faster, lasts a shorter time, and recovers more quickly in these muscles. This is important clinically for two reasons. First, since the neuromuscular block develops more rapidly in the airway than in the thumb, tracheal intubation can be performed when the response of the thumb is only beginning to show visible signs of weakening. Second, since the recovery of the airway musculature is faster than in the thumb, once monitored responses in the thumb have been correctly diagnosed as having returned to normal, the identical responses in the airway musculature have already reached that point (i.e., return of thumb responses to normal suggests that the protective airway reflexes are intact). Also important is the observation that the pattern of blockade in the orbicularis oculi is similar to that in the larynx. This means that the orbicularis can be employed as a reliable indicator of the status of the laryngeal responses *(Miller: Anesthesia, ed 4, p 421)*.

228. **(D)** A general rule for the changeover from one drug to another when the durations are dissimilar is a matter of simple kinetics. Three half-lives will be required for a clinical changeover so that 95 percent of the first drug has been cleared and for the block duration to begin to take on the characteristics of the second drug. When the short-acting muscle relaxant, mivacurium, is given for tracheal intubation with the intention of continuing maintenance of relaxation with a longer drug, it will be observed that the duration of effect of the maintenance dose will be much shorter than usual. Only after two or three maintenance doses of the longer acting agent will the expected longer duration establish itself *(Miller: Anesthesia, ed 4, p 466)*.

229. **(A)** Recent studies have documented that antagonism of residual block is actually retarded by anesthetizing concentrations of an anesthetic gas. This does make sense since the depolarizers are potentiated by the volatile anesthetic agents. The clinical lesson from this is that the anesthetic vapor concentrations should be reduced as much as possible at the end of the case to help ensure that reversal will take place as promptly as possible *(Miller: Anesthesia, ed 4, p 468).*

230. **(D)** The cardiovascular management goals for patients with aortic stenosis are: 1) maintain a sinus rhythm at a normal rate, 2) maintain systemic diastolic blood pressure and coronary perfusion, and 3) maintain cardiac output by appropriately high preload and by avoidance of myocardial depressants. Because of the propensity of pancuronium to moderately block the cardiac muscarinic receptors, it is relatively contraindicated in patients with aortic stenosis. Please see the following table for the effects of various muscle relaxants on the cardiac muscarinic receptors (Table 14-10, p 441) *(Miller: Anesthesia, ed 4, pp 441 & 1775).*

Autonomic Effects of Neuromuscular Blocking Drugs

Drug Type	Autonomic Ganglia	Heart Muscarinic Receptors	Histamine Release
Benzylisoquinoline class			
Atracurium	None	None	Slight
d-Tubocurarine	Blocks	None	Moderate
Doxacurium	None	None	None
Metocurine	Blocks weakly	None	Slight
Mivacurium	None	None	Slight
Steroid class			
Pancuronium	None	Blocks moderately	None
Pipecuronium	None	None	None
Rocuronium	None	Blocks weakly	None
Vecuronium	None	None	None
Other			
Gallamine	None	Blocks strongly	None

*From Miller (ed): Anesthesia, ed 4. New York, Churchill Livingstone, 1994, p 441.
Used with permission.

231. **(C)** Doxacurium is the only non-depolarizing neuromuscular drug in the benzoisoquinoline class of drugs that does not cause the release of histamine. Please see the above table for reference *(Miller: Anesthesia, ed 4, p 441).*

232. **(A)** Etomidate, an imidazole derivative, is used both for the induction of anesthesia and the maintenance of anesthesia. Etomidate provides stable hemodynamics and minimal respiratory depression. However, it is associated with several adverse effects when used for induction. These adverse effects include nausea and vomiting, pain on injection, myoclonic movements, and hiccups. Nausea and vomiting constitute the most common reason for patients to rate anesthesia with etomidate as unsatisfactory. The addition of fentanyl to etomidate further increases the incidence of nausea and vomiting *(Miller: Anesthesia, ed 4, p 268).*

233. **(A)** Pancuronium inhibits reuptake of norepinephrine by adrenergic nerves. This mechanism may also contribute to exaggerated cardiovascular responses after pancuronium administration *(Miller: Anesthesia, ed 4, p 442)*.

234. **(B)** Dantrolene produces skeletal muscle relaxation by a direct action on excitation-contraction coupling. Its effect is presumably by decreasing the amount of calcium release from the sarcoplasmic reticulum. This property is useful in the management of patients with skeletal muscle spasticity owing to upper motor neuron lesions. It is also effective in the prevention and treatment of malignant hyperthermia. The most common side effect of dantrolene administration is skeletal muscle weakness *(Stoelting: Pharmacology and Physiology in Anesthetic Practice, ed 2, pp 546 & 547)*.

235. **(A)** The observation of myoclonus can be seen following the administration of etomidate, propofol, or thiopental. However, myoclonus occurs more frequently following propofol than thiopental but less frequently than etomidate *(Miller: Anesthesia, ed 4, p 274)*.

236. **(D)** Disulfiram and naltrexone are occasionally used as drug deterrent adjuncts to therapy in the early months of drug rehabilitation. Specifically, naltrexone is an oral medication that demonstrates pure opioid antagonist action. Patients taking naltrexone at the time of surgery will have markedly elevated opioid requirements if opioids are chosen for pain relief. Naltrexone may be continued up to the day of surgery; however, in hospital continuance of this drug is probably not advisable since opioid antagonism is counterproductive *(Rogers: Principles and Practice of Anesthesiology, p 554)*.

237. **(B)** For rapid intubation of the trachea (rapid sequence induction) succinylcholine is still the preferred muscle relaxant for this critical maneuver. However, there are certain clinical situations in which the rapid sequence induction maneuver must be performed and that succinylcholine is absolutely contraindicated. There are suitable alternatives among the non-depolarizing relaxants. When using non-depolarizing muscle relaxants for rapid intubation of the trachea, there are five caveats which must be followed: 1) preoxygenation, 2) adequate dosage of i.v. drugs must be administered to ensure that the patient is adequately anesthetized, 3) intubation within 60 to 90 seconds is considered acceptable, 4) "priming" should be considered to shorten the onset of action of non-depolarizing muscle relaxants, and 5) cricoid pressure should be applied subsequent to the injection of the induction agent. Rocuronium is unique because a priming dose is not necessary for intubating conditions within 60 to 90 seconds following its administration. Therefore, rocuronium is probably most suitable for rapid intubation in a patient in whom succinylcholine is contraindicated *(Miller: Anesthesia, ed 4, pp 431 & 436)*.

238. **(E)** Following injection of a muscle relaxant, plasma drug concentration immediately starts to decrease. To produce paralysis, the drug must diffuse from the plasma to the neuromuscular junction after injection. The drug effect is later terminated by diffusion back into the plasma. Therefore, recovery of neuromuscular function takes place as the muscle relaxant diffuses from the neuromuscular junction back into the plasma to be metabolized and/or eliminated from the body *(Miller: Anesthesia, ed 4, p 435)*.

239. **(D)** Respiratory depression can be seen after the administration of opioid-like substances. Of the narcotics listed, respiratory depression is rare but is serious with buprenorphine because it is not

readily reversible by the administration of naloxone *(Rogers: Principles and Practice of Anesthesiology, p 548).*

240. **(B)**   Nausea and vomiting can be associated with all of the drugs listed. However, etomidate has the highest incidence of emetic sequelae of all the drugs listed *(Rogers: Principles and Practice of Anesthesiology, p 1144).*

241. **(E)**   Naloxone acts as a competitive antagonist at all opioid receptors but has the greatest affinity for μ receptors. This block is reversible and competitive so it can be overcome by additional agonists. Naloxone probably has no effect on non-narcotic anesthetics although this remains somewhat controversial *(Rogers: Principles and Practice of Anesthesiology, p 1170).*

242. **(D)**   Nitric oxide, nitroglycerin, nitroprusside, phentolamine, amrinone, milrinone, and prostaglandin E all have a vasodilatory effect on the pulmonary arterial tree. However, it is only nitric oxide that has basically no effect on the systemic circulation. Please see the following table for comparison *(Miller: Anesthesia, ed 4, p 1798).*

Relative Efficacy of Intravenous Vasodilators on Hemodynamic Variables

Vasodilator	Venous Dilation	Pulmonary Arterial Dilation	Systemic Arterial Dilation	Cardiac Output
Nitric oxide	0	+++	0	±
Nitroglycerin IV	+++	+	+	↓↑[1]
Nitroprusside	+++	+++	+++	↓↑[1]
Phentolamine	+	+	+++	↑
Hydralazine	0	?	+++	↑
Amrinone[2]	+	+	+	↑
Prostaglandin E_1[3]	+	+++	+++	↑↓[1]

[1]Effect on cardiac output depends on net balance of effects on preload, afterload, and myocardial oxygenation.
[2]Inodilators have inotropic plus vasodilating effects; see Table 53-23.
[3]Almost always requires left atrial infusion of norepinephrine to sustain adequate systemic blood pressure.
Symbols to indicate intensity of effect: 0, none; ± small, variable; + mild; +++ strongest effect of that particular drug.
*(From Miller (ed): Anesthesia, ed 4. New York, Churchill Livingstone, 1994, p 1798. Used with permission.)

243. **(D)**   Succinylcholine mimics the action of acetylcholine producing depolarization of the postjunctional membrane. However, compared with acetylcholine, the hydrolysis of succinylcholine is slow resulting in sustained depolarization. Skeletal muscle paralysis occurs because a depolarized postjunctional membrane cannot respond to subsequent release of acetylcholine. Depolarizing neuromuscular blockade is also referred to as phase I blockade. A phase I blockade cannot be antagonized with neostigmine, there is no fade in the train-of-four response or post-tetanic potentiation *(Stoelting: Basics of Anesthesia, ed 3, p 87, table 7-1).*

244. **(A)** Maximal brain uptake of barbiturates occurs within 30 seconds after their i.v. administration which accounts for the rapid induction of anesthesia produced by these drugs. Prompt awakening following i.v. administration of barbiturates reflects redistribution of these drugs from the brain to inactive tissues such as skeletal muscle and fat. The elimination half-time of methohexital is more rapid than that of thiopental, reflecting the greater hepatic metabolism of methohexital. Barbiturates are potent cerebral vasoconstrictors producing decreases in cerebral blood flow, cerebral blood volume, and intracranial pressure. Barbiturates also decrease electroencephalographic activity. An exception is the effect of methohexital on the EEG which activates epileptic foci *(Stoelting: Basics of Anesthesia, ed 3, p 61).*

245. **(C)** Pancuronium and gallamine can produce modest (10-15%) increases in heart rate and arterial blood pressure. These cardiovascular effects are primarily due to the anticholinergic effects of these agents binding to cardiac postjunctional muscarinic receptors. Please see table used for explanation to question 189 *(Stoelting: Basics of Anesthesia, ed 3, p 89).*

246. **(E)** Moricizine is a phenothiazine derivative approved for the treatment of life-threatening ventricular arrhythmias. It is similar to type Ia antiarrhythmic agents in that it has moderate sodium channel blocking effects. It also shortens the duration of action potentials (type Ib effects) and prolongs QRS interval duration (type Ic effects). As a result, it moderately prolongs the PR and QRS intervals and slightly shortens the JT interval. It is also reported that moricizine has minimal negative inotropic effects *(Thomas: Manual of Cardiac Anesthesia, ed 2, p 352).*

247. **(A)** H_2-receptor antagonists, such as cimetidine, are used preoperatively in patients to increase gastric fluid pH before induction of anesthesia. Elevation of gastric fluid pH is desirable since the severity of aspiration pneumonitis is increased when the pH of aspirated gastric contents is <2.5. H_2-receptor antagonists have gained popular use as a premedication for parturients, patients with symptomatic gastroesophageal reflux, and obese patients (these patients tend to have very acidic gastric fluid compared to nonobese patients). H_2-receptor antagonists, in contrast to metoclopramide, has no effect on lower esophageal sphincter tone, intestinal motility, or gastric emptying. Cimetidine reduces liver blood flow and thus retards metabolism of drugs that normally undergo high hepatic extraction, such as lidocaine, propranolol, and diazepam. In addition, there is evidence that cimetidine inhibits the hepatic mixed function oxidase system by binding to the microsomal cytochrome P-450 enzymes *(Stoelting: Pharmacology and Physiology in Anesthetic Practice, ed 2, pp 400-401).*

248. **(D)** Midazolam undergoes hydroxylation by hepatic microsomal oxidative mechanisms. Very little unchanged midazolam is excreted by the kidneys. Hepatic clearance of midazolam may be decreased by concomitant administration of any enzyme inhibiting drug such as erythromycin. Unlike diazepam, metabolism of midazolam is not inhibited by H_2 receptor antagonists *(Stoelting: Pharmacology and Physiology in Anesthetic Practice, ed 2, p 127).*

249. **(B)** Metoclopramide is a dopamine antagonist that is structurally similar to procainamide. Metoclopramide produces selective cholinergic stimulation of the gastrointestinal tract, which results in increased upper gastrointestinal tract motility and lower esophageal sphincter tone, and relaxation of the pylorus of the stomach. The effect of these actions is accelerated clearance of gastric contents and shortened transient time through the small intestines. In contrast to cimetidine, metoclopramide does not alter gastric acid secretion or gastric fluid pH *(Barash: Clinical Anes-*

thesia, ed 2, pp 1175 & 1176; Stoelting: Basics of Anesthesia, ed 3, p 122; Stoelting: Pharmacology & Physiology in Anesthetic Practice, ed 2, p 459).

250. **(C)**   Of the listed opioids, alfentanil has the most rapid onset. The brief duration of action of alfentanil is a result of redistribution to inactive tissue sites and hepatic metabolism. Unlike other opioids, continuous intravenous infusions of alfentanil do not seem to produce clinically significant cumulative drug effects *(Stoelting: Basics of Anesthesia, ed 3, p 67).*

251. **(A)**   Medications that are effective in the management of acute exacerbations of bronchial asthma include ß-adrenergic receptor agonists (e.g., albuterol, terbutaline), aminophylline, a potent phosphodiesterase inhibitor, corticosteroids, and anticholinergic drugs (e.g., atropine, glycopyrrolate). Cromolyn is a membrane stabilizer that inhibits antigen-induced release of histamine and other autocoids, such as leukotrienes, from mast cells. Cromolyn does not prevent the interaction between immunoglobulin E and the antigen, nor does it alter degranulation of basophils. Cromolyn is of no value in the management of acute attacks of bronchial asthma, but is effective in the prophylactic treatment of bronchial asthma *(Stoelting: Anesthesia & Co-Existing Disease, ed 3, pp 152-154; Stoelting: Pharmacology and Physiology in Anesthetic Practice, ed 2, pp 404 & 405).*

252. **(E)**   Clonidine is an α_2-adrenergic agonist. Unlike other antihypertensive drugs such as guanethidine, propranolol, and captopril which act peripherally, clonidine effects the central release of catecholamines and activates the central α_2 adrenoreceptors. Thus, as with other drugs affecting the central release of adrenergics, clonidine not only reduces anesthetic requirements (as represented by a decrease in MAC) but also decreases extremes in arterial blood pressure during anesthesia. Clonidine also reduces the requirements for sufentanil. All α_2-agonists, including clonidine, can also prevent the muscle rigidity which is seen with the administration of narcotics *(Miller: Anesthesia, ed 4, pp 1026 & 1027).*

253. **(E)**   Chronic liver disease may interfere with the metabolism of drugs because of the decreased number of enzyme-containing hepatocytes or because of decreased hepatic blood flow or both. Prolonged elimination half-times for morphine, alfentanil, diazepam, lidocaine, pancuronium, and to a lesser extent, vecuronium, have been demonstrated in patients with cirrhosis of the liver. In addition, severe liver disease may decrease the production of cholinesterase (pseudocholinesterase) enzyme that is necessary for the hydrolysis of ester linkages in drugs such as succinylcholine, mivacurium, and ester local anesthetics such as procaine *(Stoelting: Basics of Anesthesia, ed 3, p 288).*

254. **(A)**   Pseudocholinesterase, an enzyme that hydrolyses acetylcholine and succinylcholine, has a number of well known drug interactions that may lower its activity in plasma. Among these are the standard anticholinesterases, neostigmine and pyridostigmine (but not edrophonium), pancuronium, alkalizing agents, and ecothiophate, as well as other organophosphates used as active ingredients in insecticides. Therefore, the following drugs lower the activity of pseudocholinesterase in the plasma: neostigmine, ecothiophate, and pyridostigmine *(Miller: Anesthesia, ed 4, p 425).*

255. **(C)** Neonates and infants are more sensitive than adults to nondepolarizing muscle relaxants requiring lower plasma concentrations to produce pharmacologic effects. However, the initial doses of these drugs are similar in both age groups because less drug actually reaches the neuromuscular junction. This reflects the impact of increased extracellular fluid volume and the volume of distribution in neonates and infants *(Stoelting: Basics of Anesthesia, ed 3, p 384)*.

256. **(C)** Administration of opioids, intravenously, may result in spasm of the thoracoabdominal muscles ("stiff chest" syndrome) causing hypoventilation. In extreme situations, skeletal muscle rigidity may be severe enough that it interferes with ventilation of the lungs. Administration of a muscle relaxant or an opioid antagonist such as naloxone is effective for terminating opioid-induced skeletal muscle rigidity *(Stoelting: Basics of Anesthesia, ed 3, p 67)*.

257. **(A)** Thiopental produces a mild dose-related decrease in cardiac output and mean arterial pressure. There are several direct and indirect mechanisms for these observations. Thiopental has a direct negative inotropic action on the myocardium and causes venodilation, which reduces cardiac venous return. In addition, thiopental reduces sympathetic outflow from the brain, which causes venodilation and reduces systemic vascular resistance by removal of adrenergic support *(Thomas: Manual of Cardiac Anesthesia, ed 2, pp 306 & 307)*.

258. **(E)** Propofol, an alkylphenol, is an emulsion that is used to induce and maintain anesthesia as well as sedate patients. Propofol, primarily a hypnotic, possesses unique properties that are not common to other induction agents. Some of these properties including induction of bronchodilation in patients with chronic obstructive pulmonary disease (not as effective as halothane) does not potentiate neuromuscular blockade, does not affect corticosteroid synthesis or alter the normal response to ACTH stimulation, possesses significant antiemetic activity (has been used successfully to treat postoperative nausea as well as nausea following chemotherapy), and has been reported to relieve cholestatic pruritus as well as pruritus induced by spinal opiates *(Miller: Anesthesia, ed 4, p 272)*.

259. **(C)** Neuroleptic malignant syndrome is an extremely rare complication of neuroleptic therapy. It is manifested by muscular rigidity, hyperthermia, and autonomic instability. This disease is distinguishable from malignant hyperthermia by the fact that the temperature does not rise to the same degree as MH. Treatment can be carried out with administration of dantrolene. Oral bromocriptine, because of its central dopaminergic properties, may also be a useful treatment. Acute dystonic reactions may also be associated with administration of butyrophenones, phenothiazines, and thioxanthenes. The treatment for acute dystonic reactions is the administration of an anticholinergic such as diphenhydramine and benztropine.

260. **(A)** Pseudocholinesterase is an enzyme that hydrolyzes acetylcholine, succinylcholine, and mivacurium. Pseudocholinesterase is inhibited by pancuronium and weakly inhibited by vecuronium and atracurium through the binding of the ester portion of a molecule *(Miller: Anesthesia, ed 4, p 433)*.

261. **(A)**   Sodium thiosulfate is a sulfur donor which is required for the conversion of cyanide to thiocyanate in the liver and kidneys. Administration of sodium nitrate converts hemoglobin to methemoglobin. Methemoglobin binds with cyanide to form cyanmethemoglobin. Hydroxocobalamin combines with cyanide to form cyanocobalamin. Methylene blue is not an antidote for cyanide toxicity and can actually reduce cyanide metabolism by converting methemoglobin back to hemoglobin *(Stoelting: Pharmacology and Physiology in Anesthetic Practice, ed 2, p 327).*

262. **(D)**   Atypical pseudocholinesterase is an inherited disorder that occurs in approximately 1 in every 480 patients with heterozygous genome and in approximately 1 in 3200 patients with homozygous genome. The duration of neuromuscular blockade with succinylcholine may be markedly prolonged in patients with atypical pseudocholinesterase. Dibucaine is an amide-type local anesthetic that inhibits normal pseudocholinesterase activity by approximately 80%. Conversely, pseudocholinesterase activity is inhibited by 40-60% in patients who are heterozygous for the disease and is inhibited by only 20% in patients who are homozygous for the disease. It is important to note that the dibucaine number represents a qualitative assessment of pseudocholinesterase activity and not a quantitative assessment. In diseases such as cirrhotic liver disease, where the absolute amount of pseudocholinesterase is reduced but is qualitatively normal, the dibucaine number is normal *(Stoelting: Pharmacology and Physiology in Anesthetic Practice, ed 2, p 179; Stoelting: Basics of Anesthesia, ed 3, pp 87 & 88).*

263. **(C)**   Benzodiazepines possess a number of favorable pharmacologic characteristics including 1) production of amnesia, 2) minimal respiratory and cardiovascular system depression, 3) a specific site of action as an anticonvulsant, and 4) rarity of development of significant tolerance or physical dependence. Clinically, these agents produce amnesia and sedation, and reduce anxiety and skeletal muscle tone. Benzodiazepines are thought to exert their antianxiety effects by increasing the availability of glycine, an inhibitory neurotransmitter, in the central nervous system. The sedative action of benzodiazepines most likely reflects the ability of these drugs to facilitate the inhibitory action of gamma-aminobutyric acid in the central nervous system. The site of action for production of amnesia has not been determined. Midazolam and diazepam are metabolized almost exclusively by hepatic microsomal enzymes using oxidative pathways. Indeed, the plasma clearance of these two medications is markedly reduced in patients with reduced liver function. Conversely, the pharmacokinetics of these two drugs is not altered in patients with renal failure *(Stoelting: Pharmacology and Physiology in Anesthetic Practice, ed 2, pp 121, 127, & 130 [118-133]).*

264. **(E)**   The autonomic mechanism involved in sinus bradycardia after the administration of succinylcholine is stimulation of the cardiac muscarinic receptors in the sinus node. The bradycardia may be prevented by thiopental, atropine, ganglion blocking drugs, and nondepolarizing muscle relaxants. Thus, atropine, thiopental, trimethaphan, and gallamine may all be used to prevent bradycardia associated with the administration of succinylcholine *(Miller: Anesthesia, ed 4, pp 425 & 426).*

265. **(B)**   Some of the drugs used to produce sedation in anesthesia during the perioperative period can affect ventilation by altering the tidal volume and/or the respiratory rate. Volatile anesthetic agents produce a dose-dependent increase in the respiratory rate and a decrease in the tidal volume. Ventilatory depression caused by barbiturates is characterized by a reduction in both the

respiratory rate and tidal volume. However, opioid receptor agonists cause respiratory depression by decreasing the respiratory rate with the tidal volume either slightly increasing or remaining unchanged. Additionally, some opiates may interfere with breathing by causing chest wall rigidity *(Stoelting: Basics of Anesthesia, ed 3, pp 47, 60, & 66)*.

266. **(A)** Advantages of using oral barbiturates for premedication in patients prior to surgery include sedation, minimal ventilatory depressant effects, minimal circulatory depression, rarity of nausea and vomiting, and effectiveness when administered orally. Disadvantages include lack of analgesia, disorientation, and absence of a specific pharmacologic antagonist *(Stoelting: Basics of Anesthesia, ed 3, p 114)*.

267. **(B)** Steroidal non-depolarizing muscle relaxants include pancuronium, pipecuronium, vecuronium, and rocuronium. The advantages of this class of muscle relaxants include high potency and lack of histamine release. This class also generally exhibits a vagolytic property. This side effect is moderate in pancuronium, slight to moderate in rocuronium, and absent in pipecuronium and vecuronium. All steroidal relaxants are excreted by the kidney to some degree *(Miller: Anesthesia, ed 4, p 431)*.

268. **(E)** If thiobarbiturates are injected intraarterially (especially in concentrations greater than 2.5 percent) intense arterial spasm and excruciating pain may result and can be felt from the injection site to the hand and fingers. The onset of pain and burning is immediate and can persist for hours. Within the first two hours, anesthesia or hyperesthesia of the hand, edema, or motor weakness can occur. A range of symptoms from mild discomfort to gangrene and loss of tissue in the hand can result. The presence of a pulse does not rule out later development of thrombosis. The pathology is a chemical endarteritis which destroys the endothelium, subendothelial tissues, and possibly the muscle layer. To prevent permanent sequelae, treatment is necessary to dilute the drug, relieve vascular spasm, and prevent thrombosis. Injection of papaverine or lidocaine or procaine into the artery may accomplish the first two objectives. Blocking the sympathetic nerves to the upper extremity with either a stellate ganglion block or a brachial plexus block can relieve spasm. In addition, heparin can be given intravenously to prevent thrombosis *(Miller: Anesthesia, ed 4, p 236)*.

269. **(D)** Diazepam, etomidate, thiopental, and ketamine are all intravenous drugs that can be used to induce anesthesia. However, it is only ketamine that can produce analgesia in subanesthetic doses. The barbiturates may actually be hyperalgesic in subanesthetic concentrations exaggerating a response to pain. Benzodiazepines lack analgesic properties and must be used with anesthetic agents if anesthesia is desired in addition to sedation. However, as maintenance anesthetic drugs during general anesthesia, benzodiazepines do provide hypnosis and amnesia. Likewise, etomidate has no analgesic activity. Ketamine produces dose-related unconsciousness and analgesia. The anesthetized state has been termed dissociative anesthesia because the patient who receives ketamine alone appears to be in a cataleptic state. The ketamine anesthetized patients have profound analgesia but keep their eyes open and maintain many reflexes such as corneal, cough, and swallowing. However, it should not be assumed that these reflexes are protective *(Miller: Anesthesia, ed 4, pp 236, 255, 260, & 266)*.

270. **(A)**   The effectiveness of phenothiazines in schizophrenia suggests a dopamine receptor blocking action. In addition, this drug possesses varying degrees of parasympathetic stimulation and ability to block alpha-adrenergic receptors. Phenothiazines can produce sedation, depression, and antihistaminic, antiemetic, and hypothermic responses. They are also associated with cholestatic jaundice, impotence, dystonia, and photosensitivity. Other side effects include orthostatic hypotension (partly due to alpha-adrenergic blockade) and ECG abnormalities such as prolongation of the Q-T or PR intervals, blunting of T waves, depression of the S-T segment, and, on rare occasions, PVCs and torsades de pointes. There are several important drug interactions that are noteworthy for the administration of anesthesia. The effects of CNS depressants, especially narcotics and barbiturates, are enhanced by concomitant administration of phenothiazines. Also the CNS seizure threshold is lowered by the administration of phenothiazines which should be avoided in patients who are epileptic. The antihypertensive effects of guanethidine and guanadrel are blocked by phenothiazines. These drugs have no effect on neuromuscular blockade *(Miller: Anesthesia, ed 4, p 992).*

271. **(B)**   Amrinone is a non-catecholamine, non-glycoside bipyridine derivative that produces dose-dependent positive inotropic and vasodilatory effects manifesting as increased cardiac output and decreased left ventricular and diastolic pressure. The heart rate may increase and blood pressure decrease. The positive inotropic effects are not prevented by alpha- or beta-adrenergic blockade, depletion of catecholamines, or inhibition of the sodium potassium ATPase ion transport system *(Stoelting: Pharmacology and Physiology in Anesthetic Practice, ed 2, p 293).*

272. **(C)**   Tricyclic antidepressants are often administered as the initial treatment of mental depression. Side effects of antidepressant drugs influence drug choice because all these drugs are equally effective if used in an adequate dose. Tricyclic antidepressants do not need to be discontinued before administration of anesthesia for an elective operation. However, alterations in the responses to drugs administered during the perioperative period should be anticipated. The increased availability of neurotransmitters in the central nervous system can result in increased anesthetic requirement. In addition, the increased availability of norepinephrine at postsynaptic receptors in the peripheral sympathetic nervous system can be responsible for an exaggerated blood pressure response after the administration of an indirect-acting vasopressor such as ephedrine. If a vasopressor is required, a direct-acting drug such as phenylephrine may be useful. If hypertension occurs and requires treatment, a peripheral vasodilator such as nitroprusside is effective. The potential for hypertensive crisis is greatest during the acute treatment phase (the first 14 to 21 days). Chronic treatment is associated with down regulation receptors and the decreased likelihood of exaggerated blood pressure responses after the administration of a sympathomimetic *(Stoelting: Anesthesia and Co-existing Disease, ed 3, pp 518 & 519).*

273. **(A)**   Organophosphates are insecticides that are potent inhibitors of the enzyme acetylcholinesterase. Overdose is most likely to occur when the insecticides are ingested, inhaled, or absorbed through the skin. Symptoms of organophosphate overdose reflect inhibition of acetylcholinesterase resulting in accumulation of acetylcholine at nicotinic (neuromuscular junction) and cholinergic receptor sites. Organophosphate overdose may be followed by delayed peripheral neuropathy involving the distal muscles of the extremities appearing 2 to 5 weeks after the overdose. Skeletal muscle weakness developing 1 to 4 days after organophosphate overdose involves primarily proximal limbs, flexors of the neck, and certain cranial nerves and breathing muscles. The treatment of organophosphate overdose includes the administration of anticholin-

ergics, oximes, and benzodiazepines, i.e. atropine, pralidoxime, diazepam *(Stoelting: Anesthesia and Co-existing Disease, ed 3, p 535).*

274. **(B)** The beta-adrenergic blocking agents have a wide spectrum of therapeutic uses including treatment of hypertension and angina. Variations among beta-adrenergic blocking agents result from their differing pharmacologic properties in regard to β_1-selectivity, α-adrenergic blocking activity, presence of intrinsic sympathomimetic activity or membrane stabilizing activity, potency, lipid solubility, first pass effect, half-life, and mode of metabolism and excretion. All beta-adrenergic blocking agents competitively block effects of catecholamines on receptors in the heart, lung, vasculature, kidney, and brain and their therapeutic value stems from these properties. Beta-blockers are not however without substantial side effects. These drugs may precipitate overt CHF in patients with impaired ventricular function. Patients with sinus node dysfunction or A-V block may develop symptomatic bradycardias following administration. Stimulation of β_2-receptors in lungs causes bronchodilation. Conversely, treatment with beta blockers may cause bronchospasm making their use in bronchospastic disease problematic. Even beta blockers with relative β_1-selectivity (e.g. metoprolol, atenolol, bataxolol, esmolol) may cause bronchoconstriction. However, esmolol and atenolol would be suitable for use in patients with bronchospastic disease because of their relative β_1-selectivity when compared to the other beta blockers *(Rogers: Principles and Practice of Anesthesiology, pp 1548-1551).*

Pharmacologic Properties of Beta Blockers

Agent	Relative β_1 selectivity	α activity	Elimination half-life	Elimination
Atenolol	++	–	9 min	RBC esterases
Labetalol	–	+	6-8 hr	Hepatic
Metoprolol	++	–	3-7 hr	Hepatic
Nadolol	–	–	20-24 hr	Renal
Propranolol	–	–	4 hr	Hepatic
Timolol	–	–	4-5 hr	Renal

*From Rogers MC (ed): Principles and Practice of Anesthesiology. St. Louis, Mosby–Year Book, 1993, p 1551.

275. **(A)** With the exception of cocaine, which undergoes significant hydrolysis by liver cholinesterases, ester-type local anesthetics (e.g., procaine, chloroprocaine, tetracaine) are hydrolyzed by pseudocholinesterase. Other drugs metabolized by pseudocholinesterase include succinylcholine, trimethaphan, and propanidid. Etomidate is metabolized in the liver by microsomal enzymes and plasma esterases that are different from those that metabolize succinylcholine *(Stoelting: Pharmacology and Physiology in Anesthetic Practice, ed 2, pp 153-155, 217, & 333-334).*

276. **(E)** Propofol, diazepam, etomidate, and thiopental can all be used as agents for the induction of anesthesia. A property that they all have in common is the ability to cause phlebitis and thrombosis when administered intravenously *(Miller: Anesthesia, ed 4, pp 240, 256, 268, & 274).*

277. **(D)** Rapid awakening after induction of anesthesia with thiopental reflects rapid distribution following the bolus as opposed to hepatic extraction. An induction dose of barbiturates does not significantly suppress laryngeal reflexes. Thiopental does produce a modest decrease in systemic blood pressure which is transient because of a compensatory baroreceptor-mediated increase in heart rate. Hypotension, however, may be severe in patients who are hypovolemic or who have decreased myocardial reserve. Barbiturates may be useful in providing cerebral protection from regional ischemic events but not from global ischemia which is likely to occur in patients who have experienced a cardiac arrest (*Stoelting: Basics of Anesthesia, ed 3, pp 60 & 61*).

278. **(D)** Drugs with antidopaminergic properties, such as phenothiazines (e.g., chlorpromazine) and butyrophenones (e.g., droperidol, haloperidol), may exacerbate extrapyramidal symptoms. Diphenhydramine is an H_1-receptor antagonist which has antiemetic properties. The first three drugs listed in this question may exacerbate Parkinson's disease and therefore are not appropriate for the treatment of nausea in this patient. Diphenhydramine not only has no dopaminergic properties, but in fact is sometimes used to treat Parkinson's disease (*Stoelting: Anesthesia and Co-Existing Disease, ed 3, p 210; Stoelting: Pharmacology and Physiology in Anesthetic Practice, ed 2, pp 370, 460-461; Rogers: Principles and Practice of Anesthesiology, p 49*).

279. **(E)** There are a number of drugs that can be administered to treat excessive bradycardia and/or reductions in cardiac output due to excess ß-adrenergic receptor blockade. Isoproterenol and dobutamine can be administered to overcome competitive ß-adrenergic receptor blockade. Dopamine is not recommended because the high doses required to overcome ß-adrenergic receptor blockade may cause α-adrenergic receptor-induced vasoconstriction. Calcium chloride (250-1000 mg) can be administered to increase the cytosolic ionized calcium concentration, which augments myocardial contractility. Glucagon increases myocardial contractility and heart rate by 1) enhancing cytosolic cyclic AMP formation (not *via* ß-adrenergic receptor stimulation) and 2) stimulating the release of catecholamines from prejunctional sympathetic nerve fibers. Aminophylline inhibits phosphodiesterase, the enzyme responsible for inactivation of cyclic AMP, resulting in accumulation of cytosolic cyclic AMP. Thus, like glucagon, aminophylline increases cardiac output and heart rate *via* a non ß-adrenergic receptor mediated mechanism (*Stoelting: Pharmacology and Physiology in Anesthetic Practice, ed 2, pp 293 & 305; Miller: Anesthesia, ed 4, p 56*).

280. **(A)** Dantrolene is a unique muscle relaxant. Unlike the neuromuscular blocking agents whose site of action is at the nicotinic receptor of the neuromuscular junction, dantrolene operates within the muscle cell itself by reducing intracellular levels of calcium. Most likely this results from a reduction of calcium release of sarcoplasmic reticulum or inhibition of excitation contracture coupling at the transverse tubular level. Therefore, dantrolene is a specific and effective agent in the treatment of malignant hyperthermia. In usual clinical doses, dantrolene has little effect on myocardial contractility. Some of the side effects of short-term administration include muscle weakness (that may persist for 24 hours after dantrolene therapy is discontinued), nausea and vomiting, and phlebitis. Hepatotoxicity has been demonstrated only with long-term use of oral dantrolene (*Barash: Clinical Anesthesia, ed 2, p 598*).

281. **(A)** The following table summarizes the pharmacology of some of the nondepolarizing muscle relaxants. Gallamine is excreted 100 percent by the kidney. Metocurine, d-Tubocurarine, doxacurium, pancuronium, vecuronium, and pipecuronium are partially excreted by the kidney, and their action may be prolonged in patients with renal failure. Only atracurium and mivacurium are eliminated independently of kidney function *(Miller: Anesthesia, ed 4, p 432)*.

Drug	Duration	Metabolism	Renal Elim	Hepatic Elim
Mivacurium	Short	Pseudocholinesterase	< 5%	None
Atracurium	Intermediate	Hoffman elimination & hydrolysis by non-specific esterase	10-40%	None
Vecuronium	Intermediate	Liver (30-40%)	~40%	~60%
Pancuronium	Long	Liver (10-20%)	85%	15%
d-Tubocurarine	Long	None	80%?	20%
Pipecuronium	Long	None	>90%?	<10%
Metocurine	Long	None	>98%	<2%
Gallamine	Long	None	100%	0%

*From Miller RD (ed): Anesthesia, ed 4. New York, Churchill Livingstone, 1994, p 432. Used with permission.

282. **(A)** Etomidate is a carboxylated imidazole-containing compound chemically unrelated to any other intravenous anesthetic agent. Disadvantages of etomidate include 1) pain during intravenous injection, 2) involuntary skeletal muscle movements, 3) a high incidence of postoperative nausea and vomiting, and 4) suppression of adrenocortical function. Compared with other intravenous anesthetics, such as thiopental and propofol, cardiovascular stability is maintained in patients receiving etomidate, suggesting that this drug may be useful in patients with limited cardiac reserve *(Miller: Anesthesia, ed 4, pp 267 & 268)*.

283. **(C)** Etomidate is an imidazole derivative. Etomidate is unique among the induction agents because it has the propensity to cause adrenal suppression. The specific endocrine effects by etomidate are a dose-dependent reversible inhibition of the enzyme, 11-betahydroxylase, which converts 11-deoxycortisol to cortisol, and it has a relatively minor effect on 17-alphahydroxylase. This results in an increase in the cortisol precursors as well as an increase in adrenal corticotropic hormone (ACTH). Minor adrenal cortical suppressant effects have been shown to follow even a single bolus dose *(Miller: Anesthesia, ed 4, pp 267 & 268)*.

284. **(B)** The benzodiazepines are remarkably safe drugs. They have relatively high margins of safety, especially when compared with barbiturates. They are usually free of allergenic effects and do not suppress the adrenal gland. The major side effects of diazepam are venous irritation and thrombophlebitis. The most significant problem with midazolam as well as the other benzodiazepines is respiratory depression. However, the benzodiazepines are unique because there is a specific benzodiazepine receptor antagonist available that can reverse the effects of the benzodiazepine (flumazenil) *(Miller: Anesthesia, ed 4, p 256)*.

285. **(D)** Induction of anesthesia with propofol is associated with several side effects. These side effects include pain on injection, myoclonus, thrombophlebitis, and hypotension *(Miller: Anesthesia, ed 4, p 274)*.

286. **(E)** Contraindications for the administration of ketamine relate to specific pharmacologic actions and patient pathology. For example, patients with increased ICP and with intracranial mass lesions should not receive ketamine because it can increase the ICP and has been reported to cause apnea on this basis *(Miller: Anesthesia, ed 4, p 264).*

287. **(A)** Paralysis and death can occur if barbiturates are given to patients with acute intermittent porphyria or variegate porphyria. Barbiturates can precipitate acute and even fatal attacks of porphyria owing to the induction of delta aminolevulonic acid synthetase which catalyzes the rate limiting step in the biosynthesis of porphyrins. *(Miller: Anesthesia, ed 4, p 241).*

288. **(E)** 289. **(C)** 290. **(B)** 291. **(D)** 292. **(E)** Antihypertensive agents are used in the treatment of essential hypertension to reduce blood pressure toward normal values. These agents function primarily by selectively impairing sympathetic nervous system function at the heart and/or peripheral vasculature, or by reducing sympathetic nervous system outflow from the central nervous system. Any of these drugs produce side-effects that must be considered when planning the anesthetic management of patients with essential hypertension. For example, hypotension, associated with sudden changes in body position, hemorrhage, positive airway pressure, and volatile anesthetics, may be exaggerated because compensatory peripheral vasoconstriction may be impaired by the antihypertensive agent. Central acting sympatholytic agents, such as α-methyldopa and clonidine, reduce anesthetic requirement. In addition, abrupt discontinuation of clonidine may result in severe rebound hypertension in patients who have been chronically treated. Hydralazine is a direct-acting peripheral vasodilator which interferes with calcium transport in vascular smooth muscle. This antihypertensive agent does not alter the baroreceptor reflex, which minimizes or prevents orthostatic hypotension. Unfortunately, a systemic lupus erythematosus-like syndrome can occur in patients who take more than 200 mg of hydralazine daily. Minoxidil, like hydralazine, reduces blood pressure by a direct action on vascular smooth muscle. Side-effects associated with minoxidil include pulmonary hypertension (which most likely reflects fluid retention), pericardial effusion, cardiac tamponade, and hair growth. Labetalol is a α_1-adrenergic receptor and nonselective ß-adrenergic receptor antagonist *(Stoelting: Basics of Anesthesia, ed 3, pp 40-42; Stoelting: Pharmacology and Physiology in Anesthetic Practice, ed 2, p 317).*

293. **(B)** 294. **(C)** 295. **(D)** 296. **(E)** 297. **(D)** Norepinephrine is an α_1-adrenergic and $ß_1$-adrenergic receptor agonist. However, norepinephrine does not increase cardiac output or heart rate because the α_1-adrenergic receptor effects significantly overshadow the $ß_1$-adrenergic receptor effects. Indeed, cardiac output may actually be reduced. Isoproterenol is a nonspecific $ß_1$-adrenergic and $ß_2$-adrenergic receptor agonists and thus, in contrast to norepinephrine, epinephrine, and dopamine, does not increase systemic vascular resistance. Indeed, isoproterenol may actually reduce systemic vascular resistance and hence increase cardiac output because the $ß_2$-adrenergic effects decrease the smooth muscle tone of skeletal muscle blood vessels, which reduces systemic vascular resistance. In addition, isoproterenol may lower mean arterial pressure because it lacks α-adrenergic receptor properties *(Stoelting: Basics of Anesthesia, ed 3, pp 36-38).*

298. (E) 299. (A) 300. (C) 301. (D) Opioid receptor agonists produce analgesia by binding to opioid receptors in the central nervous system and other tissues. The clinical pharmacology of opioid receptor agonists is mediated by a complex interaction between μ, δ, κ, and σ opioid receptor subtypes. For example, euphoria, miosis, urinary retention, and pruritus are mediated by μ_1 receptors whereas hypertonia and dysphoria are mediated by sigma receptors. K receptors mediate miosis, sedation, and spinal analgesia and μ_2 receptors mediate respiratory depression, sedation, and bradycardia. In general, binding of opioid receptor agonists to specific receptors results in inhibition of adenylate cyclase activity. Opioids also affect cytosolic ionized calcium homeostasis, and interfere with the release of neurotransmitters, such as acetylcholine, norepinephrine, and substance P *(Stoelting: Basics of Anesthesia, ed 3, p 65)*.

302. (D) 303. (D) 304. (B) 305. (B) Phase II depolarizing blockade occurs when succinylcholine has been administered in doses 2-4 mg/kg or greater. The characteristics of a phase II depolarizing block are very similar to those of a nondepolarizing block. Anticholinesterases will inhibit both acetylcholinesterase and plasma cholinesterase, thereby prolonging phase I blockade *(Miller: Anesthesia, ed 4, p 429)*.

306. (B) 307. (A) 308. (A) 309. (E) 310. (C) 311. (C) 312. (B) 313. (A) 314. (C) 315. (C) The pharmacokinetics of anesthetics (uptake and distribution) can be linked to pharmacodynamics (effect of the drug on the body) by consideration of anesthetic potency. This linkage exists because the desired alveolar concentration is what one strives to achieve and maintain during anesthesia. For the inhaled anesthetics, potency is commonly expressed as MAC (minimum alveolar concentration) of the anesthetic. This is the alveolar concentration of the volatile anesthetic at one atmosphere of pressure, which prevents movement in 50 percent of subjects in response to a painful stimulus. Various physiologic or pharmacologic factors can increase or decrease MAC. See the following tables for various physiologic or pharmacologic factors and their effects on MAC *(Barash: Clinical Anesthesia, ed 2, p 443)*. Tables 17-4, 17-5, and 17-6.

316. (A) 317. (C) 318. (E) 319. (B) 320. (D) The goals for pharmacologic premedication must be individualized to meet each patient's requirements. Some of these goals include relief of anxiety, sedation, analgesia, amnesia, reduction of oral and respiratory secretions, reduction of gastric fluid volume, elevation of gastric fluid pH, and prophylaxis against allergic reactions. The drugs most commonly used to achieve these goals include barbiturates, opioid receptor antagonists, benzodiazepines, butyrophenones, such as droperidol and metoclopramide, antihistamines, H_2-receptor antagonists, nonparticulate antacids, and anticholinergic agents. Anticholinergic agents, such as atropine, glycopyrrolate, and scopolamine, are administered to 1) reduce oral and upper airway secretions, 2) prevention of bradydysrhythmias, and 3) to produce sedation and amnesia. This table summarizes the ability of these anticholinergic agents to achieve the aforementioned pharmacologic effects *(Stoelting: Basics of Anesthesia, ed 3, pp 119 & 120)*.

Comparative Pharmacology of Anticholinergic Agents

	Atropine	Scopolamine	Glycopyrrolate
Antisialagogue effect	Mild	Marked	Moderate
Sedation effect	Mild	Marked	None
Amnesia effect	Mild	Marked	None
Ocular effects	Mild	Marked	None
Increased gastric fluid pH	None	None	None
CNS toxicity	Mild	Moderate	None

*From Stoelting RK, Miller RD (eds): Basics of Anesthesia, ed 3. New York, Churchill Livingstone, 1994, p 119. Used with permission.

Pharmacology and Pharmacokinetics of Volatile Anesthetics

DIRECTIONS (Questions 321 through 357): Each of the questions or incomplete statements in this section is followed by answers or by completions of the statement, respectively. Select the ONE BEST answer or completion for each item.

321. N_2O, when administered in combination with which of the following anesthetic agents, can result in synergistic cardiac depression?

  A. Halothane
  B. Isoflurane
  C. Enflurane
  D. Diazepam
  E. Morphine

322. The rate of increase in the alveolar concentration of a volatile anesthetic relative to the inspired concentration (F_A/F_I) plotted against time is steep during the first moments of inhalation with all volatile anesthetics. The reason for this observation is that

  A. Volatile anesthetics decrease blood flow to the liver
  B. There is minimal anesthetic uptake from the alveoli into pulmonary venous blood
  C. Volatile anesthetics increased cardiac output
  D. The volume of the anesthetic breathing circuit is small
  E. Volatile anesthetics reduce V_A

323. During spontaneous breathing, volatile anesthetics

  A. Increase V_T and decrease respiratory rate
  B. Increase V_T and increase respiratory rate
  C. Decrease V_T and decrease respiratory rate
  D. Decrease V_T and increase respiratory rate
  E. None of the above

324. Each of the following volatile anesthetics is an ether derivative **EXCEPT**

  A. Halothane
  B. Enflurane
  C. Isoflurane
  D. Desflurane
  E. Sevoflurane

325. Attenuation of each of the following physiologic responses is observed during halothane anesthesia **EXCEPT**

    A. Ventilatory response to hypoxemia
    B. Ventilatory response to hypercarbia
    C. Hypoxic pulmonary vasoconstriction
    D. CBF/CMRO$_2$ coupling
    E. Cerebral vasoconstriction to hypocarbia

326. The output of which of the following vaporizers would approximate the setting shown on the dial if it were filled with sevoflurane?

    A. Halothane vaporizer
    B. Enflurane vaporizer
    C. Isoflurane vaporizer
    D. Desflurane vaporizer
    E. Methoxyflurane vaporizer

327. N$_2$O

    A. Decreases blood pressure
    B. Decreases systemic vascular resistance
    C. Decreases heart rate
    D. Decreases cardiac output
    E. None of the above

328. Which of the following volatile anesthetics decrease systemic vascular resistance?

    A. Halothane, enflurane, and isoflurane
    B. Halothane and enflurane
    C. Desflurane and halothane
    D. Enflurane and isoflurane
    E. Halothane only

329. Which of the following inhalation anesthetics causes the greatest ventilatory depression at 1 MAC?

    A. N$_2$O
    B. Halothane
    C. Isoflurane
    D. Enflurane
    E. Desflurane

330. Select the **FALSE** statement about isoflurane ($\leq$1 MAC).

    A. May attenuate bronchospasm
    B. Produces a 2-3 fold increase in skeletal muscle blood flow
    C. Decreases mean arterial pressure
    D. Decreases cardiac output
    E. Has intrinsic sympathomimetic properties

331. Select the correct order from greatest to least for the increase in cerebral blood flow (CBF) caused by volatile anesthetics.

    A. Enflurane > isoflurane > halothane
    B. Enflurane > halothane > isoflurane
    C. Isoflurane > enflurane > halothane
    D. Halothane > enflurane > isoflurane
    E. Halothane > isoflurane > enflurane

332. Discontinuation of 1 MAC of which volatile anesthetic followed by **immediate** introduction of 1 MAC of which second volatile anesthetic would temporarily result in the greatest combined anesthetic potency?

    A. Halothane followed by desflurane
    B. Halothane followed by enflurane
    C. Halothane followed by isoflurane
    D. Isoflurane followed by desflurane
    E. Isoflurane followed by halothane

333. Cardiogenic shock has the **LEAST** impact on the rate of increase in F_A/F_I for which of the following volatile anesthetics?

    A. Halothane
    B. Isoflurane
    C. Enflurane
    D. Desflurane
    E. The impact will be about the same for all agents

334. The vessel-rich group receives what percent of the cardiac output?

    A. 45
    B. 60
    C. 75
    D. 90
    E. 95

335. Which of the following volatile anesthetics undergoes the greatest degree of metabolism?

    A. Enflurane
    B. Isoflurane
    C. Halothane
    D. Desflurane
    E. Sevoflurane

336. An increase in the serum concentration of which of the following metabolites implies reductive metabolism of halothane?

    A. Fluoride
    B. Chloride
    C. Bromide
    D. Trichloroacetic acid
    E. Trichloroacetaldehyde

337. How would a right mainstem intubation affect the rate of increase in arterial partial pressure of volatile anesthetics?

    A. It would be reduced to the same degree for all volatile anesthetics
    B. It would be accelerated to the same degree for all volatile anesthetics
    C. There would be no change if $P_aO_2 \geq 60$ mm Hg
    D. It would be reduced the most for poorly soluble agents
    E. It would be reduced the most for highly soluble agents

338. Halothane, unlike enflurane and isoflurane, does not cause tachycardia. The most reasonable explanation for this observation is that halothane

    A. Lacks intrinsic sympathomimetic properties
    B. Lacks vagolytic properties
    C. Causes direct cardiac depression
    D. Has intrinsic parasympathomimetic properties
    E. Inhibits baroreceptor reflexes

339. Isoflurane, when administered to healthy patients in concentrations of <1.0 MAC, will decrease all the following **EXCEPT**

    A. Cardiac output
    B. Myocardial contractility
    C. Stroke volume
    D. Systemic vascular resistance
    E. Ventilatory response to changes in P_aCO_2

340. Increased V_A will accelerate the rate of rise of the F_A/F_I ratio the most for

    A. Desflurane
    B. Enflurane
    C. Isoflurane
    D. Halothane
    E. Sevoflurane

341. Select the correct order from greatest to least for anesthetic requirement.

    A. Adults > infants > neonates
    B. Adults > neonates > infants
    C. Neonates > infants > adults
    D. Neonates > adults > infants
    E. Infants > neonates > adults

342. Select the correct order from greatest to least for the depressant effect of volatile anesthetics on stroke volume.

    A. Desflurane > isoflurane > halothane
    B. Desflurane > halothane > isoflurane
    C. Halothane > isoflurane > desflurane
    D. Isoflurane > desflurane > halothane
    E. Halothane > desflurane > isoflurane

343. A 31-year-old moderately obese white female with Down's syndrome is receiving a general anesthetic for cervical spinal fusion. After induction and intubation, the patient is mechanically ventilated with isoflurane at a vaporizer setting of 2.4%. The nitrous oxide flow is set at 500 ml/min and the oxygen flowmeter is at 250 ml/min. The mass spectrometer shows an inspired isoflurane concentration of 1.7% and an expired isoflurane concentration of 0.6%. Approximately how many MAC of anesthesia would be represented by the alveolar concentration of anesthetic gases?

    A. 0.5 MAC
    B. 0.85 MAC
    C. 1.1 MAC
    D. 1.8 MAC
    E. 2.1 MAC

344. The graph in the figure depicts

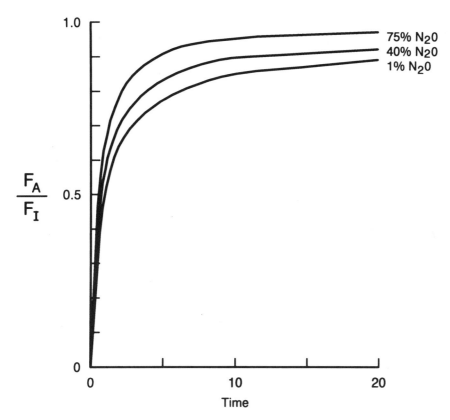

    A. The second gas effect
    B. The concentration effect
    C. The concentrating effect
    D. The effect of solubility on the rate of increase in F_A/F_I
    E. Diffusion hypoxia

345.   The rate of induction of anesthesia with volatile anesthetics would be slower than expected in patients

   A.   With anemia
   B.   With chronic renal failure
   C.   In shock
   D.   With cirrhotic liver disease
   E.   With a right-to-left intracardiac shunt

346.   A right-to-left intracardiac shunt would have the greatest impact on the rate of inhalation induction with which of the following inhalation anesthetics?

   A.   Halothane
   B.   Enflurane
   C.   Isoflurane
   D.   Sevoflurane
   E. N_2O

347.   The volatile anesthetic which causes the greatest increase in heart rate at 1.5 MAC and the volatile anesthetic which causes the greatest myocardial depression at 1.5 MAC, respectively, are

   A.   Enflurane and halothane
   B.   Enflurane and isoflurane
   C.   Isoflurane and halothane
   D.   Enflurane and enflurane
   E.   Isoflurane and isoflurane

348.   A fresh-gas flow rate of 2 L/min or greater is recommended for administration of sevoflurane because

   A.   The vaporizer cannot accurately deliver the volatile at lesser flow rates
   B.   It prevents the formation of fluoride ions
   C.   It prevents formation of Compound A
   D.   It diminishes rebreathing
   E.   None of the above

349.   Metabolism plays an important role on the rate of rise of F_A/F_I during induction of anesthesia for which of the following volatile anesthetics?

   A.   Isoflurane
   B.   Enflurane
   C.   Halothane
   D.   Desflurane
   E.   None of the above

350.   The partition coefficients for desflurane at 37°C are: blood/gas, 0.42; brain/blood, 1.3; liver/blood, 1.4; kidney/blood, 1.0; fat/blood, 27. The rate of rise of F_A/F_I of desflurane would most closely resemble that of

   A.   Sevoflurane (blood/gas partition coefficient, 0.69)
   B.   Isoflurane (brain/blood partition coefficient, 1.6)
   C.   Enflurane (liver/blood partition coefficient, 2.1)
   D.   Halothane (kidney/blood partition coefficient, 1.2)
   E.   Methoxyflurane (fat/blood partition coefficient, 38)

351. Which of the following reasons best explains the more rapid alveolar washout of halothane compared with enflurane?

    A. Differences in blood solubility
    B. Differences in the blood/brain partition coefficient
    C. Differences in the oil/gas partition coefficient
    D. The fact that halothane is not an ether
    E. Increased metabolism of halothane

352. During administration of isoflurane to an obese 40-year-old woman undergoing foot surgery, the vaporizer dial is set at 2%. The inspired concentration of isoflurane measured by the mass spectrometer is, however, only 1.2%. The **BEST** explanation for this observation is

    A. Increased uptake into the patient's fatty tissues
    B. Absorption of volatile anesthetic by the CO_2 absorber
    C. Absorption of volatile anesthetic by the anesthesia circuit tubing
    D. Dilution by expired patient gases
    E. Absorption by the endotracheal tube

353. Which of the following anesthetics is degraded by baralyme and soda lime?

    A. Halothane
    B. Enflurane
    C. Isoflurane
    D. Desflurane
    E. Sevoflurane

354. In isovolemic normal human subjects, 1 MAC of isoflurane anesthesia depresses mean arterial pressure by approximately 25 percent. The single **BEST** explanation for this is

    A. Reduction in heart rate
    B. Venous pooling
    C. Myocardial depression
    D. Decreased systemic vascular resistance
    E. Tachycardia

355. If cardiac output and alveolar ventilation are doubled, the effect on the rate of rise of F_A/F_I compared with that which existed immediately prior to these interventions would be

    A. Doubled
    B. Somewhat increased
    C. Unchanged
    D. Somewhat decreased
    E. Halved

356. Which of the following characteristics of inhaled anesthetics most closely correlates with recovery from inhaled anesthesia?

    A.   Blood:gas partition coefficient
    B.   Brain:blood partition coefficient
    C.   Fat:blood partition coefficient
    D.   MAC
    E.   Vapor pressure

357. A left-to-right tissue shunt, e.g. arteriovenous fistula, physiologically most resembles which of the following?

    A.   A left-to-right intracardiac shunt
    B.   A right-to-left intracardiac shunt
    C.   Ventilation of unperfused alveoli
    D.   A pulmonary embolism
    E.   None of the above

DIRECTIONS (Questions 358 through 373): For each of the items in this section, ONE or MORE of the numbered options is correct. Select the answer:

Select A if options *1, 2 and 3* are correct,
Select B if options *1 and 3* are correct,
Select C if options *2 and 4* are correct,
Select D if only option *4* is correct,
Select E if *all* options are correct.

358. Which of the following factors would have an impact on the F_A/F_I ratio of halothane during an inhalation anesthetic?

    1.   Presence of a right-to-left intracardiac shunt
    2.   Presence of a left-to-right intracardiac shunt
    3.   Doubling the cardiac output
    4.   Ventilation of unperfused alveoli

359. Sevoflurane

    1.   Does not contain preservatives
    2.   May significantly increase plasma fluoride concentrations when used for longer procedures
    3.   Decreases systemic vascular resistance
    4.   Is less soluble in the blood than desflurane

360. Inhalational anesthetics which decrease systemic vascular resistance include

    1.   Enflurane
    2.   Halothane
    3.   Isoflurane
    4. N_2O

Select A if options *1, 2 and 3* are correct,
Select B if options *1 and 3* are correct,
Select C if options *2 and 4* are correct,
Select D if only option *4* is correct,
Select E if *all* options are correct.

361. The ratio of delivered-to-alveolar concentration (F_D/F_A) is greater under which of the following conditions?

    1. If halothane is used instead of isoflurane (at the same fresh-gas flow rates)
    2. At low fresh-gas inflow rates vs higher ones
    3. If sevoflurane is used instead of desflurane (at the same fresh-gas flow rates)
    4. In a non-rebreathing vs a rebreathing system

362. Factors which lower MAC include

    1. Female gender
    2. Hypothyroidism
    3. P_aCO_2 65 mmHg
    4. Acute ethanol ingestion

363. Which of the following factors can influence the rate of increase in F_A/F_I?

    1. Inspired anesthetic concentration
    2. Cardiac output
    3. V_A
    4. The volume of the anesthetic breathing circuit

364. Which of the following volatile anesthetics contain no preservative?

    1. Enflurane
    2. Halothane
    3. Isoflurane
    4. Methoxyflurane

365. Which of the following statements concerning the effect of volatile anesthetics on resting P_aCO_2 during spontaneous breathing is true?

    1. The effect on resting P_aCO_2 increases with time
    2. Assisted ventilation is highly effective in maintaining normocapnia
    3. Surgical stimulation is usually sufficient to return the P_aCO_2 to normal
    4. The effect decreases with time

366. Anesthetic loss to plastic and soda lime is little to non-existent with which of the following anesthetics?

    1. Desflurane
    2. Nitrous oxide
    3. Sevoflurane
    4. Halothane

Select A if options *1, 2 and 3* are correct,
Select B if options *1 and 3* are correct,
Select C if options *2 and 4* are correct,
Select D if only option *4* is correct,
Select E if *all* options are correct.

367. Abnormally high serum [F⁻] occurs when enflurane is administered to patients who

    1. Are taking isoniazid
    2. Are obese
    3. Are taking hydralazine
    4. Are on chronic long-term phenobarbital therapy

368. Which of the following properties are **NOT** shared by both desflurane and isoflurane at concentrations of 1 MAC?

    1. Reduction of mean arterial pressure
    2. Reduction of cardiac index
    3. Reduction of systemic vascular resistance
    4. Acceleration of heart rate

369. Inhalational anesthetics that slow conduction of cardiac impulses through the His-Purkinje system include which of the following?

    1. Isoflurane
    2. N_2O
    3. Enflurane
    4. Halothane

370. Wash-in of the anesthesia circuit refers to the process of filling which of the following components with anesthetic?

    1. The inspiratory limb
    2. The expiratory limb
    3. The anesthesia bag
    4. The CO_2 absorber

371. The rate of rise of F_A to F_I during an inhalation induction could be increased by which of the following?

    1. Increasing alveolar ventilation
    2. Substitution of sevoflurane for halothane
    3. Administration of esmolol
    4. Carrying out the induction in Denver vs San Diego

372. In the first few hours following cessation of halothane anesthesia, halothane concentration in the blood falls because it

    1. Is excreted via the lungs
    2. Is taken up by the vessel poor group
    3. Is metabolized by the liver
    4. Is excreted unchanged by the kidney

373. N_2O increases

    1. Arterial blood pressure
    2. Heart rate
    3. Stroke volume
    4. Cardiac output

DIRECTIONS (Questions 374 through 382): Each group of questions consists of several numbered statements followed by lettered headings. For each numbered statement, select the ONE lettered heading that is most closely associated with it. Each lettered heading may be selected once, more than once, or not at all.

	Heart rate	Stroke volume	Cardiac output
374.	Increased	decreased	no change
375.	Increased	no change	increased
376.	No change	decreased	decreased
377.	Increased	decreased	decreased

    A. Halothane
    B. Enflurane
    C. Isoflurane
    D. N_2O
    E. None of the above

378. Enflurane

379. N_2O

380. Methoxyflurane

381. Isoflurane

382. Halothane

    A. 0.004% metabolized
    B. 0.17% metabolized
    C. 2.4-8.5% metabolized
    D. 20-50% metabolized
    E. 50-75% metabolized

PHARMACOLOGY AND PHARMACOKINETICS OF VOLATILE ANESTHETICS ANSWERS, REFERENCES, AND EXPLANATIONS

321. **(E)** No significant effect is seen on the cardiovascular system when N_2O is administered either alone or in combination with one of the volatile anesthetics halothane, isoflurane, or enflurane. However, significant changes can be seen in patients with coronary artery disease who receive 60% N_2O in combination with 1 mg/kg morphine sulphate which include reductions in cardiac index, mean arterial pressure, and heart rate, as well as increases in systemic and pulmonary vascular resistance *(Stoelting: Basics of Anesthesia, ed 3, pp 51-55; Stoelting: Anesthesia and Co-existing Disease, ed 3, p 26).*

322. **(B)** Alveolar partial pressure of a volatile anesthetic, which ultimately determines the depth of general anesthesia, is determined by the relative rates of input to removal of the anesthetic gases to and from the alveoli. Removal of anesthetic gases from the alveoli is accomplished by uptake into the pulmonary venous blood which is most dependent upon an alveolar partial pressure difference. During the initial moments of inhalation of an anesthetic gas, there is no volatile anesthetic in the alveoli to create this partial pressure gradient. Therefore, uptake for all volatile anesthetic gases will be minimal until the resultant rapid increase in alveolar partial pressure establishes a sufficient alveolar-to-venous partial pressure gradient to promote uptake of the anesthetic gas into the pulmonary venous blood. This will occur in spite of other factors which are discussed in the explanation to question 333 *(Miller: Anesthesia, ed 4, pp 101 & 102).*

323. **(D)** At concentrations at or below 1 MAC volatile anesthetics as well as the inhaled anesthetic N_2O will produce dose-dependent increases in the respiratory rate in spontaneously breathing patients. This trend continues at concentrations above 1 MAC for all of the inhaled anesthetics except isoflurane. With the exception of N_2O, the evidence suggests this effect is caused by direct activation of the respiratory center in the central nervous system rather than by stimulating pulmonary stretch receptors. Additionally, volatile anesthetics decrease tidal volume and significantly alter breathing pattern from the normal awake pattern of intermittent deep breaths separated by varying time intervals, to one of rapid, shallow, regular, and rhythmic breathing *(Stoelting: Basics of Anesthesia, ed 3, p 47).*

324. **(A)** Halothane is derived from the hydrocarbon ethane by substitution with the halogens fluorine, bromine, and chlorine. The structure of this halogenated hydrocarbon makes halothane non-flammable, and provides for low blood solubility, molecular stability, and anesthetic potency *(Stoelting: Basics of Anesthesia, ed 3, pp 5-7).*

325. **(E)** At anesthetic concentrations, halothane will abolish ventilatory response to arterial hypoxemia. Halothane, as well as other volatile anesthetics, will inhibit hypoxic pulmonary vasoconstriction, although it will not impair arterial oxygenation by this mechanism in most patients. Halothane causes a rightward shift in the position of as well as a dose-dependent decrease in the slope of the P_aCO_2 ventilatory response curve. The sensitivity of cerebral vasculature to changes in P_aCO_2 is unaffected by volatile anesthetics. However, administration of halothane,

enflurane, and perhaps isoflurane will result in a higher cerebral blood flow (CBF) while decreasing the cerebral metabolic rate (CMRO$_2$). This can be important, as increased cerebral blood flow tends to increase the total amount of blood in the head and can result in increased intracranial pressure *(Stoelting: Basics of Anesthesia, ed 3, pp 47-57; Barash: Clinical Anesthesia, ed 2, pp 875, 878, & 879).*

326. **(B)** A vaporizer's specificity is based on the vapor pressure of the anesthetic agent for which it is made. Filling a vaporizer with an agent with a higher vapor pressure results in a higher concentration in the vaporizer's output. Similarly, a volatile agent with a lower vapor pressure produces an output with a lower concentration than seen on the dial. Enflurane vapor pressure of 172 mmHg (20°C) most closely approximates the vapor pressure of sevoflurane which is 160 mmHg *(Stoelting: Pharmacology and Physiology in Anesthetic Practice, ed 2, pp 35 & 36; Miller: Anesthesia, ed 4, pp 195-197).*

327. **(E)** When administered alone, N$_2$O does not alter arterial blood pressure, stroke volume, systemic vascular resistance, or baroreceptor reflexes. Administration of N$_2$O increases heart rate slightly which may result in a mild increase in cardiac output. *In vitro* N$_2$O has a dose-dependent direct depressant effect on myocardial contractility which is probably overcome in vivo by sympathetic activation *(Miller: Anesthesia, ed 4, p 145; Stoelting: Basics of Anesthesia, ed 3, p 55).*

328. **(D)** Because of their ability to produce a 2-3 fold increase in skeletal muscle blood flow, systemic vascular resistance is decreased by isoflurane, desflurane, and, to a lesser extent enflurane. Although halothane increases cutaneous blood flow, it does not decrease systemic vascular resistance *(Miller: Anesthesia, ed 4, p 144).*

329. **(D)** At levels of 1 MAC, enflurane exerts the greatest ventilatory depression, although all volatiles will cause some degree of depression. However, at levels greater than 1 MAC, desflurane may cause greater inhibition of the ventilatory response to increasing P$_a$CO$_2$ than enflurane. The magnitude of ventilatory depression caused by volatile anesthetics may be accentuated by the presence of chronic obstructive pulmonary disease, and may be attenuated by the substitution of N$_2$O for equivalent MAC levels of the volatile anesthetic. The beneficial effect of substituting N$_2$O for volatile anesthetic is most apparent with enflurane *(Stoelting: Basics of Anesthesia, ed 3, pp 47-50).*

330. **(D)** At concentrations of 1 MAC, isoflurane may attenuate antigen-induced bronchospasm, presumably by decreasing vagal tone. At similar concentrations, isoflurane will not reduce cardiac output in patients with normal left ventricular function. Additionally, isoflurane will decrease stroke volume, mean arterial pressure, and systemic vascular resistance in a dose-dependent manner. Cardiac output remains unchanged because decreases in systemic vascular resistance result in a reflex increase in heart rate which is sufficient to offset the decrease in stroke volume. However, dose-dependent decreases in both stroke volume and cardiac index can be seen when isoflurane is administered in concentrations greater than 1 MAC *(Stoelting: Basics of Anesthesia, ed 3, pp 50-55).*

331. **(D)** Volatile anesthetics are cerebral vasodilators that cause dose-dependent increases in cerebral blood flow. At concentrations of 1.1 MAC with the P$_a$CO$_2$ held constant at 40 mm Hg, cerebral

blood flow is mildly increased by isoflurane, increased by 30-50% by enflurane, and increased nearly 200% by halothane *(Stoelting: Pharmacology & Physiology of Anesthetic Practice, ed 2, p 39).*

332. **(A)** Of all the options listed, desflurane has the lowest solubility constant which results in a very rapid rise in F_A/F_I. The rate of rise is very similar to that seen with nitrous oxide, and results in the most rapid attainment of 1 MAC concentration once the new volatile anesthetic has been initiated. Halothane has the highest blood:gas solubility coefficient of all the options, reflecting the largest quantity of gas stored in the blood. This reservoir will result in the slowest decline in the alveolar concentration of this gas upon discontinuation. The combination of these different solubilities will ultimately result in the highest combined MAC when 1 MAC of halothane is discontinued and 1 MAC of desflurane is introduced *(Miller: Anesthesia, ed 4, p 104; Stoelting: Basics of Anesthesia, ed 3, pp 20-22).*

333. **(D)** The alveolar partial pressure of an anesthetic is determined by the rate of input relative to removal of the anesthetic from the alveoli as explained in question number 322. During induction, the anesthetic gas is removed from the alveoli by uptake into the pulmonary venous blood. The rate of uptake is influenced by cardiac output, the blood:gas solubility coefficient, and the alveolar-to-venous partial pressure difference of the anesthetic. At a lower cardiac output, a slower rate of uptake of volatile anesthetic from the alveoli into the pulmonary venous blood results in a faster rate of increase in the alveolar concentration. This will result in an increased alveolar inspired gas concentration (F_A/F_I). Uptake of poorly soluble anesthetic gases from the alveoli is minimal and the rate of rise of F_A/F_I is rapid and virtually independent of cardiac output. Uptake of the more soluble anesthetics, e.g. halothane, from the alveoli into the pulmonary venous blood can be considerable and will be reflected by a slower rate of rise of the F_A/F_I ratio. Cardiogenic shock will have the smallest impact on the most insoluble agent desflurane, while the impact on the rate of rise of F_A/F_I of the relatively soluble anesthetic gases will be more profound *(Miller: Anesthesia, ed 4, pp 109 & 110).*

334. **(C)** The vessel-rich group which receives approximately 75 percent of the cardiac output is composed of the brain, heart, spleen, liver, splenic bed, kidneys, and endocrine glands. It constitutes, however, only 10 percent of the total body weight. Because of this large blood flow relative to tissue mass, these organs take up a large volume of volatile anesthetic and equilibrate with the partial pressure of the volatile anesthetic in the blood and alveoli during the earliest moments of induction *(Miller: Anesthesia, ed 4, pp 103 & 104).*

335. **(C)** Of the choices listed, halothane undergoes oxidative metabolism to the greatest extent (approximately 20%), followed by enflurane and sevoflurane (approximately 2%), isoflurane (approximately 0.2%), and desflurane (approximately 0.02%). Enflurane and sevoflurane may produce fluoride ions, which can be of concern during longer cases because of their potential for nephrotoxicity. Fluoride ion induced nephrotoxicity is characterized by the inability of the kidneys to concentrate urine, presumably by direct inhibition of adenylate cyclase activity which is necessary for normal function antidiuretic hormone at the distal convoluted tubules. This results in ADH resistant diabetes insipidus, i.e., nephrogenic diabetes insipidus characterized by polyuria, dehydration, hypernatremia, and increased serum osmolarity (see explanation to question 336) *(Stoelting: Basics of Anesthesia, ed 3, p 6; Barash: Clinical Anesthesia, ed 2, pp 456-457).*

336. **(A)** Volatile anesthetics are metabolized primarily by the liver. Other sites of metabolism include the gastrointestinal tract, kidneys, and lungs. Hepatic metabolism of volatile anesthetics requires activity of the cytochrome P-450 system which is found in the endoplasmic reticulum of the hepatocytes and mediates both oxidative and reductive metabolism. Under normal physiologic conditions halothane undergoes oxidative metabolism to yield inorganic bromide, chloride, and trichloroacetic acid. However, inorganic fluoride as well as reactive intermediary metabolites may be formed by reductive metabolism which occurs with hypoxia or hypoperfusion *(Stoelting: Basics of Anesthesia, ed 3, pp 5-7 & 294; Barash: Clinical Anesthesia, ed 2, pp 469 & 470).*

337. **(D)** The situation described in this question is that of a transpulmonary shunt. In patients with transpulmonary shunting, blood emerging from unventilated alveoli contains no anesthetic gas. This anesthetic-deficient blood mixes with blood from adequately ventilated, anesthetic containing, alveoli producing an arterial anesthetic partial pressure considerably less than expected. Since uptake of anesthetic gas from the alveoli into pulmonary venous blood will be less than normal, transpulmonary shunting accelerates the rate of rise in the F_A/F_I ratio, but reduces the rate of increase in the arterial partial pressure of all volatile anesthetics. The degree to which these changes occur depends on the solubility of the given volatile anesthetic. For poorly soluble anesthetics, such as N_2O, transpulmonary shunting only slightly accelerates the rate of rise in F_A/F_I ratio, but significantly reduces the rate of increase in arterial anesthetic partial pressure. The opposite occurs with highly soluble volatile anesthetics, such as halothane and methoxyflurane *(Miller: Anesthesia, ed 4, pp 110-112).*

338. **(E)** In unanesthetized subjects, a reduction in arterial blood pressure will elicit an increase in heart rate via the carotid and aortic baroreceptor reflexes. In contrast to isoflurane and enflurane, halothane profoundly inhibits these baroreceptor reflex responses. Therefore, despite reductions in arterial blood pressures by halothane, heart rate usually remains unchanged *(Stoelting: Basics of Anesthesia, ed 3, pp 51-52).*

339. **(A)** *(Stoelting: Basics of Anesthesia, ed 3, pp 47-55).*

340. **(D)** The rate of input of volatile anesthetics from the anesthesia machine to the alveoli is influenced by three factors: V_A, the inspired anesthetic partial pressure, and the characteristics of the anesthetic breathing system (see explanation to question 352). Increased V_A will accelerate the rate of increase in F_A/F_I for all volatile anesthetics. However, the magnitude of this effect is dependent on the solubility of the volatile anesthetic. The rate of increase in F_A/F_I depends very little on V_A for poorly soluble anesthetics because the uptake of these is minimal. In contrast, the rate of increase in F_A/F_I for highly soluble volatile anesthetics depends significantly on V_A. Halothane is the most soluble volatile anesthetic listed in this question. Therefore, an increase in V_A will accelerate the rate of increase in F_A/F_I the most for this agent *(Miller: Anesthesia, ed 4, pp 102-103).*

341. **(E)** Anesthetic requirement increases from birth until approximately 3-6 months of age. Then, with the exception of a slight increase at puberty, anesthetic requirement progressively declines with aging. For example, the MAC for halothane in neonates is approximately 0.87%, the MAC for halothane in infants is approximately 1.2%, and the MAC for halothane in young adults is

approximately 0.75% *(Stoelting: Basics of Anesthesia, ed 3, pp 382-383; Barash: Clinical Anesthesia, ed 2, pp 1318 & 1338).*

342. **(C)**   When administered to healthy volunteers, inhalational anesthetics (except for N_2O) cause a dose-dependent decrease in stroke volume. This depressant effect of volatile anesthetics on stroke volume is greatest with halothane, less with isoflurane, and least with desflurane *(Stoelting: Basics of Anesthesia, ed 3, p 52).*

343. **(C)**   Two principles of MAC must be considered in this situation. First, MAC is additive, so the fraction of MAC of each individual gas must be added to arrive at total MAC. The second is that alveolar concentrations of soluble agents are more accurately reflected by end-expiratory concentrations rather than either inspiratory concentrations or gradients between inspiratory and expiratory concentrations. Since nitrous oxide is very insoluble, it is reasonable to assume equilibrium will be established early. The inspiratory concentration of nitrous oxide, approximately 0.6 MAC, should approximate the alveolar concentration. However, the expiratory concentrations of the more soluble volatile anesthetics should be used to estimate the alveolar concentration. The end-expiratory isoflurane concentration of 0.6 reflects approximately 0.5 MAC, which in addition to 0.6 MAC of nitrous oxide would be closest to answer C, 1.1 MAC *(Stoelting: Pharmacology and Physiology in Anesthetic Practice, ed 3, pp 24 & 25; Barash: Clinical Anesthesia, ed 2, pp 739 & 740).*

344. **(B)**   The figure shown in this question depicts the concentration effect. Note that the inspired anesthetic concentration not only influences the maximum alveolar concentration that can be attained but also the rate at which the maximum alveolar concentration can be attained. The greater the inhaled anesthetic concentration, the faster the increase in F_A/F_I *(Stoelting: Pharmacology and Physiology of Anesthetic Practice, ed 2, p 21).*

345. **(E)**   The depth of general anesthesia is directly proportional to the alveolar anesthetic partial pressure. The faster the rate of increase in F_A/F_I, the faster the induction of anesthesia. With the exception of a right-to-left intracardiac shunt (see explanation to question 337 on effect of shunt on the rate of increase in F_A/F_I and explanation to question 346 on the effect of shunt on arterial anesthetic partial pressure and rate of induction of anesthesia), all of the conditions listed in this question will accelerate the rate of increase in F_A/F_I and thus, the rate of induction of anesthesia *(Stoelting: Pharmacology and Physiology of Anesthetic Practice, ed 2, pp 26 & 27).*

346. **(E)**   In general, a right-to-left intracardiac shunt or transpulmonary shunt will slow the rate of induction of anesthesia. This occurs because of a dilutional effect of shunted blood which contains no volatile anesthetic on the arterial anesthetic partial pressure coming from ventilated alveoli. The impact of a right-to-left shunt on the rate of increase in pulmonary arterial anesthetic partial pressure and, ultimately, the rate of induction of anesthesia is greatest for poorly soluble volatile anesthetics. This occurs because uptake of poorly soluble volatile anesthetics into pulmonary venous blood is minimal, thus, the dilutional effect of the shunt on pulmonary venous anesthetic partial pressure is essentially unopposed. In contrast, the uptake of highly soluble volatile anesthetics is sufficient to partially offset the dilutional effect. Of the anesthetics listed in the question, N_2O is the least soluble *(Miller: Anesthesia, ed 4, pp 110-112).*

347. **(D)** Enflurane is the only volatile anesthetic that causes a dose-dependent increase in heart rate in healthy volunteers. Isoflurane causes a maximum increase in heart rate of 20% above that of awake levels. Conversely, heart rate remains relatively unchanged by halothane and is only minimally increased by N_2O. All volatile anesthetics cause a dose-dependent decrease in myocardial contractility which is greatest for enflurane and least for isoflurane *(Stoelting: Basics of Anesthesia, ed 3, pp 51-53)*.

348. **(D)** Sevoflurane is a highly insoluble volatile anesthetic which combines with carbon dioxide absorbents to form a vinyl ether known as Compound A. The blood:gas partition coefficient for sevoflurane is 0.69. The vaporizer manufactured by Ohmeda is capable of delivering concentrations ranging from 0.2% to 8% at fresh-gas flow rates of 0.2 to 15 L/min. Its vapor pressure is 160 mm Hg at 20°C which is similar to the vapor pressure for the other volatile anesthetics with the exception of desflurane (664 mm Hg at 20°C). Gas flows greater than 2 L/min prevent rebreathing of compound A thus reducing the incidence of renal toxicity associated with it *(Stoelting: Pharmacology and Physiology in Anesthetic Practice, ed 2, pp 34-36; Rogers: Principles and Practice of Anesthesiology, p 1081; bulletin from Ohmeda, Medical Systems Division, distributed on 2/5/96)*.

349. **(E)** Metabolism may play an important role in emergence from anesthesia when one of the more soluble agents is used. However, this is not the case on induction. Factors that affect the rate of induction include the inspiratory concentration of anesthetic gas, alveolar ventilation, the characteristics of the anesthetic breathing system, solubility of the anesthetic gas, cardiac output, and the alveolar venous partial pressure difference *(Stoelting: Basics of Anesthesia, ed 3, pp 19-23)*.

350. **(A)** Greater uptake of an anesthetic gas from the alveoli decreases the rate of rise of F_A/F_I. A higher blood/gas solubility coefficient reflects a larger reservoir in the blood and promotes uptake from the alveoli, thereby decreasing the rate of rise. A lower blood/gas partition coefficient reflects a smaller reservoir resulting in a more rapid rate of rise of F_A/F_I. Sevoflurane with a blood/gas partition coefficient of 0.69 most closely approximates that of desflurane the coefficient of which is 0.42. Therefore the rate of rise of F_A/F_I most closely resembles that of sevoflurane *(Miller: Anesthesia, ed 4, p 102)*.

351. **(E)** Halothane undergoes significant metabolism compared to enflurane (15-20% vs 2-3%). Metabolism increases total elimination of halothane (which mainly occurs in the liver, but occurs in the lung as well) resulting in a more rapid alveolar washout *(Miller: Anesthesia, ed 4, p 120)*.

352. **(D)** Inspired gases consist of fresh-gas flow from the vaporizer plus expired gases contained in the anesthesia circuit. Expired gases will have a lower concentration of volatile anesthetic due to uptake that has already occurred. This will result in a lower total concentration of inspired volatile anesthetic compared to the setting on the vaporizer. The extent of the dilution will vary with the rate of the fresh-gas flow *(Miller: Anesthesia, ed 4, p 114)*.

353. **(E)** Although no toxic metabolites are formed, sevoflurane is degraded in a temperature-dependent fashion by both soda lime and baralyme. This process does not seem to be clinically significant in semi-open systems at moderate or low flows *(Barash: Clinical Anesthesia, ed 2, p 658)*.

354. **(D)** At 1 MAC concentrations isoflurane depresses mean arterial pressures primarily by decreasing systemic vascular resistance. The decrease in mean arterial pressure may be greater than that seen with the administration of halothane. However, heart rate will be increased, and stroke volume will decrease to a lesser extent than seen with administration of 1 MAC halothane *(Miller: Anesthesia, ed 4, p 144; Stoelting: Basics of Anesthesia, ed 3, pp 51 & 52)*.

355. **(B)** Changes in both cardiac output and alveolar ventilation will affect the rates of rise of F_A/F_I but in opposite directions. An increase in cardiac output will decrease the rate of F_A/F_I while an increase in alveolar ventilation will increase the rate of F_A/F_I. However, these two opposing options do not completely offset each other because the increased cardiac output also accelerates the equilibrium of the anesthetic between the blood and the tissues. This equilibrium results in a narrowing of the alveolar to venous partial pressure difference, and attenuate the impact of the increased cardiac output on uptake. The net result will be a slight increase in the rate of rise of F_A/F_I *(Miller: Anesthesia, ed 4, p 110)*.

356. **(A)** Blood:gas partition coefficient is the option listed which most closely correlates with recovery from inhaled anesthesia. A higher blood:gas partition coefficient reflects a larger quantity of gas dissolved in the blood for a given alveolar concentration. Other factors which affect emergence from anesthesia include alveolar ventilation, cardiac output, tissue concentrations, and metabolism *(Stoelting: Basics of Anesthesia, ed 3, p 23)*.

357. **(A)** Both a left-to-right intracardiac shunt and a left-to-right tissue shunt such as an arteriovenous fistula will result in a higher partial pressure of anesthetic gas in the blood returning to the lungs, ultimately resulting in a more rapid rise in F_A/F_I. However, this effect is minimal and in most cases clinically insignificant *(Stoelting: Basics of Anesthesia, ed 3, p 23)*.

358. **(B)** A right-to-left shunt will slow induction by the dilutional effect of shunted blood which contains no anesthetic gas. Doubling cardiac output will also slow the rate of rise of F_A/F_I. The presence of a left-to-right intracardiac shunt will have minimal impact on the F_A/F_I ratio. Ventilation of unperfused alveolar will not affect the F_A/F_I *(Stoelting: Basics of Anesthesia, ed 3, p 23)*.

359. **(A)** Sevoflurane is supplied in preservative-free solution. Metabolites of sevoflurane include inorganic fluoride, and plasma fluoride levels may rise measurably when this agent is used for longer cases. Sevoflurane decreases systemic vascular resistance in a dose-dependent manner. Although sevoflurane is highly insoluble similar to desflurane and N_2O, it is relatively more soluble than either of these other two gases with a blood:gas partition coefficient of 0.69 as compared to desflurane and N_2O with partition coefficients of 0.42 and 0.46 respectively *(Rogers: Principles and Practice of Anesthesiology, pp 1054 & 1081)*.

360. **(B)** Both enflurane and isoflurane decrease systemic vascular resistance. Halothane and N_2O have no significant effect of systemic vascular resistance *(Stoelting: Basics of Anesthesia, ed 3, pp 53-55)*.

361. **(E)** Factors that affect the ratio of delivered-to-alveolar concentrations (F_D/F_A) include the solubility of the anesthetic gas delivered and the inflow rate. Gases with higher solubility will have a greater delivered-to-alveolar concentration gradient; however, this ratio will be the greatest

early in the anesthetic administration for all gases regardless of solubility. Secondly, the inflow rate affects the delivered-to-alveolar concentration in the inverse manner. Higher inflow rates result in a lower ratio for the same anesthetic gas. Therefore, the use of halothane which is more soluble than isoflurane or using sevoflurane which is more soluble than desflurane results in a higher delivered-to-alveolar concentration gradient. Use of low fresh-gas inflow rates or a non-rebreathing system will also result in a higher gradient *(Miller: Anesthesia, ed 4, pp 117 & 118)*.

362. **(D)**   Acute ethanol ingestion is the only factor listed which will affect MAC. Acute ethanol ingestion decreases MAC. Gender, thyroid function, and P_aCO_2 between 15 and 95 mmHg have no effect on MAC *(Stoelting: Basics of Anesthesia, ed 3, p 25)*.

363. **(E)**   This table summarizes the factors that influence the rate of increase in F_A/F_I *(Stoelting: Basics of Anesthesia, ed 3, pp 18-23)*.

Summary of Factors That Influence the Rate of Increase in F_A/F_I

Input From Anesthesia Machine to Alveoli	Uptake From Alveoli to Pulmonary Blood	Uptake From Arterial Blood to Brain
Inspired anesthetic concentration	Blood:gas partition coefficient	Brain:blood partition coefficient
Alveolar ventilation	Cardiac output	Cerebral blood flow
Characteristics of the anesthesia breathing system	Alveolar-to-venous partial pressure difference	Arterial-to-venous partial pressure difference

364. **(B)**   In contrast to isoflurane and enflurane, commercial preparations of methoxyflurane and halothane contain preservatives, are not stable in soda lime, and react with the metal components of the anesthesia delivery system *(Stoelting: Basics of Anesthesia, ed 2, p 12)*.

365. **(D)**   During spontaneous breathing, volatile anesthetics cause a dose-dependent increase in resting P_aCO_2. Interestingly, this effect decreases with the duration of anesthesia. Although surgical stimulation increases V_E, this increase is not sufficient to return the resting P_aCO_2 to normal. Because the apneic threshold (i.e., the maximum P_aCO_2 that will not stimulate spontaneous breathing) is only 5 mm Hg below resting P_aCO_2, assisted ventilation of the lungs during inhalation anesthesia is not be effective in maintaining a normal P_aCO_2 *(Stoelting: Basics of Anesthesia, ed 3, pp 47-49)*.

366. **(A)**   Anesthetic agents are soluble in the rubber and plastic components found in the anesthesia machine. This fact can actually impede the development of anesthetic concentrations of these drugs. The worst offender is methoxyflurane. However, both isoflurane and halothane are soluble in rubber and plastic but to a lesser degree. Sevoflurane, desflurane, and nitrous oxide have little or no solubility in rubber or plastic. It should, however, be born in mind that sevoflurane can be destroyed in appreciable quantities by both wet and dry soda lime. It is therefore recommended that fresh gas flow rates exceed 2 L/min when sevoflurane is administered *(Miller: Anesthesia, ed 4, p 114)*.

367. **(A)**   Isoniazid, obesity, and hydralazine are all associated with increased serum $[F^-]$ in patients who receive enflurane anesthesia. Phenobarbital, however, does not increase defluorination of enflurane *(Stoelting: Basics of Anesthesia, ed 3, p 6; Stoelting: Pharmacology and Physiology of Anesthetic Practice, ed 2, pp 64, 317, & 498)*.

368. **(C)**

1 MAC	Mean arterial pressure	Cardiac index	Systemic vascular resistance	Heart rate
Isoflurane	Decreased	Normal	Decreased	Increased
Desflurane	Decreased	Decreased	Decreased	Normal

Both isoflurane and desflurane decrease systemic vascular resistance and cause reductions in blood pressure at concentrations less than 1 MAC. Desflurane decreases cardiac index at concentrations less than 1 MAC whereas isoflurane does not decrease cardiac index at concentrations less than 1 MAC. Isoflurane in contradistinction to desflurane does increase heart rate in a non-dose dependent fashion *(Stoelting: Basics of Anesthesia, ed 3, p 52)*.

369. **(D)**   All of the volatile anesthetics listed in this question slow conduction of cardiac impulses through the atrioventricular node, but only halothane slows conduction through both the atrioventricular node and the His-Purkinje system. Halothane increases the sensitivity of the myocardium to catecholamines, which can augment sympathomimetic-induced dysrhythmias. The mechanism for this effect is not clear; however, it is thought to be related to the direct depressant effect of halothane on transmission of electrical cardiac impulses through the His-Purkinje system, which can cause re-entry circuits or premature ventricular depolarizations. The dysrhythmia-producing dose of epinephrine is independent of the concentration of halothane between alveolar concentrations of 0.5-2.0% *(Stoelting: Basics of Anesthesia, ed 3, pp 51 & 55)*.

370. **(E)**   By definition, the wash-in of the anesthesia circuit refers to the filling of the components of the circuit with anesthetic gases. All of the components listed are part of the anesthesia circuit *(Miller: Anesthesia, ed 4, p 114)*.

371. **(A)**   Increasing minute ventilation is one of two methods of manipulating ventilation that increases the rate of rise of F_A/F_I. The other method is increasing the inspired concentration. Substituting a less soluble anesthetic, such as sevoflurane for halothane, also increases the rate of rise of F_A/F_I. Administration of esmolol reduces cardiac output which also increases the rate of rise. Carrying out the induction in Denver vs San Diego constitutes administering the anesthetic at lower atmospheric pressures which would decrease the F_A/F_I ratio

$$uptake = \frac{\lambda \dot{Q}(P_A - P_V)}{BP}$$

where λ = blood gas partition coefficient, $\dot{Q}$ = cardiac output, (P_A-P_V) = the alveolar to pulmonary venous blood partial pressure difference, and BP is the barometric pressure *(Miller: Anesthesia, ed 4, pp 101 & 102)*.

372. **(A)** Upon termination of an anesthetic, volatile concentrations in the vessel rich group may approximate alveolar concentrations. However, equilibrium may not be reached in the muscle group until several hours of anesthetic administration have elapsed. Considerably more time is necessary for equilibrium to occur in fat. Upon termination of anesthesia, higher concentrations of anesthetic will be seen in the blood relative to the concentrations in fat and other poorly perfused tissues. The concentration gradient therefore will be favorable to continue uptake into the vessel-poor tissues even as halothane is excreted via the lungs and metabolized by the liver. Excretion of unchanged drug by the kidney is insignificant *(Miller: Anesthesia, ed 4, pp 119 & 120)*.

373. **(C)** In general, N_2O produces signs of mild sympathomimetic stimulation characterized by mild increases in pulmonary vascular resistance (particularly when administered to patients with co-existing pulmonary hypertension), cardiac output, heart rate, and circulating levels of catecholamines. Although the mechanism is not known, there is evidence from animal studies that this sympathomimetic effect is due to direct activation of the sympathetic nervous system in the suprapontine areas of the brain. N_2O has no effect on arterial blood pressure, stroke volume, or systemic vascular resistance, and like isoflurane, enflurane, and halothane, has a direct depressant effect on myocardial contractility *in vitro (Stoelting: Basics of Anesthesia, ed 3, p 55)*.

374. **(C)** 375. **(D)** 376. **(A)** 377. **(B)** The cardiovascular effects of volatile anesthetics are summarized in the table *(Stoelting: Basics of Anesthesia, ed 3, pp 51-55; Stoelting: Pharmacology and Physiology in Anesthetic Practice, ed 2, pp 43-46)*.

Summary of the Cardiovascular Effects of Volatile Anesthetics

	Halothane	Enflurane	Isoflurane	N_2O
Heart rate	N	I	I	I
Cardiac output	D	D	N	I
Stroke volume	D	D	D	N
Myocardial contractility	D	D	D	D
Systemic vascular resistance	N	D	D	N
Pulmonary vascular resistance	N	N	N	I
Right atrial pressure	I	I	I	I
Dysrhythmogenic potential	I	I	I	N

*I = increase, D = decrease, N = no change

378. **(C)** 379. **(A)** 380. **(E)** 381. **(B)** 382. **(D)** There have been a number of studies performed to determine the extent to which volatile anesthetics are metabolized. Previous studies have measured trace concentrations of metabolites (e.g., inorganic bromide and F^-, and organic fluorine) to define the pharmacokinetics of fluorinated anesthetics, such as methoxyflurane, enflurane, isoflurane, and sevoflurane. More recent studies that take into account the differences between estimates of quantities of anesthetic absorbed during exposure and that which is exhaled unaltered following exposure (called the mass balance technique) have indicated that a significantly greater fraction of volatile anesthetic undergoes liver metabolism than previously measured. A summary of the amount of volatile anesthetic metabolized as measured utilizing

these two techniques are shown in the table *(Barash: Clinical Anesthesia, ed 2, p 470; Stoelting: Pharmacology and Physiology in Anesthetic Practice, ed 2, p 62).*

Summary of the % Metabolism of Volatile Anesthetics

	% Metabolized (mass balance)	% Metabolized (metabolites as a % of total uptake)
Methoxyflurane	75.3	48
Halothane	46.1	11-25
Enflurane	8.5	2.4
Isoflurane	0.0	0.2
N_2O	0.0	0.0

*From Barash PG, Cullen BF, Stoelting RK (eds): Clinical Anesthesia, ed 2. Philadelphia, JB Lippincott, 1992, p 470. Used with permission.

PART II / CLINICAL SCIENCES

Blood Products, Transfusion, and Fluid Therapy

DIRECTIONS (Questions 383 through 407): Each of the questions or incomplete statements in this section is followed by answers or by completions of the statement, respectively. Select the ONE BEST answer or completion for each item.

383. Difficulty crossmatching blood due to concurrent medication occurs most frequently in patients treated with

   A. α-Methyldopa (Aldomet)
   B. Prazosin (Minipress)
   C. Clonidine (Catapress)
   D. Labetalol (Normodyne)
   E. Nadolol (Corgard)

384. Which of the following would be the most likely cause of oozing in a patient transfused with 10 units of whole blood?

   A. Citrate toxicity
   B. Low factor V
   C. Hemolytic transfusion reaction
   D. Dilutional thrombocytopenia
   E. Low factor VIII

385. In a 70-kg patient, one unit of platelet concentrate should increase the platelet count by

   A. $2,000/mm^3$
   B. $5,000/mm^3$
   C. $10,000/mm^3$
   D. $20,000/mm^3$
   E. $30,000/mm^3$

386. The most common transfusion-associated infection in the United States is

   A. Syphilis
   B. Hepatitis B
   C. Non-A, non-B hepatitis
   D. Human immunodeficiency virus
   E. Cytomegalovirus

387. The likelihood of a clinically significant transfusion reaction resulting from administration of type-specific blood is

    A. 1 in 10
    B. 1 in 250
    C. 1 in 500
    D. 1 in 1,000
    E. 1 in 10,000

388. Frozen erythrocytes can be stored for

    A. 180 days
    B. 1 year
    C. 3 years
    D. 5 years
    E. They can be stored indefinitely

389. Which of the following clotting factors has the shortest half-life?

    A. Factor II
    B. Factor V
    C. Factor VII
    D. Factor IX
    E. Factor X

390. Which of the following clotting factors is not synthesized by the liver?

    A. Factor II
    B. Factor VII
    C. Factor VIII
    D. Factor IX
    E. Factor X

391. The half-time of albumin in the plasma is

    A. 6 hours
    B. 2 days
    C. 8 days
    D. 21 days
    E. 90 days

392. From which of the following blood products would patients be most likely to become infected with syphilis?

    A. Platelets
    B. Fresh frozen plasma
    C. Whole blood
    D. Packed red blood cells
    E. Cryoprecipitate

393. The blood volume of a 10-kg, 1-year-old infant is

    A. 650 mL
    B. 800 mL
    C. 1100 mL
    D. 1300 mL
    E. 1500 mL

394. A patient with a prosthetic aortic valve and who is anticoagulated with coumadin is scheduled for a radical retropubic prostatectomy. What is the most appropriate management of this patient's anticoagulation?

    A. Continue coumadin and replace blood loss intraoperatively with whole blood
    B. Continue coumadin and give 4 units of fresh frozen plasma prior to surgery
    C. Stop coumadin on the evening prior to surgery and administer vitamin K 4 hours prior to surgery
    D. Stop coumadin one week prior to surgery and resume coumadin 3 days after surgery
    E. Change to heparin SQ one week prior to surgery and continue the heparin until 6 hours prior to surgery

395. A 23-year-old patient with hemophilia A is scheduled for wisdom tooth extraction under general anesthesia. After the second molar is extracted the patient begins to bleed profusely. Which of the following would be the best therapy to improve hemostasis in this patient?

    A. Cryoprecipitate
    B. Fresh frozen plasma
    C. Platelets
    D. Whole blood
    E. Vitamin K

396. A 38-year-old male is undergoing a total colectomy under general anesthesia. Urine output has been 20 mL/hr for the last two hours. Volume replacement has been adequate. The rationale for administering 5 mg of furosemide to this patient is to

    A. Offset the effects of increased antidiuretic hormone (ADH)
    B. Improve renal blood flow
    C. Convert oliguric renal failure to non-oliguric renal failure
    D. Offset the effects of increased renin
    E. Promote renal venodilation

397. A 65-year-old male involved in a motor vehicle accident is brought to the emergency room with a blood pressure of 60 mm Hg systolic. He is transfused with 4 units of type O, Rh negative whole blood and 3 L of lactated ringers. After the patient is brought to the operating room his blood type is determined to be type A, Rh positive. Which of the following is the most appropriate blood type for further intraoperative transfusions?

    A. Type A, Rh positive whole blood
    B. Type A, Rh positive erythrocytes
    C. Type O, Rh positive whole blood
    D. Type O, Rh negative whole blood
    E. Type O, Rh negative erythrocytes

398. The criteria used to determine how long blood can be stored prior to transfusion is

    A. 90% of transfused erythrocytes must remain in circulation for 24 hours
    B. 70% of transfused erythrocytes must remain in circulation for 24 hours
    C. 70% of transfused erythrocytes must remain in circulation for 72 hours
    D. 70% of transfused erythrocytes must remain in circulation for 7 days
    E. 50% of transfused erythrocytes must remain in circulation for 7 days

399. Platelets are stored at room temperature because

    A. It increases platelet half-life
    B. It improves platelet function
    C. The chance for infection is reduced
    D. It decreases the incidence of allergic reactions
    E. There is less splenic sequestration

400. An 18-year-old female involved in a motor vehicle accident is brought to the emergency room in shock where she is transfused with 10 units of type O, Rh negative whole blood over 30 minutes. After infusion of the first 5 units, bleeding is controlled and her blood pressure rises to 85/51 mm Hg. During the next 15 minutes, as the remaining 5 units are infused, her blood pressure slowly falls to 60 mm Hg systolic. The patient remains in sinus tachycardia at 120 beats/min, but the QT interval is noted to increase from 310 msec to 470 msec, and the central venous pressure increases from 9 mm Hg to 20 mm Hg. Her breathing is rapid and shallow. The most likely cause of this scenario is

    A. Citrate toxicity
    B. Hyperkalemia
    C. Hemolytic transfusion reaction
    D. Cardiac tamponade
    E. Tension pneumothorax

401. A 20-kg, 3-year-old child with a hematocrit of 40% could lose how much blood and still maintain a hematocrit of 30%?

    A. 120 mL
    B. 240 mL
    C. 360 mL
    D. 460 mL
    E. 600 mL

402. A 100-kg, male patient has a measured serum sodium concentration of 120 mEq/L. What is his total body sodium deficit?

    A. 600 mEq
    B. 1,200 mEq
    C. 1,800 mEq
    D. 2,400 mEq
    E. 3,000 mEq

403. The likelihood of a clinically significant transfusion reaction resulting from administration of erythrocytes to a patient with a negative antibody screen is

    A. 1 in 100
    B. 1 in 1,000
    C. 1 in 10,000
    D. 1 in 100,000
    E. 1 in 1,000,000

404. A 23-year-old female who has been receiving total parenteral nutrition (15% dextrose and intralipids) for 3 weeks is scheduled for surgery for severe Crohn's disease. Induction of anesthesia and tracheal intubation were uneventful. After establishing peripheral intravenous access, the old central line is removed and a new one is placed at a new site. At the end of the operation, a large volume of fluid is discovered in the chest cavity on chest x-ray. Arterial blood pressure is 110/70 mm Hg, heart rate is 150 beats/min, and S_aO_2 is 100% (pulse oximeter). The most appropriate **initial** step in the management of this patient is to

    A. Place a chest tube
    B. Reintubate the trachea with a double lumen tube
    C. Start a dopamine infusion
    D. Check a blood glucose
    E. Administer esmolol 20 mg IV

405. When type O, Rh negative blood is not available, type O, Rh positive blood is acceptable for transfusion for each of the following patients **EXCEPT**

    A. A 23-year-old male with diabetes who was involved in a motor vehicle accident
    B. A 10-year-old girl with a history cystic fibrosis who sustained a gunshot wound to the upper abdomen
    C. An 84-year-old male with a ruptured abdominal aortic aneurysm
    D. A 2-year-old boy involved in a pedestrian automobile accident
    E. A 21-year-old, gravida 2, para 1 female with placenta previa and bleeding profusely

406. The advantage of infusing Hetastarch (hydroxyethyl starch) over dextran for volume replacement is that hetastarch

    A. Is not associated with allergic reactions
    B. Is less likely to cause hypervolemia
    C. Does not interfere with coagulation
    D. Does not need to be administered through a 170 micron filter
    E. Does not interfere with blood typing and crossmatching

407. All of the following characterize blood that has been stored for 28 days at 4°C in citrate-phosphate-dextrose (CPD) anticoagulant-preservative **EXCEPT**

A. Potassium concentration of 23 mEq/L
B. pH of 6.78
C. 70% erythrocyte viability 24 hours after transfusion
D. P_{50} of 25
E. Erythrocyte 2,3-DPG concentration of 1 µg/mL

DIRECTIONS (Questions 408 through 415): For each of the items in this section, ONE or MORE of the numbered options is correct. Select the answer:

Select A if options *1, 2 and 3* are correct,
Select B if options *1 and 3* are correct,
Select C if options *2 and 4* are correct,
Select D if only option *4* is correct,
Select E if *all* options are correct.

408. Blood is routinely screened for which of the following?

1. Antibodies against hepatitis A
2. Antibodies against hepatitis B
3. Antibodies against cytomegalovirus
4. Antibodies against human T-cell leukemia virus type I

409. Drugs useful in the treatment of hemolytic transfusion reactions include

1. Furosemide
2. Bicarbonate
3. Mannitol
4. Diphenhydramine

410. Viral hepatitis is a possible risk with administration of which of the following?

1. Fresh frozen plasma
2. Cryoprecipitate
3. Platelets
4. Albumin

411. Which of the following are classic signs of a hemolytic transfusion reaction in patients under general anesthesia?

1. Hypotension
2. Oozing in the surgical field
3. Hemoglobinuria
4. Fever

Select A if options *1, 2 and 3* are correct,
Select B if options *1 and 3* are correct,
Select C if options *2 and 4* are correct,
Select D if only option *4* is correct,
Select E if *all* options are correct.

412. Which of the following intravenous fluids can be administered with blood (1:1 ratio) at room temperature without causing hemolysis or clotting of the erythrocytes in the intravenous tubing?

    1. 5% dextrose in water
    2. 5% dextrose in lactated ringers
    3. Lactated ringers
    4. 5% dextrose in 0.45 saline

413. Which of the following body fluid volumes in the adult (based on percentage of total body weight) is correct?

    1. Total body water 60%
    2. Extracellular water 20%
    3. Plasma volume 7%
    4. Intracellular water 40%

414. Treatment(s) for von Willebrand's disease include

    1. Cryoprecipitate
    2. Factor IX concentrate
    3. DDAVP
    4. Factor VIII concentrate

415. During an emergency cesarean section, a 25-year-old primiparous female begins to bleed briskly. Blood is brought to the operating room which has undergone the first phase of crossmatch. A transfusion reaction involving which of the following antibodies is possible if this blood were transfused at this time?

    1. ABO
    2. Rh
    3. MN, P, and Lewis
    4. Kell, Duffy, and Kidd

DIRECTIONS (Questions 416 through 417): This group of questions consists of several numbered statements followed by lettered headings. For each numbered statement, select the ONE lettered heading that is most closely associated with it. Each lettered heading may be selected once, more than once, or not at all.

416. What is the storage life of blood stored in citrate-phosphate-dextrose (CPD)?

417. What is the storage life of blood stored in citrate-phosphate-dextrose-adenine (CPDA)?

    A. 14 days
    B. 21 days
    C. 35 days
    D. 42 days
    E. 49 days

BLOOD PRODUCTS, TRANSFUSION, AND FLUID THERAPY
ANSWERS, REFERENCES, AND EXPLANATIONS

383. **(A)** Alpha-methyldopa can combine with the red blood cell membrane and produce a complex that can elicit an antibody response. These antibodies are directed toward the erythrocyte membrane and can make crossmatching of blood difficult *(Barash: Clinical Anesthesia, ed 2, p 575).*

384. **(D)** Platelets become damaged when stored at 4°C and are therefore readily cleared from the circulation soon after transfusion. For this reason, dilutional thrombocytopenia is the most likely cause of bleeding in patients who have received multiple transfusions. With the exception of factors V and VIII, most coagulation factors are stabled in stored blood. Factors V and VIII gradually decrease to approximately 15% and 50% of normal, respectively, after 21 days of storage. Because only 5% of factor V and 30% of factor VIII are needed for adequate hemostasis during surgery, administration of fresh frozen plasma to replace these factors is not recommended either on a therapeutic or prophylactic basis. Other potential causes of a bleeding diathesis in patients who have received multiple transfusions include disseminated intravascular coagulation and hemolytic transfusion reaction. Because the serum ionized calcium concentration necessary for adequate hemostasis and coagulation are far less than that required for normal cardiovascular function, citrate toxicity (citrate chelates ionized calcium) will cause profound depression of cardiovascular function before any evidence of hypocalcemia-induced hypocoagulation is seen *(Miller: Anesthesia, ed 4, pp 1626-1632).*

385. **(C)** After whole blood has been stored at 4°C for 24 to 48 hours, platelet activity is reduced to less than 10% of normal. Therefore, dilutional thrombocytopenia is the most frequent cause of hemorrhagic diathesis following multiple transfusions. Previous studies have indicated that when the platelet count acutely falls to 75,000/mm^3 or lower, a hemorrhagic diathesis is likely to occur. For this reason, platelet concentrates should be transfused to increase the platelet count above approximately 100,000/mm^3. In general, the platelet count is increased by approximately 10,000/mm^3 for every unit of platelet concentrate transfused *(Miller: Anesthesia, ed 4, p 1640).*

386. **(C)** In addition to alterations in O_2 transport, coagulation, acid-base status, and body temperature, the potential for transfusion-associated infections, such as hepatitis, acquired immunodeficiency syndrome, cytomegalovirus, syphilis, and malaria, must be considered when administering blood products to patients. Non-A, non-B hepatitis is the most common transfusion-associated infection in the United States primarily because there previously was no screening test available for this virus *(Miller: Anesthesia, ed 4, pp 1636-1637).*

387. **(D)** Compatibility testing of blood and blood components is performed to reduce the chance of an immune-associated transfusion reaction. Compatibility testing includes determining both the recipient's and the donor's ABO-Rh type, antibody screening, and crossmatching. Blood is type-specific when the ABO-Rh type of both the donor and recipient are the same. When ABO-Rh compatible blood is transfused, the likelihood of a clinically significant immune-associated transfusion reaction is approximately 1 in 1,000 *(Miller: Anesthesia, ed 4, p 1622).*

388. **(C)** Frozen erythrocytes are stored at −55°C to −79°C in glycerol. These cells can be stored for up to three years but must be transfused within 24 hours of thawing. Glycerol must be washed from the erythrocytes prior to transfusion. This is a complex and expensive process which limits the use of this preparation. The most significant advantages of using frozen and thawed erythrocytes are that 1) blood of rare types can be stored for long periods, 2) frozen erythrocytes are believed to be safer in patients who are especially susceptible to allergic reaction (because the freezing and washing process removes leukocytes), 3) frozen erythrocytes appear to carry a reduced risk of transfusion-associated hepatitis, and 4) because normal levels of 2,3-DPG are retained in frozen erythrocytes, they are desirable in clinical conditions that require prompt tissue oxygenation *(Miller: Anesthesia, ed 4, pp 1623-1624; Stoelting: Pharmacology and Physiology in Anesthetic Practice, ed 2, pp 570 & 571).*

389. **(C)** Factor VII has a biologic half-life of 4-6 hours, the shortest of all the soluble clotting factors *(Kaplan: Cardiac Anesthesia, ed 3, p 954).*

390. **(C)** Factors IV (ionized calcium), VIII, and XII are not synthesized by the liver. Factor VIII is a glycoprotein with many functionally heterogeneous subunits. Factor VIII is synthesized by vascular endothelial cells and is involved in promoting coagulation via the intrinsic clotting pathway *(Barash: Clinical Anesthesia, ed 2, pp 252-259; Stoelting: Pharmacology and Physiology in Anesthetic Practice, ed 2, pp 815 & 816).*

391. **(D)** Albumin is synthesized exclusively by the liver. Normal plasma concentrations of albumin are 3.5 g/dl to 5.5 g/dl. In addition to hepatocellular damage, plasma albumin concentrations may be reduced in association with conditions characterized by excessive protein loss, such as nephrotic syndrome, protein-losing enteropathies, thermal injuries, exfoliative dermatitis, or ascites. Because the half-time of albumin in plasma is 14-21 days, acute liver dysfunction will not be reflected by a decrease in plasma albumin concentration. Plasma albumin concentrations less than 2.5 g/dl may result in altered responses to drugs due to decreased protein binding *(Stoelting: Anesthesia and Co-existing Disease, ed 3, p 256).*

392. **(A)** Transfusion-associated infections can be caused by non-A, non-B viral hepatitis, human immunodeficiency virus, cytomegalovirus, syphilis, malaria, toxoplasmosis, and numerous types of bacteria, such as salmonella, brucella, and typhus. The only blood products capable of transmitting syphilis are those stored at room temperature. Of the choices listed, only platelets are stored at room temperature *(Miller: Anesthesia, ed 4, p 1637).*

393. **(B)** Blood volume decreases with age. In neonates, blood volume is 85 mL/kg; in infants and small children, blood volume is 80 mL/kg; in children 5 years of age, blood volume is 75 mL/kg; in adults, blood volume is 65 mL/kg *(Stoelting: Basics of Anesthesia, ed 3, p 382).*

394. **(D)** In patients with prosthetic heart valves, coumadin therapy should be discontinued in sufficient time to allow return of the prothrombin time to within 20% of normal. This usually requires 7 to 10 days. Coumadin should be resumed 2 to 3 days after surgery. The therapeutic efficacy of low-dose heparin is controversial. Low-dose heparin may increase the incidence of hemorrhagic complications during and after surgery. For these two reasons, low-dose heparin is not recommended in these patients *(Stoelting: Pharmacology and Physiology in Anesthetic Practice, ed 2, pp 468-473).*

395. **(A)**   Hemophilia A occurs in approximately 1 in 12,000 male patients in the United States and is caused by reduced factor VIII activity. Because the gene for factor VIII activity is carried on X chromosomes, hemophilia A is only clinically manifested in males while females usually remain asymptomatic carriers. The primary goal of preoperative preparation of these patients is to increase plasma factor VIII activity to a level that will ensure adequate hemostasis. Because the biologic half-life of factor VIII is 10 hours to 12 hours, activity levels of factor VIII should be raised to 100% before elective surgery to make sure that the activity does not decrease below 30% of normal during surgery. If bleeding occurs in these patients, cryoprecipitate or factor VIII concentrates should be transfused to increase factor VIII activity. Fresh frozen plasma is no longer recommended for therapy of factor VIII deficiency in patients with hemophilia A. Cryoprecipitate contains 5 to 10 units of factor VIII/mL and factor VIII concentrates contain up to 40 units/mL. Cryoprecipitate should be used within 3 hours after thawing *(Stoelting: Pharmacology and Physiology in Anesthetic Practice, ed 2, pp 572 & 573).*

396. **(A)**   Serum antidiuretic hormone levels increase during painful stimulation associated with surgery as well as during positive pressure mechanical ventilation. Small doses of furosemide will counteract this effect during surgery *(Stoelting: Basics of Anesthesia, ed 3, pp 328 & 329; Stoelting: Anesthesia and Co-existing Disease, ed 3, p 318).*

397. **(E)**   Type O, Rh negative whole blood contains high titers of anti-A and anti-B antibodies. After emergency transfusion of two or more units of Type O, Rh negative, uncrossmatched whole blood, the patient should not be transfused with his own blood type. Intravascular hemolysis of the donor erythrocytes may occur because of the high titers of anti-A and anti-B antibodies acquired during the previous transfusions *(Miller: Anesthesia, ed 4, p 1623).*

398. **(B)**   The duration that blood can be stored is determined by the requirement that at least 70% of the erythrocytes must remain in circulation for 24 hours after transfusion. Erythrocytes that survive greater than 24 hours after transfusion are removed from circulation at a normal rate. Based on this criteria, blood stored in citrate-phosphate-dextrose (CPD) anticoagulant-preservative can be stored at 1 to 6°C for up to 28 days, while blood stored in citrate-phosphate-dextrose with adenine (CPDA) anticoagulant-preservative can be stored at 1 to 6°C for up to 35 days. The adenine (0.25 to 0.5 mM) increases erythrocyte survival by allowing the erythrocytes to resynthesize the adenosine triphosphate needed to fuel metabolic reactions *(Miller: Anesthesia, ed 4, p 1623).*

399. **(A)**   Platelets stored at room temperature can remain in circulation for up to 8 days after transfusion versus 2-3 days for those stored at 1-6°C *(Stoelting: Pharmacology and Physiology in Anesthetic Practice, ed 2, pp 574 & 575).*

400. **(A)**   Stored blood contains citrate, an anticoagulant that binds ionized calcium. When blood is transfused at rates greater than 50 mL/min, hypocalcemia may occur. However, because the serum ionized calcium concentration necessary for adequate hemostasis is far less than that required for normal cardiovascular function, hypocalcemia will cause cardiovascular depression long before coagulation abnormalities occur *(Stoelting: Pharmacology and Physiology in Anesthetic Practice, ed 2, pp 561 & 562).*

401. **(D)** A 20-kg, 3-year-old child has an estimated blood volume of 80 mL/kg (1,600 mL). The acceptable blood loss can be determined using the following formula:

$$ABL = Wt \cdot EBV \cdot \frac{(Hct_0 - Hct_1)}{\overline{Hct}},$$

where ABL is the calculated acceptable blood loss (mL), Wt is the patient's weight (kg), EBV is the patient's estimated blood volume (mL/kg), Hct_0 is the original hematocrit, Hct_1 is the lowest acceptable hematocrit, and $\overline{Hct}$ is the mean hematocrit (mean of the difference between the original and lowest acceptable hematocrit). For this patient, the acceptable blood loss is:

$$1600 \cdot \frac{(40 - 30)}{35} = 460 \; ml$$

(Barash: Clinical Anesthesia, ed 2, p 1345).

402. **(B)** Hyponatremia is defined as serum sodium concentration < 135 mEq/L. When the serum sodium concentration decreases below 120 mEq/L, signs and symptoms of water intoxication, ranging from confusion to drowsiness, is likely to manifest. A serum sodium concentration less than 110 mEq/L may cause seizures and coma, and therefore require emergency treatment. Emergency therapy for severe hyponatremia is to administer hypertonic saline to replace the sodium deficit or mannitol to reduce the water content of the brain. As a general rule of thumb, total body sodium deficit can be calculated using the following equation:

$$Na^+ \; deficit = (140 - [Na^+]) \cdot TBW,$$

where Na^+ deficit is the total body sodium deficit (mEq), $[Na^+]$ is the current serum sodium concentration (mEq/L), and TBW is the patient's total body water (l). Therefore, in this patient, the total body sodium deficit is:

$$(140 - 120) \cdot 60 = 1,200 \; mEq$$

(Stoelting: Anesthesia and Co-existing Disease, ed 3, pp 320 & 321).

403. **(C)** Antibody screening is a trial transfusion between the recipient's serum and commercially supplied erythrocytes that contain optimal numbers of common erythrocyte antigens. These antigens are those which will react with antibodies commonly implicated in causing hemolytic transfusion reactions. The likelihood of a clinically significant hemolytic transfusion reaction resulting from administration of erythrocytes to patients with a negative antibody screen is less than 1 in 10,000 *(Miller: Anesthesia, ed 4, pp 1621 & 1622).*

404. **(D)** Abrupt discontinuation of total parenteral nutrition that contains 10% to 20% dextrose may result in profound rebound hypoglycemia. Tachycardia in this patient may signify hypoglycemia. Prompt diagnosis and treatment of severe hypoglycemia is essential if neurologic damage is to be avoided *(Stoelting: Anesthesia and Co-existing Disease, ed 3, pp 389 & 390).*

405. **(E)** Transfusion of type O, Rh positive erythrocytes in Rh negative patients is acceptable in an emergency but should be avoided in women who have been pregnant or anybody who has been immunized against the D (Rh) antibody because of the increased risk for severe hemolytic transfusion reactions. Rh negative individuals who received Rh positive blood may be treated with Rhogam to prevent formation of anti-D antibodies *(Faust: Anesthesiology Review, ed 2, p 473).*

406. **(E)** Hetastarch (hydroxyethyl starch) and dextrans (branched polysaccharides with molecular weights ranging from 40,000 to 70,000 daltons) are synthetic colloid solutions that are used for intravascular fluid volume expansion. Both hetastarch and dextran have been associated with allergic reactions and interfere with coagulation. Hetastarch, unlike dextrans, does not interfere with crossmatching of blood. Neither compound needs to be administered through a filter *(Stoelting: Anesthesia and Co-existing Disease, ed 3, p 420).*

407. **(D)** Erythrocytes that have been stored at 1 to 6°C for 28 days have decreased concentrations of 2,3-DPG, which results in a leftward shift in the oxyhemoglobin dissociation curve and an increased affinity of hemoglobin for O_2. The P_{50} of erythrocytes stored for 28 days at 1 to 6°C is 17 *(Stoelting: Anesthesia and Co-existing Disease, ed 3, pp 422-424).*

408. **(C)** The infectivity of homologous blood transfusion has received a great deal of attention for many years. In the past, blood banks screened blood primarily for syphilis and hepatitis B surface antigen. However, since 1985, six tests have been added, including alanine aminotransferase, anti-hepatitis B core antibody, anti-human immunodeficiency virus (anti-HIV), anti-human T-cell leukemia virus, anti-hepatitis C antibody, and anti-HIV-2. Screening for antibodies against homologous blood for antibodies against cytomegalovirus is not routinely done. However, patients who are immunocompromised should be transfused with blood which is seronegative for CMV. Other patients who should receive cytomegalovirus seronegative blood include pre-term and newborn babies. Human T-cell leukemia virus type I can be transmitted through homologous blood transfusions and recently has been associated with human or adult T-cell leukemia and progressive myelopathy. In general, there is a very small risk of human T-cell leukemia virus from transfused blood in blood products that have been screened for antibodies against human immunodeficiency virus *(Miller: Anesthesia, ed 4, pp 1636-1637).*

409. **(A)** The incidence of hemolytic transfusion reaction is in the range of 1:4,000 to 1:6,000. The incidence of a fatal hemolytic transfusion reaction is approximately 1:100,000. Intravascular hemolysis is one of the most catastrophic events arising from hemolytic transfusion reactions. This occurs when there is a direct attack on transfused donor red blood cells by the recipient's immune system. When such a reaction occurs, 20 to 60 percent of those patients with severe symptoms (e.g., as a result from ABO blood group incompatibility) will die. Under general anesthesia, the only signs of a hemolytic transfusion reaction may be hemoglobinuria, bleeding diathesis, or intractable hypotension. The first step in treating a hemolytic transfusion reaction is to stop the transfusion. The primary emphasis of therapy should be directed toward maintaining the urine output by generous administration of intravascular fluids and diuretics. Alkalinization of the urine by administration of sodium bicarbonate may prevent precipitation of acidic hematin in the distal tubules, improving urine output. Additionally, the administration of mannitol or a more potent diuretic such as furosemide may be useful by increasing blood flow to the renal cortex. Platelet count, partial thromboplastin time, and serum fibrinogen level

should be determined since disseminated intravascular coagulation may occur *(Miller: Anesthesia, ed 4, pp 1633-1635)*.

410. **(A)**   Except for albumin, each of the blood products listed in this question has the potential to be infective. Coagulation factors and blood group antibodies are not present in albumin since it is obtained by fractionating human plasma that is nonreactive for hepatitis B service antigen. Additionally, albumin is heated for 10 hours at 60°C thereby removing the hazard of viral hepatitis *(Stoelting: Pharmacology and Physiology in Anesthetic Practice, ed 2, pp 574 & 575)*.

411. **(A)**   A hemolytic transfusion reaction occurs when specific antibodies in the plasma of the recipient bind to specific antigens on the cell membrane of the donor erythrocytes, causing intravascular hemolysis, activation of the complement system, and increased capillary permeability. The classic signs of a hemolytic transfusion reaction in patients undergoing general anesthesia include hypotension, oozing, and hemoglobinuria. Fever is masked by general anesthesia and is therefore not a reliable sign. Precipitation of stromal and lipid contents of hemolyzed erythrocytes in the distal renal tubules, decreased renal cortical blood flow (due to histamine-induced vasomotor changes), and deposition of fibrin in the microcirculation are the predominant factors that contribute to renal dysfunction in these patients. The severity of the hemolytic transfusion reaction is directly proportional to the amount of incompatible blood transfused into the recipient. Therefore, the initial treatment of acute hemolytic transfusion reactions is discontinuation of the transfusion. To maintain renal function, urine output should be increased by liberal intravenous infusion of crystalloid solution and by the administration of mannitol or furosemide. The efficacy of alkalinization of the urine to prevent deposition of foreign material in the distal renal tubules has not been determined *(Stoelting: Basics of Anesthesia, ed 3, p 242; Stoelting: Anesthesia and Co-existing Disease, ed 3, p 422)*.

412. **(D)**   Five percent dextrose in water causes hemolysis when mixed with blood in a 1:1 ratio. Lactated ringers solution contains calcium and therefore may cause clotting when mixed with blood in a 1:1 ratio *(Miller: Anesthesia, ed 4, pp 1639 & 1640)*.

413. **(E)**   In the adult, total body water is approximately 60% of the total body weight. Of this, approximately two-thirds is located in the intracellular space (40% of the total body weight) and one-third is located in the extracellular space (20% of total body weight). Plasma volume comprises approximately 7% to 8% of the total body weight in adults *(Barash: Clinical Anesthesia, ed 2, pp 203 & 204)*.

414. **(B)**   Von Willebrand's disease is a deficiency of von Willebrand's factor, a protein that is important for adequate factor VIII activity and platelet function. This disease is transmitted as an autosomal dominant trait. Thus, unlike hemophilia A, it affects both sexes. Hemorrhagic diathesis associated with this disease can be readily corrected by administration of cryoprecipitate, which contains both factor VIII and von Willebrand's factor. The synthetic analogue of antidiuretic hormone, desmopressin (DDAVP), causes the release of von Willebrand's factor and is therefore also effective in treating bleeding in these patients. Factor VIII concentrates alone are not effective therapy for von Willebrand's disease *(Stoelting: Anesthesia and Co-existing Disease, ed 3, pp 412 & 413)*.

415. **(C)** Crossmatch for compatibility of recipient and donor erythrocytes and plasma is performed in three phases. This process can be thought of as a "trial transfusion" in which donor erythrocytes are mixed with recipient serum. The first phase occurs at room temperature and detects ABO, MN, P, and Lewis antigen incompatibilities. The second phase involves incubation of the donor erythrocytes in albumin for 30 to 45 minutes at 37°C and detects Rh antigen incompatibilities. The third phase involves the indirect antiglobulin test which detects incompatibilities to the Kidd, Duffy and Kell antigens *(Miller: Anesthesia, ed 4, pp 1620 & 1621)*.

416. **(B)** 417. **(C)** The only compound which can increase the storage life of packed erythrocytes to 42 days is ADSOL (adenine-glucose-mannitol-sodium chloride) *(Miller: Anesthesia, ed 4, p 1623)*.

General Anesthesia

DIRECTIONS (Questions 418 through 507): Each of the questions or incomplete statements in this section is followed by answers or by completions of the statement, respectively. Select the ONE BEST answer or completion for each item.

418. A 78-year-old patient with a history of hypertension and adult onset diabetes for which she takes chlorpropamide (Diabinase) is admitted for elective cholecystectomy. On the day of admission, blood glucose is noted to be 270 mg/dL and the patient is treated with 15 units of regular insulin SQ in addition to her regular dose of chlorpropamide. Twenty-four hours later after overnight fasting, the patient is brought to the OR without her daily dose of chlorpropamide and is anesthetized. A serum glucose is measured and found to be 35 mg/dL. The most likely explanation for this is

  A. Insulin
  B. Chlorpropamide
  C. Hypovolemia
  D. Effect of general anesthesia
  E. It is a normal finding in fasting patients

419. Select the true statement.

  A. Dibucaine is an ester-type local anesthetic
  B. A dibucaine number of 20 is normal
  C. The dibucaine number represents the quantity of normal pseudocholinesterase
  D. Neuromuscular blockade with succinylcholine would last several hours in a patient with a dibucaine number of 80
  E. None of the above

420. A 56-year-old patient with a history of liver disease and osteomyelitis is anesthetized for tibial debridement. After induction and intubation the wound is inspected and debrided with a total blood loss of 300 ml. The patient is transported intubated to the recovery room at which time the systolic blood pressure falls to 50 mm Hg. Heart rate is 120/minute, arterial blood gases are P_aO_2 103, P_aCO_2 45, pH 7.3 with a 97% O_2 saturation with 100% F_IO_2. Mixed venous blood gases are: P_vO_2 60, P_vCO_2 50, pH 7.25, with 90% O_2 saturation. Which of the following diagnoses is most consistent with this clinical picture.

  A. Myocardial infarction
  B. Congestive heart failure
  C. Cardiac tamponade
  D. Sepsis with ARDS
  E. Hypovolemia

421. Normal tracheal capillary pressure is

  A. 12 mm Hg
  B. 23 mm Hg
  C. 32 mm Hg
  D. 41 mm Hg
  E. 53 mm Hg

422. What percent of asymptomatic patients younger than 40 years will have positive findings on a preoperative screening chest x-ray?

    A. <1.5%
    B. 2% to 5%
    C. 5% to 10%
    D. 10% to 15%
    E. >15%

423. Which of the following peripheral nerves is most likely to become injured in patients who are under general anesthesia?

    A. Ulnar nerve
    B. Median nerve
    C. Radial nerve
    D. Common peroneal nerve
    E. Sciatic and peroneal nerve

424. Renal failure associated with fluoride toxicity anesthesia most closely resembles

    A. Papillary necrosis
    B. Acute tubule necrosis
    C. Hepatorenal syndrome
    D. Central diabetes insipidus
    E. Nephrogenic diabetes insipidus

425. A 45-year-old obese male is in the intensive care unit after an elective open lung biopsy. Which of the following would provide the best prophylaxis against deep-vein thrombosis in this patient?

    A. Pneumatic compression boots
    B. Heparin, 5,000 units subcutaneously every 8 hours
    C. Early ambulation
    D. Dextran, 10 mL/kg IV during surgery
    E. Incentive spirometry

426. A patient with which of the following eye diseases would be at greatest risk for retinal damage from hypotension during surgery?

    A. Strabismus
    B. Cataract
    C. Glaucoma
    D. Severe myopia
    E. Open eye injury

427. Naltrexone is

    A. A narcotic with local anesthetic properties
    B. An opioid agonist-antagonist similar to nalbuphine
    C. A pure opioid antagonist with a shorter duration of action than naloxone
    D. An opioid antagonist used in the treatment of previously detoxified heroin addicts
    E. A synthetic opioid derived from oxymorphone

428. Which of the following mechanisms is most frequently responsible for hypoxia in the recovery room?

    A. Ventilation/perfusion mismatch
    B. Hypoventilation
    C. Hypoxic gas mixture
    D. Intracardiac shunt
    E. Abnormal gas diffusion

429. Hypoparathyroidism secondary to inadvertent surgical resection of the parathyroid glands during total thyroidectomy usually results in symptoms of hypocalcemia within

    A. 1 to 2 hours
    B. 3 to 12 hours
    C. 12 to 24 hours
    D. 24 to 72 hours
    E. greater than 72 hours

430. Damage to which nerve may lead to wrist drop?

    A. Radial
    B. Axillary
    C. Median
    D. Musculocutaneous
    E. Ulnar

431. The most common cause of bronchiectasis is

    A. Cigarette smoking
    B. Air pollution
    C. α_1-antitrypsin deficiency
    D. Recurrent bronchial infections
    E. Squamous cell carcinoma

432. A 6-year-old child is transported to the recovery room after a tonsillectomy. The patient was anesthetized with isoflurane, fentanyl, and N_2O. Twenty minutes prior to emergence and tracheal extubation, droperidol was administered. The anesthesiologist is called to the recovery room because the patient is "making strange eye movements." The patient's eyes are rolled back into his head and his neck is twisted and rigid. The most appropriate drug for treatment of these symptoms is

    A. Dantrolene
    B. Thiopental
    C. Glycopyrrolate
    D. Chlorpromazine
    E. Diphenhydramine

433. A 32-year-old military officer is unable to oppose the left thumb and left little finger after an 8-hour exploratory laparotomy under general anesthesia. Damage to which of the following nerves would most likely account for this deficit?

    A. Radial
    B. Ulnar
    C. Median
    D. Musculocutaneous
    E. Median antebrachial cutaneous nerve

434. A 73-year-old obese patient is anesthetized for a radical mastectomy. The patient has a 200-pack-year history of cigarette smoking. After anesthetic induction and tracheal intubation, bilateral breath sounds are noted. The peak airway pressure, however, is 40 cm H_2O. The operation is performed uneventfully. The trachea is extubated and the patient is taken to the recovery room where she complains of difficulty breathing. Chest x-ray is remarkable only for changes consistent with chronic obstructive pulmonary disease (COPD). Breath sounds are present and equal on both sides. After a nebulizer treatment with albuterol, she states that breathing is less difficult. The following ABGs are noted on 100% O_2 by facemask: P_aO_2 80 mm Hg, pCO_2 65, pH 7.25, HCO_3^- 23. The most appropriate treatment for this patient is

    A. Intubate and mechanically ventilate
    B. D/C supplemental O_2
    C. Administer sodium bicarbonate
    D. Place a chest tube
    E. Titrate F_IO_2 down

435. The plasma concentration of which of the following liver enzymes is increased in patients with biliary obstruction?

    A. Serum glutamic-oxaloacetic transaminase
    B. Serum glutamic-pyruvic transaminase
    C. Lactate dehydrogenase
    D. Alkaline phosphatase
    E. Alcoholic dehydrogenase

436. The onset of delirium tremens following abstinence from alcohol usually occurs in

    A. <24 hours
    B. 2 to 3 days
    C. 3 to 4 days
    D. 4 to 7 days
    E. >7 days

437. A 78-year-old retired coal miner with an intraluminal tracheal tumor is scheduled for tracheal resection. Which of the following is a relative contraindication for tracheal resection?

    A. Need for postoperative mechanical ventilation
    B. Tumor located at the carina
    C. Documented liver metastases
    D. Ischemic heart disease with a history of congestive heart failure
    E. Tracheal diameter of 0.5 cm at the level of the tumor

438. A 78-year-old patient with multiple myeloma is admitted to the intensive care unit for treatment of hypercalcemia. The primary risk associated with anesthetizing patients with hypercalcemia is

    A. Coagulopathy
    B. Cardiac dysrhythmias
    C. Hypotension
    D. Laryngospasm
    E. Fluid imbalance

439. What is the mortality rate for patients with a previous myocardial infarction who have a perioperative myocardial infarction during a subsequent operation?

    A. 5% to 10%
    B. 15% to 20%
    C. 25% to 40%
    D. 50% to 70%
    E. 75% to 95%

440. Patients with a history of previous myocardial infarction would have the greatest risk of mortality should they undergo an operation involving the

    A. Coronary arteries
    B. Great vessels
    C. Abdomen
    D. Lungs
    E. Left ventricle

441. A 62-year-old male undergoes an emergency craniotomy for subdural hematoma. Two years earlier a VVI pacemaker was inserted for third-degree heart block. The patient received vancomycin, 1 g IV, prior to arriving in the operating room. General anesthesia is induced with thiopental, 300 mg IV and the lungs are hyperventilated to a P_aCO_2 of 25 mm Hg by mask. Just prior to tracheal intubation, the patient's heart rate decreases from 70 to 40 beats/min and the pacemaker spikes previously present in lead II on the electrocardiogram disappear. The most likely cause of bradycardia in this patient is

    A. Hypocarbia
    B. Vancomycin allergy
    C. Acute increase in intracranial pressure
    D. A side effect of thiopental
    E. Pacemaker battery failure

442. A 28-year-old obese patient has diminished breath sounds bilaterally at the lung bases 18 hours after an emergency appendectomy under general anesthesia. Which of the following maneuvers would be **LEAST** effective in preventing postoperative pulmonary complications in this patient?

    A. Coughing
    B. Voluntary deep breathing
    C. Performing a forced vital capacity
    D. Use of incentive spirometry
    E. Sitting up in bed

443. Below what value of cerebral blood flow will signs of cerebral ischemia first begin to appear on the EEG?

    A. 6 mL/100 g/min
    B. 15 mL/100 g/min
    C. 22 mL/100 g/min
    D. 31 mL/100 g/min
    E. 40 mL/100 g/min

444. A 67-year-old patient is mechanically ventilated in the intensive care unit two days after repair of a ruptured abdominal aortic aneurysm. Ten cm H_2O PEEP is added to the ventilator cycle to maintain the P_aO_2 in the 60-65 range. The patient's blood pressure has averaged 110/65 prior to the addition of PEEP. After the addition of PEEP, the blood pressure is noted to slowly fall to an average of approximately 95/50. The best explanation for this decrease in blood pressure is:

    A. Tension pneumothorax
    B. Decreased venous return to the heart
    C. Increased afterload on the right side of the heart
    D. Increased afterload on the left side of the heart
    E. Decreased cardiac output from global myocardial ischemia

445. A 64-year-old male undergoes an elective cholecystectomy. Other than essential hypertension, for which he takes propranolol, he is in good health. The patient is anesthetized with isoflurane, N_2O, and fentanyl, and paralyzed with d-tubocurarine. At the end of the operation neuromuscular blockade is antagonized with pyridostigmine and atropine, the trachea is suctioned, and the patient is extubated and taken to the recovery room. Oxymorphone is administered IV for analgesia. One hour after arrival in the recovery room, the patient's heart rate decreases from 70 to 40 beats/min. Which of the following would most likely account for bradycardia in this patient?

    A. Recurarization
    B. Oxymorphone
    C. Pyridostigmine
    D. Propranolol
    E. Paradoxical effect of atropine

446. Which of the following is most closely associated with MAC?

    A. Blood:gas partition coefficient
    B. Oil:gas partition coefficient
    C. Vapor pressure
    D. Brain:blood partition coefficient
    E. Molecular weight

447. A 15-year-old, 65-kg patient with Cushing's disease is to undergo a hypophysectomy to remove a pituitary adenoma. General anesthesia is induced with thiopental IV and tracheal intubation was facilitated with vecuronium, 0.25 mg/kg IV. Anesthesia is maintained with enflurane and N$_2$O. Mannitol, 1 gm/kg, is administered IV to reduce intracranial pressure. At the end of the operation the patient is extubated and taken to the intensive care unit. Over the next 6 hours the patient has a total urine output of 8.3 L. Serum sodium concentration is 154 mEq/L, serum potassium concentration is 4.8 mEq/L, and serum glucose concentration is 160 mg/dL. Urine specific gravity is 1.003 and urine osmolality is 125 mOsm/L. The most likely cause of the large urine output is

    A. Osmotic diuresis from mannitol
    B. Excess mineralocorticoid activity
    C. Hyperglycemia
    D. Nephrogenic diabetes insipidus
    E. Central diabetes insipidus

448. Scopolamine should be avoided as a premedication in patients with which of the following neurologic diseases?

    A. Parkinson's disease
    B. Alzheimer's disease
    C. Multiple sclerosis
    D. Narcolepsy
    E. Amyotrophic lateral sclerosis

449. A 63-year-old male patient is scheduled to undergo a right hemicolectomy under general anesthesia. Anesthesia is induced with thiopental, 4 mg/kg IV, and fentanyl, 100 µg IV. Succinylcholine, 1.5 mg/kg IV is administered to facilitate tracheal intubation. Anesthesia is maintained with enflurane and N$_2$O. After all four twitches of the train-of-four stimulus have returned to baseline values, pancuronium, 5 mg IV is administered. Gentamicin, 80 mg, and cefazolin, 1 gm, are administered IV as a prophylactic treatment. At the end of surgery two of four thumb twitches can be elicited to train-of-four stimulation of the ulnar nerve and neuromuscular blockade is antagonized with neostigmine, 0.05 mg/kg IV, and atropine, 0.015 mg/kg IV. The patient, however, begins to move before the incision is completely closed and succinylcholine, 20 mg IV, is given. Fifteen minutes later all anesthetics are discontinued and the patient is ventilated with 100% O$_2$, but the patient remains apneic. The most likely cause of apnea is

    A. Fentanyl
    B. Recurarization
    C. Succinylcholine
    D. Thiopental
    E. Gentamicin

450. A 53-year-old female with endometrial cancer is undergoing an abdominal hysterectomy under general anesthesia with enflurane. During the first hour of anesthesia, the urine output is 100 mL. Blood loss is minimal. When the patient is placed in the Trendelenburg position, the urine output declines to virtually zero. The most likely explanation for this sudden decrease in urine output in this patient is

    A. Pooling of urine in the dome of the bladder
    B. Kinking of the urinary catheter
    C. Fluoride toxicity from enflurane
    D. Increased ADH production from surgical stimulation
    E. Hypovolemia

451. Which of the following tests obtained preoperatively is most predictive of pulmonary hypertension?

    A. FEV_1/FVC ratio
    B. Maximum breathing capacity
    C. Arterial blood gases
    D. DL_{CO}
    E. FEF_{25-75}

452. Each of the following postoperative complications of thyroid surgery can result in upper airway obstruction **EXCEPT**

    A. Tracheomalacia
    B. Tetany
    C. Cervical hematoma
    D. Bilateral recurrent laryngeal nerve injury
    E. Bilateral superior laryngeal nerve injury

453. The most sensitive early sign of malignant hyperthermia during general anesthesia is

    A. Tachycardia
    B. Hypertension
    C. Fever
    D. Hypoxia
    E. Increased end-expiratory CO_2 tension (P_ECO_2)

454. A 78-year-old female is anesthetized for a right hemicolectomy for 3 hours. At the end of the operation the patient's blood pressure is 130/85 mm Hg, heart rate is 84 beats/min, core body temperature is 35.4°C, and P_ECO_2 on the mass spectrometer is 38 mm Hg. Which of the following would be the least plausible reason for prolonged apnea in this patient?

    A. Residual neuromuscular blockade
    B. Narcotic overdose
    C. Cerebral hemorrhage
    D. Unrecognized obstructive pulmonary disease and high baseline P_aCO_2
    E. Persistent intraoperative hyperventilation

455. A 68-year-old woman with severe rheumatoid arthritis undergoes pulmonary function evaluation prior to a total knee arthroplasty. The FEV_1 and FVC are within normal limits; however, the MVV is only 40% of predicted. The next step in the pulmonary function evaluation of this patient should be to

   A. Obtain arterial blood gases on room air
   B. Obtain a flow-volume loop
   C. Obtain a measurement of peak flow
   D. Obtain a ventilation/perfusion scan
   E. Assume, in the face of normal FEV_1, poor effort on the part of the patient and proceed

456. A 29-year-old male is admitted to the intensive care unit after a drug overdose. The patient is placed on a ventilator with a set tidal volume of 750 ml at a rate of 10. The patient is making no inspiratory effort whatsoever. The measured minute ventilation is 6 L and the peak airway pressure is 30 cm H_2O. What is the compression factor for this ventilator delivery circuit?

   A. 1 ml $(cm\ H_2O)^{-1}$
   B. 2 ml $(cm\ H_2O)^{-1}$
   C. 3 ml $(cm\ H_2O)^{-1}$
   D. 4 ml $(cm\ H_2O)^{-1}$
   E. 5 ml $(cm\ H_2O)^{-1}$

457. During emergency repair of a mandibular jaw fracture in an otherwise healthy 19-year-old male the patient's temperature is noted to rise from 37°C on induction to 38°C after 2 hours of surgery. Which of the following informational items would be **LEAST** useful in ruling out malignant hyperthermia in this patient:

   A. Normal heart rate and blood pressure
   B. History of negative caffeine-halothane contracture test carried out six months earlier
   C. History of a uncomplicated general anesthetic at age 16 with halothane and succinylcholine
   D. Normal arterial blood gases drawn when the patient's temperature reached 38°C
   E. No increase in respiration rate while spontaneous breathing

458. An oximetric pulmonary artery catheter is placed in a 69-year-old male patient who is undergoing surgical resection of an abdominal aortic aneurysm under general anesthesia. Before the aortic cross-clamp is placed, the mixed venous O_2 saturation decreases from 75% to 60%. Each of the following could account for the fall in mixed venous O_2 saturation **EXCEPT**

   A. Hypovolemia
   B. Bleeding
   C. Hypoxia
   D. Sepsis
   E. Congestive heart failure

459. A 68-year-old, 100-kg patient is undergoing a transurethral resection of the prostate gland under general anesthesia. In the recovery room the serum [Na$^+$] is 115 mEq/L. How much 5% saline should be administered to this patient to raise the serum [Na$^+$] to 125 mEq/L?

   A. 300 mL
   B. 400 mL
   C. 500 mL
   D. 600 mL
   E. 700 mL

460. Trismus after administration of succinylcholine IV signals the onset of malignant hyperthermia in what percent of patients?

   A. <50
   B. 50
   C. 75
   D. 80
   E. >80

461. A 45-year-old male is brought to the operating room emergently for repair of a ruptured abdominal aortic aneurysm. The patient is pretreated with 3 mg of d-tubocurarine, anesthesia is induced with ketamine, 2 mg/kg IV, and tracheal intubation is facilitated with succinylcholine, 1.5 mg/kg IV. Immediately following tracheal intubation the patient's blood pressure falls from 110/80 mm Hg to 50/20 mm Hg. What is the most likely cause of severe hypotension in this patient?

   A. Hypovolemia
   B. Direct myocardial depression from ketamine
   C. Vasovagal response to direct laryngoscopy
   D. Arteriolar vasodilation from succinylcholine-mediated histamine release
   E. Ganglionic blockade from d-tubocurarine

462. Malignant hyperthermia is believed to involve a generalized disorder of membrane permeability to

   A. Sodium
   B. Potassium
   C. Calcium
   D. Magnesium
   E. Phosphate

463. A 25-year-old male with a history of testicular cancer is scheduled to undergo an exploratory laparotomy under general anesthesia. He has received bleomycin for metastatic disease. Which of the following is an important consideration concerning the pulmonary toxicity of bleomycin?

   A. N$_2$O should not be used
   B. Preoperative pulmonary function tests should be obtained
   C. The patient should be ventilated at a slow rate and I:E ratio of 1:3
   D. Aminophylline should be started preoperatively
   E. The F$_I$O$_2$ should be less than 0.3

464. A 39-year-old obese female undergoes an abdominal hysterectomy under general anesthesia. Induction of anesthesia is uneventful. The S_aO_2 is 98% during the first 15 minutes of the operation. However, when her head is flexed and she is placed in the Trendelenburg position to improve surgical exposure, the S_aO_2 falls to 90%. The most likely explanation for this desaturation is

A. Diffusion hypoxia
B. Decreased functional residual capacity
C. Mainstem intubation
D. Decreased cardiac output
E. Venous air embolism

465. How long after intravitreal injection of sulfur hexafluoride and air can N_2O be used without risk of increasing intraocular pressure?

A. 1 hour
B. 24 hours
C. 10 days
D. 1 month
E. Never

466. A 54-year-old female is undergoing a total thyroidectomy under general anesthesia. The patient is awakened in the operating room, the mouth and pharynx are suctioned, and after intact laryngeal reflexes are demonstrated, the endotracheal tube is removed. Two days later the anesthesiologist is consulted because the patient has severe stridor and upper airway obstruction. The most likely cause of airway obstruction in this patient is

A. Damage to the recurrent laryngeal nerve
B. Damage to the superior laryngeal nerve
C. Tracheomalacia
D. Hypocalcemia
E. Hematoma

467. A 27-year-old obese woman is scheduled to undergo foot surgery under general anesthesia. She underwent a subtotal thyroidectomy 3 years ago and takes levothyroxine (Synthroid). Which of the following laboratory tests would be the most useful in evaluating whether this patient is euthyroid?

A. Total plasma thyroxine (T_4)
B. Total plasma triiodothyronine (T_3)
C. Thyroid-stimulating hormone (TSH)
D. Resin triiodothyronine uptake
E. Radioactive iodine uptake

468. An 85-year-old black male with no previous medical history except for cataracts is undergoing a transurethral resection of the prostate gland under spinal anesthesia. Twenty minutes into the procedure the patient becomes restless. Over the next 20 minutes his blood pressure increases from 110/70 mm Hg to 140/90 mm Hg and his heart rate slows from 90 to 50 beats/min. The patient is also noted to have some difficulty breathing. The most likely cause of these symptoms in this patient is

A. Volume overload
B. Hyponatremia
C. High spinal
D. Bladder perforation
E. Autonomic hyperreflexia

469. A 17-year-old patient with third degree burns over 25% of his body is scheduled for debridement and skin grafting 12 days after sustaining a thermal injury. Select the true statement regarding the use of depolarizing and nondepolarizing muscle relaxants in this patient compared with normal patients.

A. Sensitivity to both depolarizing and nondepolarizing muscle relaxants is increased
B. Sensitivity to both depolarizing and nondepolarizing muscle relaxants is decreased
C. Sensitivity to depolarizing muscle relaxants is increased while sensitivity to nondepolarizing muscle relaxants is decreased
D. Sensitivity to depolarizing muscle relaxants is decreased while sensitivity to nondepolarizing muscle relaxants is increased
E. Sensitivity to nondepolarizing is unchanged while sensitivity to depolarizing muscle relaxants is increased

470. A 72-year-old male is brought to the intensive care unit after elective repair of an abdominal aortic aneurysm. His vital signs are stable, but he requires a sodium nitroprusside infusion at a rate of 5 µg/kg/min to keep the systolic blood pressure below 140 mm Hg. The S_aO_2 is 98% with controlled ventilation at 12 breaths/min and an F_IO_2 of 0.60. After 2 days his S_aO_2 falls to 85% on the pulse oximeter. Chest x-ray and physical examination are normal. Which of the following would most likely account for this desaturation?

A. Cyanide toxicity
B. Thiocyanate toxicity
C. O_2 toxicity
D. Thiosulfate toxicity
E. Methemoglobinemia

471. A 65-year-old patient with a history of chronic obstructive pulmonary disease and coronary artery disease undergoes an appendectomy uneventfully under general anesthesia. In the recovery room, arterial blood gases are as follows: P_aO_2 60 mm Hg, P_aCO_2, 50 mm Hg, pH 7.35, and hemoglobin 8.1 g/dL. Which of the following steps would produce the greatest increase in O_2 delivery to the myocardium?

A. Administration of 100% O_2 with a close-fitting mask
B. Administration of 35% O_2 with a Venturi mask
C. Withhold narcotics
D. Transfuse with 2 units of packed RBCs
E. Administer 1 ampule of HCO_3^-

472. Which of the following lung parameters is the most important from the standpoint of postoperative pulmonary complications?

    A. Tidal volume
    B. Inspiratory reserve volume
    C. Vital capacity
    D. Functional residual capacity
    E. Inspiratory capacity

473. Succinylcholine should be avoided in patients with Huntington's chorea because

    A. They are at increased risk for malignant hyperthermia
    B. Potassium release may be excessive
    C. They may have a decreased concentration of pseudocholinesterase
    D. There may be adverse interactions between succinylcholine and phenothiazine
    E. Succinylcholine increases intracranial pressure

474. An 83-year-old woman is admitted to the ICU after coronary artery surgery. A pulmonary artery catheter is in place and yields the following data: central venous pressure (CVP) 5 mm Hg, cardiac output 4.0 L/min, mean arterial pressure 90 mm Hg, mean pulmonary artery pressure 20 mm Hg, pulmonary artery occlusion pressure 12 mm Hg and heart rate 90. Calculate this patient's pulmonary vascular resistance

    A. 40 dynes-sec-cm^{-5}
    B. 80 dynes-sec-cm^{-5}
    C. 160 dynes-sec-cm^{-5}
    D. 200 dynes-sec-cm^{-5}
    E. 240 dynes-sec-cm^{-5}

475. The fact that high atmospheric pressure partially antagonizes volatile anesthetics supports which theory of anesthesia?

    A. Inhibition of gamma-aminobutyric acid (GABA) breakdown hypothesis
    B. Increased endorphin production hypothesis
    C. Inhibition of neural transmission via dorsal root ganglia
    D. Protein receptor hypothesis
    E. Critical-volume hypothesis

476. Which of the following preoperative pulmonary function tests is **NOT** associated with an increased operative risk for pneumonectomy?

    A. FEV_1 < 50% of the FVC
    B. FEV_1 < 2 L
    C. Maximum breathing capacity < 50% of predicted
    D. Residual volume/total lung capacity < 50%
    E. Hypercarbia on room air arterial blood gases

477. A 26-year-old male patient is undergoing an emergency exploratory laparotomy under general anesthesia with enflurane. The S_aO_2 is 89% on the pulse oximeter. The P_aO_2 on arterial blood gases is 77 mm Hg. The patient's core body temperature is 35°C. What is the corrected P_aO_2?

    A. 68 mm Hg
    B. 72 mm Hg
    C. 77 mm Hg
    D. 86 mm Hg
    E. 92 mm Hg

478. A 27-year-old patient with a 10-year history of Crohn's disease is scheduled to undergo drainage of a rectal abscess under general anesthesia. His preoperative medications include prednisone, sulfasalazine, and cyanocobalamin. He has no known allergies and is otherwise healthy. Prior to induction of anesthesia the pulse oximeter shows an S_aO_2 of 89%, which does not increase after administration of 100% O_2 for 2 minutes. Arterial blood gases are as follows: P_aO_2 490 mm Hg, P_aCO_2 32 Hg, pH 7.43, S_aO_2 89%. The most likely cause of these findings is

    A. The presence of sulfhemoglobin
    B. The presence of methemoglobin
    C. The presence of cyanohemoglobin
    D. The presence of carboxyhemoglobin
    E. Blood gas error

479. The muscle relaxant of choice during resection of a pheochromocytoma is

    A. Mivacurium
    B. Pancuronium
    C. Curare
    D. Metocurine iodide
    E. Vecuronium

480. The most frequently damaged nerve in the lower extremity in anesthetized patients is the

    A. Obturator nerve
    B. Femoral nerve
    C. Anterior tibial nerve
    D. Saphenous nerve
    E. Common peroneal nerve

481. A 72-year-old male patient with a history of myocardial infarction 12 months earlier is scheduled to undergo elective repair of a 6-cm abdominal aortic aneurysm under general anesthesia. When would this patient be most likely to have a reinfarction?

    A. On induction of anesthesia
    B. During placement of the aortic crossclamp
    C. Upon release of the aortic crossclamp
    D. 24 hours postoperatively
    E. On the third postoperative day

482.   A 55-year-old male is to undergo a transurethral resection of the prostate gland under general anes-
       thesia. The patient has a 40-pack-year smoking history and a history of congestive heart failure. The
       patient receives metoclopramide and scopolamine preoperatively. General anesthesia is induced with
       ketamine and the patient undergoes the procedure uneventfully. However, in the recovery room the
       patient complains of not being able to see objects "up close". Which of the following would be the
       most likely cause of this complaint?

       A.   Emergence delirium from ketamine anesthesia
       B.   Effect of scopolamine
       C.   Effect of glycine in the irrigating solution
       D.   Corneal abrasion
       E.   Hyponatremia

483.   Malignant hyperthermia and neuroleptic malignant syndrome share each of the following characteris-
       tics **EXCEPT**

       A.   Generalized muscular rigidity
       B.   Hyperthermia
       C.   Effectively treated with dantrolene
       D.   Tachycardia
       E.   Flaccid paralysis following administration of pancuronium

484.   A 23-year-old male involved in a motor vehicle accident is brought to the operating room for open
       reduction and internal fixation of multiple fractures under general anesthesia. During the surgery, the
       patient is transfused with 7 units of type AB, Rh-negative packed RBCs and 3 units of platelets. At
       the end of the procedure the endotracheal tube is removed and the patient taken to the intensive care
       unit. Several hours later the patient complains of shortness of breath. His temperature is 38°C, heart
       rate is 146 beats/min, blood pressure is 105/69 mm Hg, and respiratory rate is 36 breaths/min. In addi-
       tion, the patient is noted to have a fine petechial rash on his arms and shoulders. Which of the fol-
       lowing is the most likely cause of these signs and symptoms?

       A.   Pulmonary embolism
       B.   Transfusion reaction from packed RBCs
       C.   Transfusion reaction from platelets
       D.   Fat embolism
       E.   Sepsis

485.   An 83-year-old, 100-kg patient with a serum sodium of 140 mEq/L undergoes a transurethral resec-
       tion of the prostate gland under spinal anesthesia. At the end of the operation serum [Na^+] is 105
       mEq/L. What is the total excess of free water in this patient?

       A.   5 L
       B.   10 L
       C.   15 L
       D.   20 L
       E.   25 L

486. A 3-year-old child is brought to the operating room after aspiration of a peanut. The patient is anesthetized, the trachea is intubated, and the lungs are mechanically ventilated. The peanut is extracted through a rigid bronchoscope but is then lost in the upper airway. The anesthesiologist notes that he can no longer ventilate the patient's lungs. What should be the next step in the management of this problem?

    A. Needle cricothyroidotomy
    B. Emergency tracheotomy
    C. Placement of a chest tube
    D. Pushing the peanut more distally
    E. Attempting jet ventilation

487. Patients who undergo extracorporeal shock-wave lithotripsy are at increased risk for

    A. Venous air embolism
    B. Pneumothorax
    C. Peripheral neuropathies
    D. Postdural puncture headache
    E. Hypotension with regional anesthesia

488. The most common reason for admitting outpatients to the hospital following general anesthesia is

    A. Hypotension
    B. Respiratory complications
    C. Inability to ambulate
    D. Surgical pain
    E. Nausea and vomiting

489. A 37-year-old male with myasthenia gravis arrives in the emergency room confused and agitated after a 2-day history of weakness and increased difficulty breathing. Arterial blood gases on room air are: P_aO_2 60 mm Hg, P_aCO_2 51 mm Hg, HCO_3^- 25 mEq/L, pH 7.3, S_aO_2 of 90%. His respiratory rate is 30 breaths/min and V_T is 4 mL/kg. After administration of edrophonium, 5 mg IV, his V_T declines to 2 mL/kg. What should be the most appropriate step in the management of this patient at this time?

    A. Tracheal intubation and mechanical ventilation
    B. Repeat the test dose of edrophonium
    C. Administer neostigmine, 1 mg IV
    D. Administer atropine, 0.4 mg IV
    E. Emergency tracheostomy and mechanical ventilation

490. A 3-year-old child is scheduled to undergo a voiding cystourethrogram. Which of the following agents is least likely to interfere with urodynamic studies?

    A. Atropine
    B. Diazepam
    C. Morphine
    D. Thiopental
    E. N_2O

491. Which of the following patients would not be a good candidate for outpatient inguinal hernia repair under general anesthesia?

    A. A 62-year-old pharmacist who lives 10 miles away
    B. A 20-year-old healthy college student who had a renal transplant 3 years earlier
    C. A 38-year-old housewife with a hiatal hernia
    D. A premature infant that is 43 weeks postconceptual age
    E. A 29-year-old diabetic that is well controlled on insulin

492. A 72-year-old male undergoes emergency repair of an abdominal aortic aneurysm. In the first hour after release of the suprarenal crossclamp urine output is only 10 mL. After administration of furosemide, 20 mg IV, urine output increases to 100 mL/hr. Urine [Na^+] is 43 mEq/L and urine osmolality is 210 mOsm/L. The most likely cause of the initial oliguria is

    A. Fluoride toxicity
    B. Renal hypoperfusion
    C. Acute tubular necrosis
    D. Increased ADH
    E. Impossible to differentiate

493. Which of the following is not associated with an increased incidence of postoperative pulmonary complications in patients with normal pulmonary function?

    A. Obesity
    B. History of cigarette smoking
    C. Operation in the upper abdomen
    D. Age of 68 years
    E. S_aO_2 of 87% in the recovery room on room air 30 minutes after surgery

494. A 58-year-old male is undergoing a left inguinal hernia repair under general anesthesia in San Diego, California. N_2O is administered at 3 L/min, O_2 at 1 L/min, and isoflurane at 0.85%. What minimum alveolar concentration (MAC) is this patient receiving?

    A. 0.8
    B. 1.25
    C. 1.50
    D. 1.75
    E. 2.0

495. An otherwise healthy 140-kg, 24-year-old male is scheduled for thyroid surgery under general anesthesia. Which of the following statements concerning his cardiac output at 140 kg compared to his cardiac output at his ideal body weight (70 kg) is correct?

    A. Cardiac output is diminished by factor of 2
    B. Cardiac output is diminished by 10%
    C. Cardiac output is the same
    D. Cardiac output is increased by 10%
    E. Cardiac output is doubled

496. Potential complications associated with total parenteral nutrition (TPN) include all of the following **EXCEPT**

    A. Ketoacidosis
    B. Hyperglycemia
    C. Hypoglycemia
    D. Hypophosphatemia
    E. Increased work of breathing

497. A 58-year-old hemophiliac is scheduled for total knee arthroplasty. His factor VIII levels are shown to be 35% of normal. Which of the following would be the most appropriate therapy prior to surgery?

    A. Administer sufficient cryoprecipitate to raise factor VIII levels to 50% normal
    B. Administer sufficient factor VIII concentrate to raise levels to 50% normal
    C. Transfuse fresh-frozen plasma until factor VIII levels are 100% normal
    D. Administer factor VIII concentrates until levels are 100% normal
    E. None of the above

498. A 16-year-old boy whose maternal uncle has hemophilia A is scheduled for wisdom-tooth extraction. Which test below would be the best screening test for hemophilia A?

    A. Partial thromboplastin time (PTT)
    B. Prothrombin time (PT)
    C. Thrombin time
    D. Platelet count
    E. Bleeding time

499. The reason four twitches are used in the train-of-four to determine degree of neuromuscular blockade versus 5 (or more) is

    A. Additional twitches will exhaust the neurotransmitter regardless of degree of blockade
    B. Four twitches informs the user of the degree of blockade in the useful clinical range, i.e. 75% to 100% blockade
    C. Post-tetanic facilitation will begin to appear after four twitches
    D. Additional twitches may damage the nerve by overstimulation
    E. There would be no additional decrement in twitch height after four twitches

500. A 57-year-old male is undergoing a right hemicolectomy under general anesthesia. The patient has no history of cardiac disease. During the operation 5 mm ST segment elevation is noted in lead II and the patient develops complete heart block. The coronary artery most likely affected is

    A. Circumflex coronary artery
    B. Right coronary artery
    C. Left main coronary artery
    D. Left anterior descending coronary artery
    E. Branch to obtuse margin

501. Each of the following may increase MAC for volatile anesthetics **EXCEPT**

    A. Cocaine
    B. Hyperthyroidism
    C. Monoamine oxidase inhibitor therapy
    D. Tricyclic antidepressants
    E. Hypernatremia

502. A 37-year-old patient with history of manic-depressive illness is scheduled to undergo surgery for removal of an intramedullary rod in the left tibia. Which of the following statements regarding potential untoward effects of lithium therapy is **NOT** true?

    A. Long-term administration may be associated with nephrogenic diabetes insipidus
    B. Administration of succinylcholine to patients treated with lithium may result in hyperkalemia
    C. Long-term therapy may be associated with hypothyroidism
    D. The duration of action of pancuronium may be prolonged
    E. Administration of furosemide may increase plasma lithium concentrations

503. A 32-year-old male is found unconscious by the fire department in a room where he has inhaled 0.1% carbon monoxide for a prolonged period. His respiratory rate is 42 breaths/min, but he is not cyanotic. Carbon monoxide has increased this patient's minute ventilation by which of the following mechanisms?

    A. Shifting the O_2 hemoglobin dissociation curve to the left
    B. Increasing CO_2 production
    C. Causing lactic acidosis
    D. Decreasing P_aO_2
    E. Producing methemoglobin

504. A 75-year-old male patient is scheduled to undergo elective orchiectomy for prostate cancer. The patient has selected spinal anesthesia. What is the minimum dermatomal level that must be achieved to carry out this operation?

    A. T_1
    B. T_4
    C. T_{10}
    D. L_3
    E. S_1

505. A 31-year-old patient has been in the intensive care unit on a ventilator for 24 hours after a motor vehicle accident. The patient does not open his eyes to any stimulus and has no verbal response and no motor response. The Glasgow coma scale corresponding to this patient would be:

    A. 0
    B. 1
    C. 2
    D. 3
    E. 4

506. Hypoglycemia is more likely to occur in the diabetic surgical patient with which of the following diseases?

   A. Renal disease
   B. Rheumatoid arthritis requiring high-dosage prednisone
   C. Chronic obstructive lung disease treated with a terbutaline inhaler and aminophylline
   D. Manic depressive disorder treated with lithium
   E. Congestive heart failure

507. Which of the following is most likely to be associated with a falsely elevated S_aO_2 as measured by pulse oximetry?

   A. Hemoglobin F
   B. Carboxyhemoglobin
   C. Bilirubin
   D. Fluorescein dye
   E. Methylene blue dye

508. The diagram below depicts which mode of ventilation?

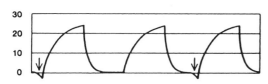

   A. Spontaneous ventilation?
   B. Controlled ventilation
   C. Assisted ventilation
   D. Assisted/controlled ventilation
   E. Synchronized intermittent mandatory ventilation

DIRECTIONS (Questions 509 through 554): For each of the items in this section, ONE or MORE of the number options is correct. Select the answer:

Select A if options *1, 2 and 3* are correct,
Select B if options *1 and 3* are correct,
Select C if options *2 and 4* are correct,
Select D if only option *4* is correct,
Select E if *all* options are correct.

509. A 48-year-old patient with insulin-dependent diabetes mellitus is anesthetized for coronary revascularization. He takes 15 units regular insulin and 20 units NPH insulin daily. Anesthetic implications of this disease include

   1. Reduced heart-rate response to propranolol
   2. Increased incidence of protamine allergy
   3. Reduced heart-rate response to atropine
   4. Increased incidence of hypoglycemia during cardiopulmonary bypass

Select A if options *1, 2 and 3* are correct,
Select B if options *1 and 3* are correct,
Select C if options *2 and 4* are correct,
Select D if only option *4* is correct,
Select E if *all* options are correct.

510. A 67-year-old patient is scheduled to undergo a right hemicolectomy. Knowledge of which of the following would prompt the administration of prophylactic antibiotics?

    1. Presence of ventricular septal defect
    2. Mitral valve regurgitation
    3. Asymmetric septal hypertrophy
    4. Presence of dialysis fistula

511. Signs of cyanide toxicity in patients receiving nitroprusside include

    1. Hemoglobinuria
    2. Resistance to the hypotensive effects of nitroprusside
    3. Decrease in mixed venous PO_2
    4. Metabolic acidosis

512. Spontaneous shivering (post-anesthetic tremor):

    1. May increase metabolism and oxygen consumption significantly
    2. May be treated with meperidine
    3. May be treated with droperidol
    4. Does not occur in the absence of hypothermia

513. Electrocardiograph (EKG) changes associated with hyperkalemia include

    1. Peaked T waves
    2. Increased PR interval
    3. Widened QRS complex
    4. Increase in U wave amplitude

514. Which of the following is associated with an increased risk of severe pulmonary dysfunction following pneumonectomy?

    1. P_aO_2 43 mm Hg with temporary occlusion of the pulmonary artery perfusing the diseased lung
    2. Increase in the mean pulmonary artery pressure of 40 mm Hg during temporary occlusion of the pulmonary artery perfusing the diseased lung
    3. Predicted postoperative FEV_1 600 ml
    4. $\dot{V}O_2$ max of 25 ml/kg/min

Select A if options *1, 2 and 3* are correct,
Select B if options *1 and 3* are correct,
Select C if options *2 and 4* are correct,
Select D if only option *4* is correct,
Select E if *all* options are correct.

515. Which of the following will adversely alter the distribution of ventilation during general anesthesia and positive pressure ventilation via a double lumen tube for thoracotomy performed in the lateral decubitus position?

   1. Exposure of the pleural space to atmospheric pressure
   2. Volatile anesthetics
   3. Neuromuscular blockade
   4. Application of PEEP to the dependent lung

516. Which of the following medications may be efficacious for treating nausea in patients who have received spinal anesthesia?

   1. Droperidol
   2. Ephedrine (if hypotensive)
   3. Oxygen
   4. Atropine

517. A 58-year-old patient with a history of severe chronic obstructive pulmonary disease and pulmonary hypertension is scheduled for cholecystectomy. Which of the following would further increase pulmonary vascular resistance in this patient?

   1. Positive end-expiratory pressure
   2. Alkalosis
   3. Hypoventilation
   4. High F_IO_2

518. Gastric emptying is decreased by

   1. Pain
   2. Narcotics
   3. Ethanol
   4. Cigarette smoking

519. True statements concerning asthma include which of the following?

   1. An eosinophil count > 300/mm^3 suggests remission of an acute exacerbation
   2. The endotracheal tube should be removed when the patient is deeply anesthetized
   3. Cimetidine is useful in preventing histamine-mediated bronchoconstriction
   4. Succinylcholine may be used to facilitate tracheal intubation

Select A if options *1, 2 and 3* are correct,
Select B if options *1 and 3* are correct,
Select C if options *2 and 4* are correct,
Select D if only option *4* is correct,
Select E if *all* options are correct.

520. Patients with chronic bronchitis compared to those with pulmonary emphysema tend to develop which of the following signs or symptoms early in the natural history of the disease?

    1. Arterial hypoxemia
    2. Cor pulmonale
    3. Hypercarbia
    4. Dyspnea

521. Which of the following will increase intraocular pressure in the intact eye?

    1. Coughing
    2. Mydriasis
    3. Acute hypertension
    4. Respiratory acidosis

522. Management of patients with pulmonary emphysema should include

    1. Avoidance of systemic dehydration
    2. Liberal use of narcotics
    3. Humidification of inhaled gases
    4. Rapid ventilatory rate

523. A 48-year-old patient is scheduled to undergo a right thoracotomy. Following induction of general anesthesia and tracheal intubation, the patient is paralyzed, mechanically ventilated, and placed in the lateral decubitus position. Which of the following statements concerning the distribution of ventilation and/or perfusion in this patient is true?

    1. Perfusion to the dependent lung is decreased
    2. Ventilation to the nondependent lung is increased
    3. The ventilation/perfusion ratio in the nondependent lung is decreased
    4. The ventilation/perfusion ratio in the dependent lung is decreased

524. A 46-year-old man is scheduled to undergo a right pneumonectomy under general anesthesia. He has a 60-pack-year history of cigarette smoking, a productive cough, and dyspnea on exertion. Preoperative test(s) predictive of postoperative pulmonary function in this patients include

    1. Spirometry
    2. Ventilation/perfusion scan
    3. Arterial blood gases
    4. Chest roentgenogram

Select A if options *1, 2 and 3* are correct,
Select B if options *1 and 3* are correct,
Select C if options *2 and 4* are correct,
Select D if only option *4* is correct,
Select E if *all* options are correct.

525. The following occur in patients with obesity/hypoventilation syndrome (Pickwickian syndrome)

    1. Hypoventilation
    2. Pulmonary hypertension
    3. Right ventricular failure
    4. Delayed emergence

526. Laboratory values consistent with a prerenal cause of oliguria in a postoperative patient include

    1. Urine osmolality 521 mOsm/L
    2. Urine sodium 8 mEq/L
    3. Urine creatinine/plasma creatinine ratio 45
    4. Fractional excretion of sodium 0.8%

527. Causes of sickling in patients with sickle cell anemia include

    1. Hyponatremia
    2. Dehydration
    3. Metabolic alkalosis
    4. Hypothermia

528. Intraocular pressure may be elevated when succinylcholine is administered under which of the following conditions?

    1. Intramuscularly
    2. As a single intravenous dose
    3. As a continuous infusion
    4. After pretreatment with curare

529. The threshold for eliciting the oculocardiac reflex can be decreased by

    1. Hyperoxia
    2. Retrobulbar block
    3. Hypokalemia
    4. Hypercarbia

530. The oculocardiac reflex is

    1. Mediated through cranial nerves III and X
    2. Caused by traction of the extraocular muscles
    3. Prevented with prophylactic use of atropine
    4. Fatiguable

Select A if options *1, 2 and 3* are correct,
Select B if options *1 and 3* are correct,
Select C if options *2 and 4* are correct,
Select D if only option *4* is correct,
Select E if *all* options are correct.

531. Metabolic abnormalities that frequently occur in patients with Addison's disease include

1. Hypoglycemia
2. Hyponatremia
3. Hypotension
4. Hypokalemia

532. Thyroid storm can be treated with

1. Cortisone
2. Sodium iodide
3. Propylthiouracil
4. Propranolol

533. Measures useful for renal protection in burn patients with myoglobinuria include administration of

1   Mannitol
2. Bicarbonate
3. Furosemide
4. Fresh-frozen plasma

534. Hazards of O_2 administration include

1. Retinopathy of prematurity
2. Retention of CO_2
3. Adsorption atelectasis
4. Bronchopulmonary dysplasia

535. True statements regarding intrathecal opiates include which of the following?

1. They do not block the sympathetic nervous system
2. Delayed respiratory depression after bolus administration reflects systemic absorption
3. Analgesia is specific for visceral rather than somatic pain
4. Delayed depression occurs less often with morphine than with fentanyl

536. Normal changes in geriatric patients who maintain a physically fit lifestyle compared with their younger counterparts include

1. Decreased conduction velocity in peripheral nerves
2. 40% decrease in cardiac output by age 70
3. Decreased serum albumin
4. 50% increase in serum creatinine

Select A if options *1, 2 and 3* are correct,
Select B if options *1 and 3* are correct,
Select C if options *2 and 4* are correct,
Select D if only option *4* is correct,
Select E if *all* options are correct.

537. A 100-kg male patient is 24 hours status post four vessel coronary artery bypass graft. Which of the following pulmonary pressures and volumes would be compatible with successful extubation in this patient?

    1. Vital capacity 2.5 L
    2. P_aCO_2 44 mm Hg
    3. Maximum inspiratory pressure −38 cm H_2O
    4. P_aO_2 155 mm Hg on F_IO_2 0.40

538. A 68-year-old patient with a history of asymmetric septal hypertrophy is to undergo an elective cholecystectomy under general anesthesia. Reasonable steps in the anesthetic management of this patient include which of the following?

    1. Prompt treatment of bradycardia with an isoproterenol drip
    2. Afterload reduction with sodium nitroprusside
    3. Prophylaxis against dysrhythmias with digitalis
    4. Prompt replacement of blood loss with crystalloid solutions or blood

539. Radiographic findings consistent with chronic obstructive lung disease include

    1. Hyperinflated lungs
    2. Notching along the ribs
    3. Depressed diaphragm
    4. Increased heart size

540. A 68-year-old man undergoes a transurethral resection of the prostate gland under general anesthesia. Preoperative serum [Na^+] is 135 mEq/L and serum [K^+] is 3.5 mEq/L. After induction of anesthesia and tracheal intubation, severe bronchospasm is noted and treated with albuterol and aminophylline. At the end of the case the patient is extubated and taken to the recovery room where he is dyspneic and breathing rapidly. Serum electrolytes are as follows: [Na^+] 108 mEq/L, [K^+] 2.8 mEq/L. Possible causes of hypokalemia in this patient include

    1. Volume overload
    2. Hyperventilation
    3. Albuterol
    4. Aminophylline

Select A if options *1, 2 and 3* are correct,
Select B if options *1 and 3* are correct,
Select C if options *2 and 4* are correct,
Select D if only option *4* is correct,
Select E if *all* options are correct.

541. A 67-year-old mechanic with a 48-pack-year history of cigarette smoking is scheduled to undergo a radical cystectomy under general anesthesia. He states that he "quit" smoking 24 hours prior to admission. Beneficial effects of short-term abstinence from cigarette smoking include

   1. Improvement in ciliary function
   2. Decreased sputum production
   3. Decreased airway resistance
   4. Increased P_{50} for hemoglobin

542. A 38-year-old patient with multiple sclerosis is admitted for emergency appendectomy. Appropriate anesthetics for this operation include

   1. General anesthesia with thiopental, succinylcholine, and tracheal intubation
   2. General anesthesia with thiopental, vecuronium, and tracheal intubation
   3. Hyperbaric spinal anesthesia
   4. Lumbar epidural anesthesia

543. A 93-year-old patient with acute angle-closure glaucoma is scheduled to undergo a cervical lymph node biopsy under general anesthesia. Which of the following would increase intraocular pressure in this patient.

   1. Succinylcholine
   2. Scopolamine 0.4 mg IM
   3. P_aCO_2 of 50 mm Hg following extubation
   4. Pancuronium for neuromuscular blockade

544. A 73-year-old patient with a history of hypothyroidism is scheduled to undergo emergency cholecystectomy under general anesthesia. True statements concerning the anesthetic management of this patient include which of the following?

   1. The patient is at increased risk for developing congestive heart failure
   2. Fluid maintenance should be with 5% dextrose in water
   3. The patient is at increased risk for hypothermia
   4. Anesthetic requirement will be decreased

545. Factors associated with decreased hepatic blood flow include

   1. Positive pressure ventilation
   2. Spinal anesthesia
   3. General anesthesia with isoflurane
   4. Hyperventilation during general anesthesia

Select A if options *1, 2 and 3* are correct,
Select B if options *1 and 3* are correct,
Select C if options *2 and 4* are correct,
Select D if only option *4* is correct,
Select E if *all* options are correct.

546. In which of the following conditions would the response to atropine be diminished?

    1. Severe diabetic neuropathy
    2. Brain death
    3. Status post heart transplant
    4. High (C_8) spinal anesthesia

547. Drugs considered suitable for anesthetizing patients who are susceptible to malignant hyperthermia include

    1. Lidocaine
    2. N_2O
    3. Droperidol
    4. Vecuronium

548. Metabolic derangements associated with acute diabetic ketoacidosis include

    1. Hyponatremia
    2. Hypovolemia
    3. Hypochlorhydria
    4. Potassium depletion

549. A 65-year-old woman with rheumatoid arthritis is scheduled for total hip arthroplasty. Conditions associated with rheumatoid arthritis include

    1. Aortic regurgitation
    2. Anemia
    3. Pulmonary fibrosis
    4. Pleural effusion

550. A 68-year-old man with insulin-dependent diabetes mellitus and chronic renal failure is brought to the operating room for placement of an arterial-to-venous dialysis shunt. Medications include regular insulin 15 units SQ, and NPH insulin, 20 units SQ, daily. Preoperative laboratory tests indicate a hemoglobin level of 9 g/dL. Correct statements concerning the anesthetic management of this patient include which of the following?

    1. Hyperventilation of the lungs is recommended
    2. Mild hypothermia is recommended
    3. Anemia results in greater solubility of volatile anesthetic in blood
    4. Shivering in the postoperative period should be avoided

Select A if options *1, 2 and 3* are correct,
Select B if options *1 and 3* are correct,
Select C if options *2 and 4* are correct,
Select D if only option *4* is correct,
Select E if *all* options are correct.

551. A 4-year-old child is brought to the operating room for an elective adenoidectomy under general anesthesia. Inhalation induction of anesthesia with halothane is uneventful. After the succinylcholine is administered, however, it is very difficult to open the patient's mouth and perform direct laryngoscopy for tracheal intubation. After the airway is secured, halothane is discontinued and anesthesia is maintained with N_2O 50% in O_2, fentanyl, and midazolam, and skeletal muscle paralysis is achieved with vecuronium. The patient's core body temperature increases by approximately 1°C over the next 15 minutes and malignant hyperthermia is suspected. Correct statements concerning the anesthetic management of this patient include which of the following?

    1. Dantrolene should be administered intravenously
    2. Hyperventilation of the lungs with 100% O_2 should be initiated
    3. Mannitol, 0.5 mg/kg, should be administered intravenously
    4. HCO_3^- should be given to correct metabolic acidosis

552. A 4-year-old boy who sustained a thermal injury covering 40 percent of his body is brought to the OR 4 weeks after the initial event. A decreased dose of which of the following drugs might be anticipated for this patient's anesthetic for wound debridement?

    1. Thiopental
    2. Vecuronium
    3. Morphine
    4. Midazolam

553. In a 72-year-old male with a history of multiple myeloma and hypercalcemia is scheduled for an exploratory laparotomy for a bowel obstruction. The patient's total calcium is 15 mg/dl. The following would be effective in reducing this patient's serum calcium prior to surgery

    1. Saline hydration
    2. Salmon calcitonin
    3. Mithramycin
    4. Thiazide diuretics

554. A 7-year-old girl is brought to the emergency room by her parents unconscious and unresponsive to painful stimuli. The parents state that the child has had flu-like symptoms and a mild fever for the past week. Then two days ago, the child became sleepy and tired, difficult to arouse, stopped eating, and had three episodes of vomiting. Current medications include multivitamins and aspirin for fever. Plasma ammonia level is 100 mmol/L and PT is 18 seconds. Correct statements concerning the treatment of this patient include which of the following?

    1. Tracheal intubation and hyperventilation of the lungs should be initiated
    2. Aspirin should be discontinued
    3. Vitamin K should be administered
    4. Lactulose should be administered

DIRECTIONS (Questions 555 through 566): Each group of questions consists of several numbered statements followed by lettered headings. For each numbered statement, select the ONE lettered heading that is most closely associated with it. Each lettered heading may be selected once, more than once, or not at all.

555. Decreased FEV_1/FVC ratio

556. Decreased total pulmonary compliance

557. Increased total lung capacity

558. Decreased FRC

559. Decreased FEV_1, normal FEV_1/FVC ratio

560. Increase lung compliance

    A. Pulmonary emphysema
    B. Chronic bronchitis
    C. Restrictive pulmonary disease
    D. Pulmonary emphysema and chronic bronchitis
    E. Pulmonary emphysema and restrictive pulmonary disease

561. Weakness of all muscles below the knee

562. Foot drop; loss of dorsal extension of the toes

563. Weakness of the muscles that extend the knee

564. Inability to adduct the leg; diminished sensation over the medial side of the thigh

    A. Sciatic nerve injury
    B. Common peroneal nerve injury
    C. Femoral nerve injury
    D. Obturator nerve injury
    E. Anterior tibial nerve injury

565. The likelihood of reinfarction during the perioperative period if the operation is performed less than 3 months after an acute myocardial infarction is

566. The likelihood of reinfarction during the perioperative period if the operation is performed 3 to 6 months after an acute myocardial infarction is

    A. 0.13%
    B. 5%
    C. 16%
    D. 37%
    E. 61%

GENERAL ANESTHESIA
ANSWERS, REFERENCES, AND EXPLANATIONS

418. **(B)** Patients with insulin-dependent diabetes (IDDM) and non-insulin dependent diabetes (NIDDM) require special consideration when presenting for surgery. Geriatric age patients come to the OR in the fasting state and without having taken their morning dose of their oral diabetic agent. Chlorpropamide is the longest acting sulfonylurea and has a duration of action up to 72 hours. Accordingly, it is prudent to measure serum glucose prior to inducing anesthesia and periodically during the course of the anesthetic and surgery. Chlorpropamide is also interesting in that it is sometimes associated with the inappropriate secretion of ADH. Approximately 5 percent of patients treated with this drug have serum sodium levels less than 129 mEq/L but are usually asymptomatic. Regular insulin has a peak effect 2-4 hours after administration and a duration of action approximately 6-8 hours and would therefore not cause a serum glucose of 35 mg/dl 24 hours after it was administered *(Stoelting: Pharmacology and Physiology in Anesthetic Practice, ed 2, pp 442-443; Miller: Anesthesia, ed 4, p 906).*

419. **(E)** Dibucaine is an amide-type local anesthetic which inhibits normal pseudo-cholinesterase by approximately 80%. In patients who are heterozygous for atypical pseudocholinesterase, enzyme activity is inhibited by 40 to 60%, in patients who are homozygous for atypical pseudo-cholinesterase enzyme activity is inhibited by only 20%. The dibucaine number is a qualitative assessment of pseudocholinesterase. A quantitative as well as qualitative determination of enzyme activity should be carried out in any patient who is suspected of having a pseudo-cholinesterase abnormality *(Stoelting: Basics of Anesthesia, ed 3, pp 87-88).*

420. **(D)** All hypotension can be broadly broken down into two main categories: decreased cardiac output and decreased systemic vascular resistance. Flow or cardiac output can be further subdivided into problems related to decreased heart rate, i.e. bradycardia, vs. problems related to decreases in stroke volume. A mixed venous arterial oxygen level of 60 mm Hg in the absence of factors which would decrease peripheral uptake, e.g. cyanide, would represent a significant increase in cardiac output. The normal PO_2 in mixed venous blood is 40 mm Hg. The other choices in this question all represent conditions whereby cardiac output is diminished and consequently would not be consistent with the data given in the question *(Stoelting: Anesthesia and Co-existing Disease, ed 3, pp 474-475).*

421. **(C)** Capillary arteriolar pressure is important to keep in mind in patients who are intubated with cuffed endotracheal tubes. If the endotracheal tube cuff exerts a pressure greater than capillary arteriolar pressure, tissue ischemia may result. Persistent ischemia may lead to destruction of tracheal rings and tracheomalacia. Endotracheal tubes with low pressure cuffs are recommended in patients who are to be intubated for periods longer than 48 hours as this will minimize the chances for development of tissue ischemia *(Stoelting: Basics of Anesthesia, ed 3, pp 150-151 & 161-162).*

422. **(A)** Findings on a routine preoperative chest x-ray which would be important for the anesthesiologist include pneumothorax, mediastinal mass, pulmonary nodule, deviated trachea, thoracic aneurysm, pulmonary blebs, pneumonia, atelectasis, pulmonary edema, and fractures of the

clavicles, ribs, or vertebrae. The incidence of significant new finding on routine preoperative chest x-ray in patients under the age of 40 is in most series < 2.2%. For this reason, routine chest x-rays are not indicated in asymptomatic individuals under the age of 40. Some, in fact, question the benefit of routine preoperative chest x-rays in asymptomatic patients younger than 60 years of age *(Miller: Anesthesia, ed 4, pp 842-844)*.

423. **(A)** The principle mechanism of peripheral nerve injury is ischemia caused by stretching or compression of the nerves. Anesthetized patients are at increased risk for peripheral nerve injuries because they are unconscious and unable to complain about uncomfortable positions an awake patient would not tolerate and because of reduced muscle tone which facilitates placement of patients into awkward positions. The ulnar nerve in particular is vulnerable as it passes around the posterior aspect of the medial epicondyle of the humerus. Nerve may become compressed between the medial epicondyle and the sharp edge of the operating table leading to ischemia and possible nerve injury which may be transient or permanent *(Stoelting: Basics of Anesthesia, ed 3, p 195)*.

424. **(E)** Methoxyflurane is extensively metabolized resulting in the liberation of the fluoride anion. Fluoride and lithium in appropriate concentrations are capable of making the kidney unresponsive to antidiuretic hormone. This condition is known as nephrogenic diabetes insipidus and is the reason that methoxyflurane was withdrawn from clinical practice. Enflurane is also capable of yielding free fluoride ions particularly in patients who concurrently take a medication which results in enzyme induction. Very small amounts of free fluoride ion are produced through the metabolism of isoflurane and halothane *(Miller: Anesthesia, ed 4, pp 169-170)*.

425. **(C)** The incidence of deep-vein thrombosis can be reduced from 30% to less than 10% in patients undergoing thoracoabdominal surgery if low-dose heparin (5,000 units) is administered 2 hours prior to surgery and every 8 to 12 hours thereafter (until the patient is able to walk). Although the reduction in deep-vein thrombosis in these patients is clear, it is not certain if this therapy prevents pulmonary embolism or reduces mortality. Aspirin, warfarin, dextran, and compression boots may also be of benefit in specific clinical situations. Early ambulation, however, is the best prophylaxis against deep-vein thrombosis. Coughing does nothing to prevent deep-vein thromboses *(Stoelting: Anesthesia and Co-existing Disease, ed 2, p 191)*.

426. **(C)** Blood flow to the retina can be decreased by either a decrease in mean arterial pressure or an increase in intraocular pressure. Decreased blood flow and stasis are more likely in patients with glaucoma because the latter have elevated intraocular pressure. During periods of prolonged hypotension, the incidence of retinal artery thrombosis increases in these patients *(Stoelting: Basics of Anesthesia, ed 3, pp 346-347)*.

427. **(D)** Naloxone is the only intravenous opioid antagonist currently available. It is a competitive inhibitor at all opioid receptors but has the greatest affinity for mu receptors. Its duration of action is relatively short. For example a 0.4 mg dose of naloxone will antagonize morphine for less than 1 hour. For this reason, one must be vigilant for the possibility of renarcotization. Naltrexone is the N-cyclopropylmethyl derivative of oxymorphone. It is currently only available as an oral preparation and is used to block the euphoric effects of injected heroin in addicts who have been previously detoxified. An experimental opioid antagonist nalmefene has an extremely long duration of action. Investigators have shown that a 2 mg dose of this antagonist can block

the effects of fentanyl for up to 8 hours. Caution with the administration of this antagonist is indicated as it could block the analgesic effects of opioids for many hours *(Rogers: Principles and Practice of Anesthesiology, p 1171).*

428. **(A)**   In the recovery room, the most common cause of postoperative hypoxemia is a uneven ventilation/perfusion distribution caused by loss of lung volume resulting from small airway collapse and atelectasis. Risk factors for ventilation/perfusion mismatch in the postoperative period include old age, obstructive lung disease, obesity, increased intraabdominal pressure, and immobility. Supplemental oxygen should be administered to keep the P_aO_2 in the 80 to 100 mm Hg range as this is associated with a 95% saturation of hemoglobin. Other measures can be taken which serve to restore lung volume. These would include recovering obese patients in the sitting position, coughing, and deep breathing *(Barash: Clinical Anesthesia, ed 2, pp 1528-1529).*

429. **(D)**   Airway obstruction following total thyroidectomy may be caused by a postoperative hematoma, compressing the trachea, tracheomalacia, bilateral recurrent laryngeal nerve damage, or hypocalcemia resulting from inadvertent removal of the parathyroid glands. The airway symptoms of hypocalcemia usually manifest 24 to 48 hours postoperatively and include laryngeal stridor, labored breathing, and eventual laryngospasm. Therapy consists of the IV administration of calcium gluconate or calcium chloride *(Stoelting: Basics of Anesthesia, ed 3, p 321).*

430. **(A)**   Damage to the radial nerve is manifested by weakness in abduction of the thumb, inability to extend the metacarpophalangeal joints, wrist drop, and numbness in the webbed space between the thumb and the index finger. The radial nerve passes around the humerus between the middle and lower portion in the spiral groove posteriorly. As it wraps around the bone, the radial nerve can become compressed between it and the operating room table resulting in nerve injury *(Barash: Clinical Anesthesia, ed 2, p 717).*

431. **(D)**   Bronchiectasis is one of several obstructive lung diseases characterized by a diminished FEV_1 when pulmonary function is evaluated. It is characterized by permanently dilated bronchi which frequently contain purulent secretions. The affected bronchi are often highly vascularized giving rise to the possibility of hemoptysis. Collateral circulation through the intercostal and bronchial arteries is also possible in these patients and if these vessels connect with the pulmonary circulation, pulmonary hypertension and eventual cor pulmonale are possible sequelae. Any patient with chronic bronchial infections may develop bronchiectasis *(Stoelting: Anesthesia and Co-existing Disease, ed 3, pp 145-146).*

432. **(E)**   Drugs that block dopamine receptors may cause acute dystonic reactions in some patients. The treatment for this is the administration of a drug with anticholinergic properties such as diphenhydramine or benztropine. Although glycopyrrolate is an anticholinergic drug, it would not be useful in this setting because it does not cross the blood-brain barrier *(Stoelting: Anesthesia and Co-existing Disease, ed 3, p 524).*

433. **(C)**   The median nerve is most frequently injured at the antecubital fossa by extravasation of intravenous drugs (e.g., thiopental) that are toxic to neural tissue, or by direct injury caused by the needle during attempts to cannulate the medial cubital or basilic veins. The median nerve provides sensory innervation to the palmer surface of the lateral three and one-half fingers and

adjacent palm, and motor function to the abductor pollicis brevis, flexor pollicis brevis and opponens pollicis muscles *(Stoelting: Basics of Anesthesia, ed 3, p 198)*.

434. **(E)**	The arterial blood gas results are consistent with acute respiratory depression, possibly associated with oxygen supplementation. The major goal of oxygen therapy for hypoxia in patients with COPD is to restore the patient's arterial saturation while approximating the patient's stable baseline. This usually requires a P_aO_2 of 50-60 mm Hg. The mechanism for CO_2 retention associated with oxygen administration is not fully known. The classic explanation is that of suppression of hypoxic drive. However, more complex mechanisms may be involved including such factors as changes in the work of breathing, hypoxic vasoconstriction, denitrogenation, and hemoglobin-oxygen affinity relationships. Thus, although oxygen administration to patients with chronic obstructive pulmonary disease is clinically necessary, the risk of carbon dioxide retention increases with increasing concentrations of expired O_2. Thus, the best treatment for this patient is to decrease the inspired O_2 concentration.

435. **(D)**	Serum glutamic-oxaloacetic transaminase (aspartate aminotransferase), serum glutamic-pyruvic transaminase (alanine aminotransferase), and lactate dehydrogenase are all elevated in patients with liver disease. The serum level of alkaline phosphatase may be a specific indicator of biliary obstruction. Since this enzyme is also produced in the intestines, bone, and placenta, other serum tests must be ordered to differentiate among these potential sources. Concurrent measurement of the serum gamma glutaryl transferase (GGT), leucine aminopeptidase, or 5'-nucleotidase levels can be measured simultaneously with alkaline phosphatase to determine the origin of the latter *(Miller: Anesthesia, ed 4, pp 979-980)*.

436. **(B)**	Treatment of severe alcohol withdrawal consists of fluid replacement, electrolyte replacement, and intravenous vitamin administration with particular attention paid to thiamine. ß-blockers may also be used to suppress overactivity of the sympathetic nervous system, and lidocaine may be effective in the treatment of cardiac dysrhythmias. Aggressive administration of benzodiazepines is also indicated to prevent seizures (5-10 mg of diazepam every 5 minutes until the patient becomes sedated but not unconscious) *(Stoelting: Anesthesia and Co-existing Disease, ed 3, pp 527-528)*.

437. **(A)**	Operations on the trachea may be indicated in patients who have tracheal tumors or patients who have had a previous trauma to the trachea resulting in tracheal stenosis or tracheomalacia. Eighty percent of the operations on the trachea involve segmental resection with primary anastomosis, 10% involve resection with prosthetic reconstruction, and another 10% involve insertion of a T-tube stent. These operations are frequently very complicated and require constant communication between the surgeon and the anesthesiologist. Preoperative pulmonary function tests are indicated in all patients who are to undergo elective tracheal resection. Severe lung disease necessitating postoperative mechanical ventilation is a relative contraindication for tracheal resection since positive airway pressure may cause wound dehiscence *(Miller: Anesthesia, ed 4, p 1728)*.

438. **(B)**

	Serum Calcium	Serum Ionized Calcium
Conventional units (mEq/L)	4.5-5.5 mEq/L	2.1-2.6 mEq/L
Conventional units (mg/dl)	9.0-11.0 mg/dl	4.25-5.25 mg/dl
SI units	2.25-2.75 mmol/L	1.05-1.30 mmol/L

Hypercalcemia is associated with a number of signs and symptoms including hypertension, dysrhythmias, prolongation of the QT interval, kidney stones, seizure, nausea and vomiting, weakness, depression, personality changes, psychosis, and even coma. Generally patients with total serum calcium levels of 12 mg/dl or less do not require any intervention with the possible exception of rehydration with saline. Higher calcium levels may be associated with clinical symptoms and should be treated prior to anesthetizing the patient. Caution should be taken with digitalis administration to any patient who is hypercalcemic because some patients may exhibit extreme digitalis sensitivity *(Rogers: Principles and Practice of Anesthesiology, pp 284-285)*.

439. **(D)** The classic studies by Tarhan and Stein carried out in the 1970s have shown that patients who have suffered a myocardial infarction less than 3 months prior to surgery have about a 30% chance of reinfarction. If the operation is carried out 3 to 6 months after the myocardial infarction, the risk drops to about 15%. If surgery is delayed for six months or more after a myocardial infarction, the risk of reinfarction is around 5% to 6%. For reasons which are not fully understood, the mortality from such postoperative myocardial infarctions is 50% to 70%. This is much higher than the mortality which would be expected from repeat myocardial infarctions not complicated by surgery *(Thomas: Manual of Cardiac Anesthesia, ed 2, p 275)*.

440. **(B)** A patient with a history of previous myocardial infarction would be at the greatest risk by far for perioperative reinfarction and death with an operation involving the great vessels. A patient with a history of prior myocardial infarction who undergoes surgery for repair of an abdominal aortic aneurysm has at least a 15% chance of reinfarction; of those, 50% to 70% will die. Operations involving the upper abdomen and thorax are also associated with an increased risk of reinfarction in patients who have had a previous myocardial infarction compared with other operations *(Thomas: Manual of Cardiac Anesthesia, ed 2, p 276)*.

441. **(A)** Causes for acute pacemaker malfunction in the operating room are numerous and include threshold changes, inhibition, generator failure, and lead or electrode dislodgement or breakage. A VVI pacemaker may be inhibited by myopotentials. In this regard, administration of succinylcholine could actually inhibit a VVI pacemaker. Similarly, electrocautery can inhibit a VVI pacemaker through electromagnetic interference. Should this occur, a magnet should be placed over the pacemaker to convert it into a VOO pacemaker, eliminating the possibility of further inhibition. Pacemakers should be evaluated preoperatively to eliminate the possibility of generator failure. Lead breakage or dislodgement is an unlikely cause of pacemaker failure unless the surgeon is working in the vicinity of the electrodes. Acute threshold changes are almost always associated with changes in the serum potassium concentration. In this particular patient, hyperventilation causes a respiratory alkalosis which results in the intracellular shifting of serum

potassium. The net result is that the electrical threshold for the pacemaker is raised preventing ventricular capture *(Thomas: Manual of Cardiac Anesthesia, ed 2, pp 382-383).*

442. **(C)** Therapies aimed at increasing the functional residual capacity of the lungs are useful in reducing the incidence of postoperative pulmonary complications. Forced expiratory maneuvers may lead to airway closure, which would be of no benefit for this patient *(Stoelting: Anesthesia and Co-existing Disease, ed 3, pp 144-145).*

443. **(C)** The human brain is able to maintain neuronal function in the face of decreasing cerebral blood flow below the normal level of 50 mL/100 g/min. Since O_2 delivery is directly related to cerebral blood flow, electroencephalographic (EEG) evidence of cerebral ischemia will appear if CBF is diminished sufficiently. The CBF reserve, however, is substantial and the first signs of cerebral ischemia do not appear on EEG until cerebral blood flow has fallen to approximately 22 mL/100 g/min. When CBF has fallen to 15/100 g/min, the EEG becomes isoelectric. Irreversible membrane damage and cellular death do not occur, however, until CBF falls to 6 mL/100 g/min. Areas of the brain in which CBF fall in the 6 to 15 mL/100 g/min range are referred to as zones of ischemic penumbra. Several hours, however, may elapse in these areas of the brain before irreversible membrane damage occurs *(Miller: Anesthesia, ed 4, pp 711-713).*

444. **(B)** Positive end-expiratory pressure (PEEP) is the maintenance of positive airway pressure during the entire ventilator cycle. The addition of PEEP to the ventilator cycle is often recommended when the P_aO_2 is not maintained above 60 mm Hg, when breathing an F_IO_2 of 0.50 or greater. Although not completely understood, PEEP is thought to increase arterial oxygenation, pulmonary compliance, and functional residual capacity (FRC) by expanding previously collapsed but perfused alveoli, thereby decreasing shunt and improving ventilation-to-perfusion matching. An important adverse effect of PEEP is a decrease in arterial blood pressure caused by a decrease in venous return, left ventricular filling and stroke volume, and cardiac output. These effects are exaggerated in patients with decreased intravascular fluid volume. Other potential adverse effects of PEEP include pneumothorax, pneumomediastinum, and subcutaneous emphysema *(Stoelting: Anesthesia and Co-existing Disease, ed 3, p 171).*

445. **(C)** Reversal of neuromuscular blockade with an anticholinesterase drug requires co-administration of an anticholinergic drug to prevent the muscarinic side-effects, (e.g., bradycardia and salivation) from the neuromuscular reversal agent. The onset of neuromuscular reversal activity is most rapid with edrophonium followed by neostigmine and pyridostigmine. The durations of action of edrophonium and neostigmine are similar, but pyridostigmine has a somewhat longer duration of action. Of the anticholinergic drugs, glycopyrrolate has a longer duration of action than atropine and for this reason should be co-administered with pyridostigmine. In the question the patient received long-acting pyridostigmine in combination with short acting atropine. After the effects of the atropine wore off, the antimuscarinic effects of pyridostigmine became evident resulting in bradycardia *(Stoelting: Pharmacology and Physiology in Anesthetic Practice, ed 2, pp 233-34).*

446. **(B)**   As a rough approximation, if one divides 150 by the MAC for any given volatile anesthetic, the quotient will be approximately equal to the oil:gas partition coefficient. For example, if one were to divide the MAC of halothane (0.75) into 150, the quotient would be 200, which is very close to the actual oil:gas partition coefficient for halothane (224). Similarly, if one were to divide the MAC of enflurane (1.68) into 150, the quotient would be 89, which is very similar to the oil:gas partition coefficient for enflurane (98). The fact that anesthetics with a high oil:gas partition coefficient (i.e., lipid soluble agents) have lower MACs supports the Meyer-Overton theory (critical-volume hypothesis) *(Stoelting: Pharmacology and Physiology in Anesthetic Practice, ed 2, p 25).*

447. **(E)**   Diabetes insipidus is characterized by hypernatremia, serum hyperosmolality, polyuria, and urine hypo-osmolality. Diabetes insipidus may occur after any intracranial procedure, but is particularly common in surgery involving the pituitary gland. It may develop intraoperatively, but more commonly occurs 24 to 48 hours postoperatively. The pharmacologic treatment for diabetes insipidus is synthetic ADH, 1-(3-mercaptoproprionic acid)-D-arginine vasopressin (DDAVP). In a conscious patient it is not essential to administer DDAVP since the patient may increase his oral intake to compensate for polyuria. In the unconscious patient, however, administration of DDAVP is necessary. DDAVP may be administered subcutaneously, intravenously, or intranasally. Fortunately, diabetes insipidus related to surgery and head trauma is usually transient *(Barash: Clinical Anesthesia, ed 2, pp 219-222; Stoelting: Anesthesia and Co-existing Disease, ed 3, p 370).*

448. **(B)**   The principle feature of Alzheimer's disease is progressive dementia. The onset typically occurs after the age of 60 and may affect as many as 20% of patients over the age of 80 years. In addition to age, other risk factors include history of serious head trauma (e.g., boxing), Down's syndrome, and presence of the disease in a parent or sibling. One biochemical feature of this disease is a decrease in the enzyme choline acetyltransferase in the brain. There is a strong correlation between reduced enzyme activity and decreased cognitive function. Interestingly, administration of the anticholinergic drug scopolamine causes confusion similar to that seen in the early stages of Alzheimer's disease. Conversely, administration of anticholinesterase drugs capable of penetrating the blood:brain barrier such as physostigmine, tetrahydroaminoacridine, and ergoloid may have beneficial effects in some patients. Scopolamine is therefore a poor choice for premedication in patients with Alzheimer's disease *(Stoelting: Anesthesia and Co-existing Disease, ed 3, pp 213-224).*

449. **(C)**   At the end of any general anesthetic spontaneous ventilation must be restored before the patient can be extubated. The differential diagnosis for persistent apnea includes muscle relaxants (inadequate reversal or pseudocholinesterase deficiency), volatile anesthetics, narcotics, hypocarbia, damage to the phrenic nerves bilaterally, and the possibility of a CNS event. Succinylcholine is hydrolyzed by pseudocholinesterase to succinylmonocholine and choline. This is then further hydrolyzed by plasma cholinesterase to succinic acid and choline. All of the anticholinesterase agents used to reverse nondepolarizing neuromuscular blockade also inhibit pseudocholinesterase. Administration of succinylcholine to any patient who has already received an anticholinesterase will result in a prolonged block from the succinylcholine because it can no longer be easily hydrolyzed. In this patient, therefore, succinylcholine would be by far the most likely cause of apnea at the end of the operation *(Stoelting: Pharmacology and Physiology in Anesthetic Practice, ed 2, p 235).*

450. **(A)** Pooling of urine in the dome of the bladder should be considered as a possible cause of oliguria in a patient in the Trendelenburg position. Acute hypovolemia is an unlikely cause of oliguria in this patient in the absence of bleeding. Fluoride toxicity from the metabolism of enflurane is extremely rare and is associated with nonoliguric renal failure *(Stoelting: Anesthesia and Co-existing Disease, ed 3, pp 294-296).*

451. **(D)** Preoperative pulmonary function tests will **NOT** detect pulmonary hypertension. Pulmonary hypertension can be suspected, however, on the basis of a decreased DL_{co}. The DL_{co} is influenced by the volume of blood (hemoglobin) within the pulmonary circulation. Thus, diseases associated with a decrease in pulmonary blood volume (i.e., anemia, emphysema, hypovolemia, pulmonary hypertension) will be reflected by a decrease in the DL_{co} *(West: Respiratory Physiology—The Essentials, ed 3, pp 28-29).*

452. **(E)** Patients undergoing thyroid surgery are at risk for airway obstruction from a number of causes. Postoperative hemorrhage sufficient to cause a large hematoma could compress the trachea causing airway obstruction because of the close proximity of the thyroid gland to the trachea. Permanent hypoparathyroidism is a rare complication which may cause hypocalcemia leading to progressive stridor followed by laryngospasm. The most common nerve injury following thyroid surgery is damage to the abductor fibers of the recurrent laryngeal nerve. Unilaterally, this is manifested as hoarseness. Bilateral recurrent laryngeal nerve damage, however, may lead to airway obstruction during inspiration. Selective injury of the adductor fibers of the recurrent laryngeal nerve is also a possible complication of thyroid surgery. This injury would leave the vocal cords open because the abductor fibers would be unopposed placing the patient at great risk for aspiration. The superior laryngeal nerve has an extrinsic branch which innervates the cricothyroid muscle (which tenses the vocal cords), and an internal branch, which provides sensory innervation to the pharynx above the vocal cords. Bilateral damage to this nerve would result in hoarseness and would also predispose the patient to aspiration but would not lead to airway obstruction per se *(Stoelting: Basics of Anesthesia, ed 3, pp 320-321).*

453. **(E)** Malignant hyperthermia is a clinical syndrome that may develop rapidly or take hours to manifest, sometimes not occurring until the patient is in the recovery room. Clinical signs include hypertension, tachycardia, respiratory acidosis, metabolic acidosis, muscle rigidity, myoglobinuria, and fever. The diagnosis of malignant hyperthermia is unlikely, however, if only one of these signs is manifested. Since malignant hyperthermia is a metabolic disorder, one of the first signs is an increase in the production of CO_2 and concomitant respiratory acidosis. This is the most reliable early sign of this syndrome *(Miller: Anesthesia, ed 4, p 1085).*

454. **(E)** Hyperventilation to a P_aCO_2 of ≤ 20 mm Hg for >2 hours will result in active transport of HCO_3^- out of the central nervous system. This results in spontaneous breathing at a lower (not higher) P_aCO_2. The other choices should be included in the differential diagnosis of apnea *(Stoelting: Anesthesia and Co-existing Disease, ed 3, p 336).*

455. **(B)** Maximum voluntary ventilation (MVV) is a nonspecific pulmonary function test which may detect obstructive or restrictive pulmonary disease. A decreased MVV may be caused by impairment to inspiration or expiration. In this patient, the FEV_1 is normal which would strongly suggest that the ventilatory impairment is during inspiration. A flow-volume loop would be a very useful confirmatory test *(Barash: Clinical Anesthesia, ed 2, p 945).*

456. **(E)** A tidal volume of 750 ml delivered at a rate of 10/minute would deliver a minute ventilation of 7.5 liters. The measured minute ventilation, however, is only 6 liters; therefore, 1.5 liters must be absorbed by the distensible tubing. This volume is known as the compression volume. If one divides the volume by 10 (number of breaths/minute), then one determines the compression volume/breath. This number (ml) can be further divided by the peak inflation pressure (cm H_2O) to determine the actual compression factor which in this case is 5:

$$\frac{1,500\ ml}{(10) \cdot (30\ cm\ H_2O)} = 5\ ml \cdot (cm\ H_2O)^{-1}$$

(Stoelting: Basics of Anesthesia, ed 3, p 460).

457. **(C)** Malignant hyperthermia is a difficult diagnosis to make on clinical grounds alone. Signs of MH may be fulminant or very subtle. They may occur immediately following induction or may not be manifested until the patient has reached the recovery room or even later. Malignant hyperthermia is a disorder of metabolism and is associated with hypertension, tachycardia, dysrhythmias, respiratory acidosis, metabolic acidosis, muscular rigidity, rhabdomyolysis, and fever. Contrary to what one might believe based on the name of this disease, fever is typically a late finding. There are other diseases which may mimic malignant hyperthermia such as alcohol withdrawal, acute cocaine toxicity, bacteremia, pheochromocytoma, hyperthyroidism, and neuroleptic malignant syndrome to mention a few. An elevation in temperature alone with normal blood gases, normal heart rate and blood pressure, and no evidence of muscle breakdown would very likely not be due to malignant hyperthermia. If a patient had been previously subjected to muscle biopsy and caffeine-halothane contracture testing with negative results, malignant hyperthermia would be exceedingly rare although a false negative is possible. A history of a previous anesthetic without MH triggering would be of little reassurance in a patient in whom an MH episode is suspected. It is not uncommon for MH-susceptible individuals to not trigger when a triggering anesthetic is administered initially but develop fulminant malignant hyperthermia with a subsequent anesthetic *(Miller: Anesthesia, ed 4, pp 1084-1089).*

458. **(D)** Physiologic factors which affect mixed venous O_2 saturation include hemoglobin concentration, arterial P_aO_2, cardiac output, and O_2 consumption. Anemia, hypoxia, decreased cardiac output, and increased O_2 consumption decrease mixed venous O_2 saturation. During sepsis the cardiac output is increased (not decreased), which results in an elevated mixed-venous O_2 saturation. These factors are summarized in the equation below:

Mixed venous O_2 saturation ($S\overline{v}O_2$) is related to a number of factors, as shown in equation:

$$S\overline{v}O_2 = S_aO_2 - \frac{\dot{V}O_2}{13.9 \cdot \dot{Q} \cdot [Hb]}$$

[Hb] = hemoglobin concentration
13.9 = constant (O_2 combining power of Hb [ml/10 g])
$\dot{Q}$ = cardiac output *(Miller: Anesthesia, ed 4, p 1265).*

459. **(E)** The total body water in this patient is 60 L (100 kg • 0.6). The difference in serum sodium concentration is 10 mEq/L (125 mEq/L − 115 mEq/L). Thus, the patient needs 600 mEq of sodium (60 L • 10 mEq/L). Each liter of 5% saline contains 855 mEq of sodium. Thus, 706 mL of 5% saline should be infused to increase the serum sodium concentration from 115 mEq/L to 125 mEq/L. Replacement should be carried out slowly approximately 0.6-1 mmol/L/hr until the serum sodium reaches a concentration of 125 mEq/L at which time further correction should be carried out even more slowly. Continuous laboratory reassessment should also be carried out every 1-2 hours *(Stoelting: Anesthesia and Co-existing Disease, ed 3, pp 320-321; Miller: Anesthesia, ed 4, p 1602).*

460. **(A)** Trismus (masseter spasm) is characterized by rigidity of the jaw muscles while the limb muscles remain flaccid after administration of succinylcholine. Trismus may herald the onset of malignant hyperthermia in some patients but may be due to a number of other causes and may occur in normal patients. It had been previously held that 50% of patients who experience trismus after administration of succinylcholine would go on to develop malignant hyperthermia. Recent evidence suggests, however, that the incidence is less. If masseter spasm does occur in a patient after administration of succinylcholine, the most conservative course would be to cancel the operation. If cancellation of the operation is not feasible, then a nontriggering anesthetic should be used and the anesthesiologist should pay close attention for any signs of malignant hyperthermia *(Miller: Anesthesia, ed 4, pp 1076-77).*

461. **(B)** Ketamine is unique among the intravenous induction agents in that it usually produces cardiac stimulation manifested by increased heart rate, mean arterial pressure, and cardiac output. Ketamine is believed to have a centrally mediated sympathetic nervous system-stimulating effect. This effect is, however, not related to dose. In isolated rabbit and canine hearts and in intact dogs, ketamine has been demonstrated to produce myocardial depression. Clinically, however, the myocardial depressant properties of ketamine are overridden by its sympathetic nervous system stimulating properties. When, however, systemic catecholamines have been depleted or when the patient is under deep anesthesia, the myocardial depressant properties of ketamine may predominate *(Stoelting: Pharmacology and Physiology, ed 2, p 138).*

462. **(C)** In the normal muscle cell, depolarization results in release of calcium from the sarcoplasmic reticulum. The increased intracellular calcium concentration results in muscle contraction. The calcium is then rapidly taken up via calcium pumps back into the sarcoplasmic reticulum resulting in relaxation. Both the release and reuptake of calcium are energy-requiring processes, i.e., result in the hydrolysis of ATP. Dantrolene, the pharmacologic treatment for malignant hyperthermia, blocks release of calcium from the sarcoplasmic reticulum without affecting the reuptake process. The defect in malignant hyperthermia is thought to be decreased control of intracellular calcium stores preventing muscle relaxation *(Miller: Anesthesia, ed 4, pp 1078-79).*

463. **(E)** Approximately 10% to 25% of patients treated with bleomycin develop pulmonary toxicity, which manifests as severe pulmonary fibrosis and hypoxemia. Death from severe pulmonary toxicity occurs in approximately 1% to 2% of patients treated with bleomycin. Patients who are at greater risk for bleomycin-induced pulmonary toxicity include elderly patients, those receiving more than 200 to 400 units, and those with coexisting lung disease. In addition, there is evidence that prior radiotherapy and possibly receipt of enriched concentrations of O_2 during surgery increase risk of pulmonary toxicity. Clinically, patients gradually develop dyspnea, a

nonproductive cough, and hypoxemia, and pulmonary function tests typically demonstrate changes in gas flow and lung volumes consistent with restrictive pulmonary disease. If radiographic evidence, such as bilateral diffuse interstitial infiltrates appear, pulmonary fibrosis is usually irreversible *(Stoelting: Pharmacology and Physiology in Anesthetic Practice, ed 2, pp 515-516)*.

464. **(C)**   Head flexion can advance the tube up to 1.9 cm toward the carina and in some cases convert an endotracheal intubation into an endobronchial intubation. Extension of the head has the opposite effect and can withdraw the tube up to 1.9 cm resulting in an extubation in some patients. Turning the head laterally can move the distal tip of the endotracheal tube about 0.7 cm away from the carina *(Stoelting: Basics of Anesthesia, ed 3, p 161)*.

465. **(C)**   Sulfur hexafluoride is sometimes injected in the vitreous in patients with a detached retina to mechanically facilitate reattachment. To prevent changes in size of the gas bubble, the patients should be given 100% O_2 15 minutes prior to injection of sulfur hexafluoride. If these patients are anesthetized with general anesthesia within 10 days, N_2O should be avoided *(Barash: Clinical Anesthesia, ed 2, p 1103)*.

466. **(D)**   The symptoms of hypocalcemia, which may be manifested as laryngospasm or laryngeal stridor, usually develop within the first 24 to 48 hours after total thyroidectomy. After the airway is established and secured, the patient should be treated with intravenous calcium either in the form of calcium gluconate or calcium chloride *(Barash: Clinical Anesthesia, ed 2, p 225)*.

467. **(C)**   Since the circulating levels of T_3 and T_4 regulate TSH release from the anterior pituitary gland by a negative feedback mechanism, a normal plasma concentration of TSH confirms a euthyroid state. The pharmacologic treatment of choice for patients with hypothyroidism is sodium levothyroxine (T_4). Sodium levothyronine (triiodothyronine, T_3) and desiccated thyroid are alternate therapeutic agents *(Stoelting: Anesthesia and Co-existing Disease, ed 3, pp 347-348)*.

468. **(A)**   Large quantities of irrigating fluid can be absorbed during transurethral resection of the prostate gland because of open venous sinuses in the prostate. From 10 to 30 mL of fluid/min are absorbed on the average. During long cases, this can amount to several liters causing hypertension, reflex bradycardia, and pulmonary congestion *(Barash: Clinical Anesthesia, ed 2, pp 1161-64)*.

469. **(C)**   Patients who have sustained thermal injuries are at risk for massive potassium release and potential cardiac arrest if succinylcholine is administered to them 24 hours or more after the burn and they remain at risk until the burn has healed. This increased sensitivity to succinylcholine is thought to be related to proliferation of extrajunctional receptors. These same receptors are also thought to be related to the increased requirement for nondepolarizing neuromuscular blocking agents in these patients *(Barash: Clinical Anesthesia, ed 2, p 1422)*.

470. **(E)**   The metabolism of nitroprusside in the body requires the conversion of oxyhemoglobin (Fe^{++}) to methemoglobin (Fe^{+++}). The presence of sufficient quantities of methemoglobin in the blood will cause the pulse oximeter to read 85% saturation regardless of the true arterial saturation. Cyanide toxicity is certainly also a possibility in any patient who is receiving nitroprusside. Cyanide toxicity should be suspected when the patient becomes resistant to the hypotensive

effects of this drug despite a sufficient infusion rate. This can be confirmed by measuring the mixed venous PO_2 which would be elevated in the presence of cyanide toxicity. Thiocyanate toxicity is also a potential hazard of nitroprusside administration in patients with renal failure. Patients suffering from thiocyanate toxicity display nausea, mental confusion, and skeletal-muscle weakness *(Barash: Clinical Anesthesia, ed 2, p 375; Stoelting: Pharmacology and Physiology in Anesthetic Practice, ed 2, p 326).*

471. **(D)** One gram of hemoglobin can combine with 1.34 mL of O_2. None of the other choices in this question will do as much to increase the O_2-carrying capacity of this patient's blood than a transfusion *(Stoelting: Pharmacology and Physiology in Anesthetic Practice, ed 2, p 737).*

472. **(D)** Functional residual capacity is composed of expiratory reserve volume plus residual volume. It is essential to maximize FRC in the postoperative period to ensure that it will be greater than closing volume. Closing volume is that lung volume in which small-airway closure begins to occur. Maximizing FRC, therefore, reduces atelectasis and lessens the incidence of arterial hypoxemia and pneumonia. Maneuvers aimed at increasing FRC include early ambulation, incentive spirometry, deep breathing, and intermittent positive pressure breathing *(Stoelting: Basics of Anesthesia, ed 3, p 440).*

473. **(C)** Decreased levels of pseudocholinesterase have been reported in patients with Huntington's chorea. For this reason, the effects of succinylcholine may be prolonged in some of these patients. It has also been suggested that the sensitivity to nondepolarizing muscle relaxants is also increased *(Stoelting: Anesthesia and Co-existing Disease, ed 3, p 211).*

474. **(C)**

$$PVR = \frac{\overline{PAP} - \overline{PCWP}}{CO} \times 80,$$

where PVR is the pulmonary vascular resistance, $\overline{PAP}$ is the mean pulmonary artery pressure, PCWP is the mean pulmonary capillary wedge pressure, and CO is the cardiac output.

$$PVR = \frac{20 - 12}{4} \times 80; PVR = 160 \, dynes\text{-}sec\text{-}cm^{-5}$$

The normal range for PVR is 50 to 150 dynes-sec-cm^{-5} *(Davison: Clinical Anesthesia Procedures of the Massachusetts General Hospital, ed 4, p 339).*

475. **(E)** The Meyer-Overton theory (critical-volume hypothesis) suggests that membrane expansion is the mechanism by which volatile anesthetics produce their effect. The fact that high pressures (40 to 100 atmospheres) antagonize these anesthetic effects suggests that the disrupted membranes can be compressed back to their normal configuration *(Stoelting: Basics of Anesthesia, ed 3, pp 25-26).*

476. **(D)** Any patient who is scheduled for a pneumonectomy should undergo a series of preoperative pulmonary function tests. These tests are generally conducted in three phases. The tests listed in this question pertain to the first battery of pulmonary function tests which are whole-lung tests. Residual volume to total lung capacity > 50% (not < 50%) is associated with an increased

operative risk. If any of the initial whole-lung tests are below the acceptable limits, a second phase of testing should be carried out in which the function of each lung is evaluated separately. The predicted postoperative FEV_1 after the second phase of pulmonary function testing is carried out should be >0.85 liters. If the criteria for the second level of pulmonary function testing cannot be met and pneumonectomy is still desired, then a third level of testing should be carried out. During the third phase of testing, postoperative conditions mimicking pneumonectomy are produced by occluding pulmonary artery with a balloon on the side which is to be resected. Results of this test which are consistent with the poor outcome after pneumonectomy include mean pulmonary artery pressure > 40 mm Hg, P_aCO_2 > 60 mm Hg, or P_aO_2 < 45 mm Hg *(Miller: Anesthesia, ed 4, p 1666)*.

477. **(A)**   The measured P_aO_2 should be decreased about 6% for each degree Celsius cooler the patient's temperature is than the electrode (37°C). Since the patient is 2° cooler than the electrode, a 12% decrease (9 mm Hg) would be expected in this patient. 77 mm Hg − 9 mm Hg = 68 mm Hg *(Stoelting: Basics of Anesthesia, ed 3, p 227)*.

478. **(A)**   Sulfasalazine causes the formation of sulfhemoglobin. Sulfhemoglobin, like methemoglobin, may cause a low O_2 saturation in the face of a high P_aO_2. There is no treatment for sulfhemoglobinemia except to wait for the destruction of the erythrocytes *(Stoelting: Anesthesia and Co-existing Disease, ed 3, p 403)*.

479. **(E)**   Muscle relaxants that stimulate histamine release or cause increased sympathetic outflow should be avoided in patients with pheochromocytoma. Vecuronium has no histamine-releasing properties and does not stimulate the sympathetic nervous system. Mivacurium, curare, and metubine all release histamine to some degree. Pancuronium is associated with tachycardia and should therefore be avoided in patients with pheochromocytoma *(Stoelting: Anesthesia and Co-existing Disease, ed 3, pp 365-66)*.

480. **(E)**   Damage to the common peroneal nerve is associated with inability to evert the foot, foot drop, and loss of extension of the toes *(Stoelting: Basics of Anesthesia, ed 3, p 198)*.

481. **(E)**   For reasons which are not fully understood, patients who have sustained a myocardial infarction and subsequently undergo surgery are most likely to reinfarct on the third postoperative day *(Stoelting: Basics of Anesthesia, ed 3, p 250)*.

482. **(B)**   Scopolamine is an anticholinergic which may produce mydriasis and cycloplegia. This can result in the inability of patients to accommodate *(Stoelting: Basics of Anesthesia, ed 3, pp 119-120; Barash: Clinical Anesthesia, ed 2, p 627)*.

483. **(E)**   Neuroleptic malignant syndrome is a potentially fatal disease which affects 0.5% to 1% of all patients being treated with neuroleptic (antipsychotic) drugs. The syndrome develops gradually over 1 to 3 days in young males and is characterized by 1) hyperthermia, 2) skeletal muscle rigidity, 3) autonomic instability manifested by changes in blood pressure heart rate, and 4) fluctuating levels of consciousness. The mortality from neuroleptic malignant syndrome is 20% to 30%. Liver transaminases and creatine phosphokinase are often elevated in these patients. Treatment includes supportive care and administration of dantrolene. This disease may mimic malignant hyperthermia because of its many similarities. One difference between neuroleptic

malignant syndrome and MH is the fact that nondepolarizing muscle relaxants such as vecuronium or pancuronium will cause flaccid paralysis in patients with neuroleptic malignant syndrome but not with malignant hyperthermia *(Stoelting: Pharmacology and Physiology in Anesthetic Practice, ed 2, pp 367-368)*.

484. **(D)** The classic signs of fat embolism include tachycardia, dyspnea, mental confusion, fever, and frequently there may be a petechial rash on the upper part of the body. Fat embolism more than 72 hours after trauma is not likely *(Stoelting: Anesthesia and Co-existing Disease, ed 3, p 135)*.

485. **(D)** Total body sodium can be calculated using the following equation:

Total body sodium = sodium concentration • 0.6 • total body weight

Thus, 140 mEq/L • 0.6 L/kg • 100 kg = 8,400 mEq. In order for a patient with 8,400 mEq of sodium to have a sodium concentration of 105 mEq/L, the total body water must equal 80 L. This would represent a 20-L increase in total body water *(Stoelting: Anesthesia and Co-existing Disease, ed 3, pp 316-317)*.

486. **(D)** If a peanut or other foreign body becomes lost in the upper airway such that ventilation of the patient is impossible and retrieval is not feasible, the person performing the bronchoscopy should push the foreign body distally past the carina so that gas exchange can take place. Once the patient is stabilized, another attempt to retrieve the foreign body can be made *(Gregory: Pediatric Anesthesia, ed 3, pp 678-679)*.

487. **(E)** Anesthesia for extracorporeal shock-wave lithotripsy may be accomplished with either general anesthesia or epidural anesthesia. When a patient is submerged in the stainless steel tub, the peripheral vasculature becomes compressed by the hydrostatic pressure, resulting in an increase in preload. Removing the patient from the tank has the opposite effect. In patients who have received epidural anesthesia, there is an increased incidence of hypotension after emersion from the bath caused by epidural induced sympathectomy *(Barash: Clinical Anesthesia, ed 2, p 1166)*.

488. **(E)** Protracted nausea and vomiting are the most common reasons for hospitalization following anesthesia for outpatient surgery. Life-threatening complications are rarely a cause of hospitalization *(Stoelting: Basics of Anesthesia, ed 3, p 415)*.

489. **(A)** Cholinergic crisis can be differentiated from myasthenic crisis by administering small intravenous doses of anticholinesterases. Since this patient's tidal volume decreased with the administration of edrophonium, the diagnosis of cholinergic crisis is made. These patients should be electively intubated until strength returns *(Stoelting: Anesthesia and Co-existing Disease, ed 3, p 441)*.

490. **(E)** Deep inhalational anesthesia, atropine, sedatives, and narcotics may inhibit bladder tone and sphincter pressure to such an extent as to invalidate urodynamic studies *(Barash: Clinical Anesthesia, ed 2, p 1158)*.

491. **(D)** Premature infants are at increased risk for development of apnea until they have reached 60 weeks postconceptual age, which is defined as gestational age plus postnatal age. Apnea in these patients is central apnea, that is, apnea associated with absence of respiratory effort related to immaturity of the central nervous system. It is reasonable, therefore, to delay elective surgery until the infant is beyond the susceptible time period. If surgery must be carried out prior to 60 weeks of postconceptual age, then the patient should be admitted and monitored for apnea and bradycardia for at least 24 hours *(Stoelting: Anesthesia and Co-existing Disease, ed 3, p 589)*.

492. **(E)** In the absence of diuretics, oliguria associated with urine sodium concentration > 40 mEq/L and a urine osmolality < 400 mOsm/L is strongly suggestive of intrinsic renal disease (e.g., acute tubule necrosis). Furosemide, however, obscures the issue *(Stoelting: Basics of Anesthesia, ed 3, p 311)*.

493. **(E)** Each of the choices is associated with an increased incidence of postoperative pulmonary complication except for S_aO_2 of 87% in the recovery room. Decreased arterial oxygen saturation in postoperative patients is not unusual and is related to the impact of the anesthetics and events which occurred intraoperatively. In patients without coexisting lung disease, S_aO_2 usually returns to normal within 2 hours of emergence from anesthesia *(Stoelting: Anesthesia and Co-existing Disease, ed 3, p 142)*.

494. **(C)** MAC is the minimum alveolar concentration of anesthetic which will prevent movement of 50% of patients when a skin incision is made. MAC x 1.3 will prevent movement in 95% of patients. In this question the total gas flow is (1 L/min + 3 L/min) 4 L/min. Roughly 75% of the total gas is N_2O. The MAC of N_2O is 104%. The patient is receiving about 0.75 MAC N_2O. The MAC for isoflurane is 1.15. A concentration of 0.85% would represent 0.75 MAC. Since MACs are additive, the total MAC would be 1.5 *(Davison: Clinical Anesthesia Procedures of the Massachusetts General Hospital, ed 4, pp 143-144)*.

495. **(E)** Cardiac output increases by about 100 mL/min for each kilogram of weight gained. It is estimated that every kilogram of adipose tissue contains nearly 3,000 m of additional blood vessels. The additional cardiac output is due to increased stroke volume since resting heart rates are not increased in obese patients *(Stoelting: Anesthesia and Co-existing Disease, ed 3, p 385)*.

496. **(A)** TPN therapy is associated with electrolyte disturbances, volume overload, catheter related sepsis, renal and hepatic dysfunction, thrombosis of the central veins, and nonketotic hyperosmolar coma. Increased work of breathing is related to increased production of CO_2. Acidosis in these patients is hyperchloremic metabolic acidosis resulting from formation of HCl during metabolism of amino acids. Ketoacidosis is not associated with TPN therapy *(Stoelting: Anesthesia and Co-existing Disease, ed 3, p 389)*.

497. **(D)** Ideally, factor VIII levels should be raised to 100% predicted prior to elective surgery to ensure that the levels will not fall below 30% intraoperatively. Thirty percent of the normal factor VIII concentration or greater is thought to be necessary for a patient who is to undergo major surgery. The elimination half-time of factor VIII is 10 to 12 hours. This may be accomplished with factor VIII concentrate or cryoprecipitate. Fresh-frozen plasma is no longer considered therapy for hemophilia *(Stoelting: Anesthesia and Co-existing Disease, ed 3, p 411)*.

498. **(A)** Hemophilia A is associated with decreased levels of factor VIII. The partial thromboplastin time (PTT) tests the intrinsic coagulation cascade and would be abnormally elevated in all but the most mild disease. A normal PTT is 25 to 35 seconds *(Stoelting: Anesthesia and Co-existing Disease, ed 3, p 412).*

499. **(E)** Conventional peripheral nerve stimulators deliver 4 twitches at 2 Hz spaced 0.5 seconds apart. These devices were designed with the knowledge that successive twitches deplete acetylcholine stores. After the fourth twitch, there is no additional decrement in twitch height *(Stoelting: Basics of Anesthesia, ed 3, p 96).*

500. **(B)** Inferior ischemia is associated with blockage or spasm of the right coronary artery. The right coronary artery supplies blood to the atrioventricular node in 90% of patients. Complete heart block is therefore not unexpected in patients with severe coronary artery disease involving the right coronary artery *(Stoelting: Anesthesia and Co-existing Disease, ed 3, p 7).*

501. **(B)** Minimum alveolar concentration (MAC) is influenced by a variety of disease states, conditions, drugs, and other factors. Drugs, which increase CNS catecholamines, such as monoamine oxidase inhibitors, tricyclic antidepressants, acute amphetamine ingestion, and cocaine increase MAC. Other factors which increase MAC include hyperthermia, hypernatremia, and infancy. It is interesting that MAC values are higher for infants than neonates or older children and adults. Thyroid gland dysfunction including hyperthyroidism does not affect the minimum alveolar concentration. Below is a table summarizing the impact of various factors on minimum alveolar concentration:

Impact of Physiologic and Pharmacologic Factors on Minimum Alveolar Concentration

No change in MAC	Increase in MAC	Decrease in MAC
Duration of anesthesia	Hyperthermia	Hypothermia
Gender	Drugs that increase CNS catecholamines (monoamine oxidase inhibitors, tricyclic antidepressants, cocaine, acute amphetamine ingestion)	Preoperative medication
Anesthetic metabolism		Intravenous anesthetics
Thyroid gland dysfunction		Neonates
Hyperkalemia or hypokalemia		Elderly
P_aCO_2 15-95 mm Hg	Infants	Pregnancy
$P_aO_2 > 38$ mm Hg	Hypernatremia	Alpha-2 agonists
Blood pressure > 40 mm Hg	Chronic ethanol abuse (?)	Acute ethanol ingestion
		Lithium
		Cardiopulmonary bypass
		Neuraxial opioids (?)
		$P_aO_2 < 38$ mm Hg

*(From Stoelting RK (ed): Basics of Anesthesia, ed 3. New York, Churchill Livingstone, Inc., p 25. Used with permission).

502. **(B)** Long-term lithium therapy in patients with manic-depressive illness may be associated with nephrogenic diabetes insipidus. Hypothyroidism may develop in a small number of patients because of the ability of lithium to block the release of thyroid hormones. Lithium is almost 100% renally excreted. Reabsorption occurs at the proximal convoluted tubule and is inversely related to the concentration of sodium in the glomerular filtrate. Consequently, administration of diuretics may lead to the development of toxic lithium levels. Lithium has sedative properties and may reduce the need for intravenous and inhalational anesthetic agents. It may prolong the duration of action of both pancuronium and succinylcholine, but is not associated with an exaggerated release of potassium when succinylcholine is administered *(Stoelting: Anesthesia and Co-existing Disease, ed 3, p 523)*.

503. **(C)** Carbon monoxide inhalation is the most common immediate cause of death from fire. Carbon monoxide binds to hemoglobin with an affinity 240 times greater than that of oxygen. For this reason very small concentrations of carbon monoxide can greatly reduce the oxygen carrying capacity of blood. In spite of this, the arterial P_aO_2 is often normal. Since the carotid bodies respond to arterial P_aO_2, there would not be an increase in minute ventilation until tissue hypoxia were sufficient to produce lactic acidosis *(Stoelting: Anesthesia and Co-existing Disease, ed 3, p 536)*.

504. **(C)** Testicular innervation can be traced up to the T_{10} dermatomal level. For this reason, any operation which involves manipulation or traction on the testicles must have adequate anesthesia to prevent pain. This can be achieved with spinal or epidural anesthesia which is associated with a T_{10} level of blockade *(Barash: Clinical Anesthesia, ed 2, p 826)*.

505. **(D)** The Glasgow coma scale has three categories: eye opening for which a maximum of 4 points can be received; verbal response, a maximum of 5 points; and motor response, which a maximum of 6 points. The lowest possible score would be a 3 (1 point in each category) and the highest possible score 15. This patient is totally unresponsive and would therefore receive a score of 3 *(Barash: Clinical Anesthesia, ed 2, p 906)*.

506. **(A)** Insulin metabolism involves both the liver and kidneys. Renal dysfunction, however, has a greater impact on insulin metabolism than does hepatic dysfunction. In fact, unexpected prolonged effects of insulin are sometimes seen in patients with renal disease *(Stoelting: Pharmacology and Physiology, ed 2, p 439)*.

507. **(B)** Carboxyhemoglobin has an absorbance at 660 nm, very similar to O_2 hemoglobin. For this reason, it will produce a falsely elevated S_aO_2 when present in the blood. Hemoglobin F, bilirubin, and fluorescein dye have no effect on pulse oximetry. Methylene blue lowers the S_aO_2 measured by pulse oximetry *(Miller: Anesthesia, ed 4, p 1117)*.

508. **(D)** Mechanical ventilation of the lungs can be accomplished by various modes. These modes are categorized as controlled, assisted, assisted/controlled, controlled with positive end-expiratory pressure (PEEP), and assisted/controlled employing intermittent mandatory ventilation (IMV). Assisted/controlled modes of mechanical ventilation are best used in patients when the muscles of respiration require rest, since minimal breathing efforts are required. IMV exercises inspiratory muscles and decreases mean thoracic pressure, and is thus used most frequently when weaning patients from mechanical ventilation. With the assisted/controlled mode of ventilation,

positive pressure ventilation is triggered by small breathing efforts produced by the patient. The airway pressure tracing shown is typical of that of a patient requiring assisted/controlled ventilation *(Stoelting: Anesthesia and Co-existing Disease, ed 3, p 172).*

509. **(A)** Autonomic neuropathy leads to a decreased response to atropine and propranolol. NPH and protamine zinc insulin preparation are associated with a 50-fold higher incidence of allergic reactions to protamine. Patients are prone to hyperglycemia (not hypoglycemia) during cardiopulmonary bypass because of hypothermia-related insulin resistance *(Stoelting: Anesthesia and Co-existing Disease, ed 3, pp 341-342).*

510. **(E)** Initiation of antibiotic therapy should be begun 30 minutes to 1 hour before a known bacteremic event in accordance with American Heart Association guidelines. Patients with known valvular heart disease of any type including mitral valve prolapse are candidates for antibiotic prophylaxis. Likewise, patients with ventricular septal defect, atrial septal defect, subvalvular aortic stenosis, and intravascular shunt should be protected against bacteria with antibiotic prophylaxis *(Miller: Anesthesia, ed 4, p 951).*

511. **(C)** Signs of cyanide toxicity in patients receiving sodium nitroprusside include tachyphylaxis, metabolic acidosis, and an increase (not a decrease) in the mixed venous PO_2. Treatment for cyanide toxicity includes sodium thiosulfate, 150 mg IV, over a period of 15 minutes. Thiosulfate provides sulfur to convert cyanide into thiocyanate. If cyanide toxicity is so severe that hemodynamic deterioration has begun, then sodium nitrate, 5 mg/kg, should be considered. Sodium nitrate is administered slowly by the intravenous route and acts to oxidize hemoglobin (Fe^{++}) to methemoglobin (Fe^{+++}). Methemoglobin then combines with one cyanide molecule to form cyanmethemoglobin *(Stoelting: Pharmacology and Physiology, ed 2, pp 326-327).*

512. **(A)** Post-anesthetic tremor can occur during recovery from all types of general anesthesia. If profound, shivering can increase metabolic rate and O_2 consumption by up to 400 percent which may not be tolerated in patients with marginal cardiopulmonary function. It is believed that the shivering occurs as an attempt to generate heat in response to intraoperative hypothermia. However, although shivering usually occurs in patients with decreased body temperature, it may also occur in patients with normal body temperature after anesthesia. Postanesthesia shivering is best treated by rewarming the patient or the administration of intravenous meperidine. Other less frequently used pharmacologic treatments include magnesium sulphate, calcium chloride, chlorpromazine, droperidol, and other opioids. Application of radiant heat to the face, head, neck, chest, and abdomen has been shown to eliminate shivering within minutes in postoperative patients, despite low core body temperatures *(Rogers: Principles and Practice of Anesthesiology, p 2374).*

513. **(A)** The ECG signs of hyperkalemia include peaked T waves, prolonged PR interval, absence of P waves, and a widened QRS interval. In extreme cases, the ECG can actually appear as a sine wave. An increase in U-wave amplitude suggests hypokalemia not hyperkalemia *(Miller: Anesthesia, ed 4, p 1603).*

514. **(A)** Patients in whom pneumonectomy is contemplated must be evaluated to determine the prognosis after removal of lung tissue. A battery of initial tests is performed, and if it is determined that the patient does not meet any of these criteria, then split lung function tests are indicated.

The initial criteria include: 1) an FEV$_1$ of 2 liters or more and an FEV$_1$-FVC ratio greater than or equal to 50%, 2) a maximum breathing capacity greater than or equal to 50% of predicted, and 3) a residual volume to total lung capacity ratio less than 50%. Split function lung testing is carried out by balloon occlusion of the pulmonary artery of the lung which is to be removed. During temporary occlusion of this pulmonary artery if the P$_a$O$_2$ is less than 45 mm Hg or the mean pulmonary artery pressure is greater than 35 mm Hg, the patient is considered at high risk for pneumonectomy. By knowing the relative perfusion of each lung, the postoperative FEV$_1$ can be predicted and if it is calculated to be less than 0.8 liters, a bad outcome is predicted. Measurement of a patient's maximum oxygen uptake during exercise ($\dot{V}O_2$ max) has also been shown recently to be an accurate method for detecting postoperative morbidity with pneumonectomy. Patients with a $\dot{V}O_2$ max greater than 20 ml/kg/min have minimal morbidity whereas those with 15 ml/kg/min or less had increased cardiac and pulmonary complications. Patients who have $\dot{V}O_2$ max values less than 10 ml/kg/min have an extremely high risk of mortality from pneumonectomy *(Miller: Anesthesia, ed 4, p 899).*

515. **(A)** The vertical gradient in pleural pressure is an important determinant of alveolar ventilation. When the chest cavity is closed, gravity maintains this gradient such that alveolar ventilation is relatively increased in the dependent (lower) lung compared with the nondependent (upper) lung. General anesthesia causes a significant change in the distribution of ventilation between the two lungs because it affects the function of the chest wall such that the functional residual capacity is decreased. Opening the chest wall will influence the distribution of ventilation between the two lungs because it will expose the pleural space to atmospheric pressure, thereby eliminating the influence of the vertical gradient in pleural pressure on the distribution of alveolar ventilation. Paralysis and positive pressure ventilation also adversely affect this distribution. Application of PEEP to the dependent lung is beneficial because it increases ventilation to that lung which is well perfused thus improving the $\dot{V}Q$ relationship *(Miller: Anesthesia, ed 4, pp 1685-1689).*

516. **(E)** During spinal anesthesia, treatment of hypotension with fluids or vasopressors may often eliminate nausea. In some patients droperidol may also be effective in eliminating nausea, particularly if it is associated with opiate administration. In patients who are both nauseated and bradycardic, atropine may be useful in treating both of these. The sympathectomy associated with high spinal anesthesia will cause an imbalance in the autonomic innervation to the gastrointestinal tract. The parasympathetic limb of the autonomic nervous system acts unopposed on the gastrointestinal tract, resulting in increased activity that is frequently associated with nausea *(Barash: Clinical Anesthesia, ed 2, p 834).*

517. **(B)** The pulmonary vascular resistance depends on the collective influence of numerous metabolic, neural, hormonal and mechanical factors. Of the choices listed in the question, only positive end-expiratory pressure ventilation and hypoventilation (which causes hypercarbia, hypoxia, and acidosis) will increase pulmonary vascular resistance *(West: Respiratory Physiology, ed 3, p 110).*

518. **(A)** Other factors which may delay gastric emptying include pregnancy, high osmotic pressure, shock, myocardial infarction, diabetic autonomic neuropathy, drugs such as anticholinergics, and tricyclic antidepressants. Gastric emptying may be accelerated by gastric distention,

neostigmine, metoclopramide, and propranolol. Cigarette smoking accelerates gastric emptying as well *(Barash: Clinical Anesthesia, ed 2, pp 622-625)*.

519. (C) The absence of wheezing on physical examination and an eosinophil count < $50/mm^3$ suggests that the patient is not experiencing an acute exacerbation of asthma during the preoperative evaluation. Unless contraindicated, deep extubation of the trachea in asthmatic patients is desirable as it suppresses hyperactive airway reflexes and lessens the chance of acute bronchospasm. Cimetidine, an H_2 blocker, would theoretically worsen bronchospasm by antagonizing H_2-receptor-mediated bronchodilation and leaving the H_1-mediated bronchoconstriction unopposed. Although succinylcholine is thought to have histamine releasing properties, there is no evidence that it is associated with increased airway resistance in patients with asthma *(Stoelting: Anesthesia and Co-existing Disease, ed 3, pp 152-157)*.

520. (A) Arterial hypoxemia, cor pulmonale, and hypercarbia are early features of chronic bronchitis, but late features in patients with pulmonary emphysema. Dyspnea, however, is an early feature of pulmonary emphysema because of the increased work of breathing related to the loss of elastic recoil in the lungs *(Stoelting: Anesthesia and Co-existing Disease, ed 3, p 138)*.

521. (E) The anesthetic management of patients undergoing ophthalmologic surgery requires an understanding of the concepts that govern intraocular pressure. The normal range for intraocular pressure is from 12 to 20 mm Hg, reflecting the balance between the production rate of aqueous humor in the ciliary body and its elimination via the spaces of Fontana and the central canal of Schlemm at the iridocorneal angle. Intraocular pressure can be raised by any number of mechanisms. Drugs that produce mydriasis inhibit the elimination of aqueous humor by relaxing the ciliary muscles and closing the iridocorneal angle at the fontana spaces. Any maneuver, such as coughing or straining, that increases central venous pressure will also decrease the outflow of aqueous humor and raise intraocular pressure. Changes in choroidal blood volume (CBV) also have a significant effect on intraocular pressure. Choroidal blood flow is autoregulated over blood pressures in the physiologic range thus keeping intraocular stable. Sudden increases in systolic arterial pressure can cause a transient increase in CBV resulting in an increased intraocular pressure. Respiratory acidosis and hypercarbia also raise CBV and intraocular pressure. Likewise, hypoxia increases intraocular pressure by inducing choroidal vasodilation *(Miller: Anesthesia, ed 4, pp 2177-2178)*.

522. (B) Patients with pulmonary emphysema are at risk for developing respiratory failure in the postoperative period. Obviously every effort should be taken to avoid this complication. Humidification of inspired gases and avoidance of systemic dehydration prevent drying and inspissation of the secretions in the airway. Narcotics should be used judiciously in these patients because of the potential for postoperative respiratory depression. Because of the increased pulmonary compliance in patients with pulmonary emphysema, a slow respiratory rate is desirable *(Stoelting: Basics of Anesthesia, ed 3, pp 278-279)*.

523. (C) In an anesthetized, paralyzed, mechanically ventilated patient in the lateral decubitus position, the distribution of ventilation, but not perfusion, is altered such that ventilation is greatest in the nondependent lung and perfusion is greatest in the dependent lung. Thus, the degree of mismatching of ventilation and perfusion is adversely altered in both lungs such that the ventilation/perfusion ratio is high in the nondependent lung and low in the dependent lung *(Miller: Anesthesia, ed 4, pp 1685-1689)*.

524. **(A)** Pulmonary function tests, arterial blood gases on room air, lung volume measurement, and ventilation/perfusion scanning are all helpful in predicting the risk of postoperative pulmonary dysfunction following pneumonectomy *(Miller: Anesthesia, ed 3, p 1521)*.

525. **(A)** Pickwickian syndrome also known as obesity hypoventilation syndrome is a condition which occurs in roughly 8% of obese patients. The hallmark of this syndrome is hypoventilation, and patients affected by it may have a defect in the central control of respiration. Hypercarbia leads to pulmonary vasoconstriction and ultimately to pulmonary hypertension and right ventricular failure. Theoretically, one might think that anesthetic drugs because of their high lipid solubility, i.e. volatile anesthetics, opiates, and intravenous anesthetics, might be stored in fat and might lead to delayed awakening in Pickwickian's. This, however, is not born out in these patients and delayed awaking is not observed in these patients *(Stoelting: Basics of Anesthesia, ed 3, pp 326-327)*.

526. **(E)** Renal causes of oliguria are associated with a urine osmolality of < 350 mOsm/L, a fractional excretion of sodium > 2%, a urine creatinine/plasma creatinine ratio < 20, and a urine sodium concentration > 40 mEq/L *(Barash: Clinical Anesthesia, ed 2, p 1143)*.

Diagnostic Tests in Acute Oliguria

Test	Prerenal	Renal
Urinary osmolality (mOsm $\cdot$ kg^{-1})	>500	<350
Urine/plasma osmolality	>1.3	<1.1
Urine sodium (mEq $\cdot$ l^{-1})	<20	>40
Urine/plasma urea	>8	<3
Urine/plasma creatinine	>40	<20
FENa (%)*	<1	>2

*FENa = fractional excretion of sodium, calculated as

$$\frac{U/P_{NA}}{U/P_{Cr}} \times 100$$

where U = urinary concentration, P = plasma concentration, Na = sodium, and Cr = creatinine
(From: Barash PG, Cullen BF, Stoelting RK (eds): Clinical Anesthesia, ed 2. Philadelphia, JB Lippincott, 1992, p 1143.)

527. **(C)** Sickle-cell anemia is an inherited disease affecting approximately 0.3% to 1% of the black population in the U.S. Affected patients are homozygous for hemoglobin S such that 70% to 98% of the hemoglobin found in their RBCs is of the unstable S type, resulting in severe hemolytic anemia. Factors which favor the formation of sickle cells include arterial hypoxemia, acidosis, dehydration, and reductions in body temperature *(Stoelting: Anesthesia and Co-existing Disease, ed 3, pp 401-402)*.

528. **(E)**   The ocular hypertensive response to succinylcholine occurs regardless of the route of administration. Pretreatment with nondepolarizing neuromuscular blocking drugs reduces but does not reliably eliminate the increase in intraocular pressure associated with succinylcholine administration *(Stoelting: Basics of Anesthesia, ed 3, pp 343-344).*

529. **(D)**   Several metabolic derangements such as hypoxia, hypercarbia and acidosis lower the threshold for eliciting the oculocardiac reflex, and thus may cause persistent or recurrent episodes of bradydysrhythmias *(Stoelting: Basics of Anesthesia, ed 3, pp 343-344).*

530. **(C)**   The oculocardiac reflex is mediated by the 5th and 10th cranial nerves. The reflex is elicited by traction of the extraocular muscles and is fatiguable. Prophylactic administration of intramuscular atropine is not useful in preventing this reflex *(Barash: Clinical Anesthesia, ed 2, pp 2181-2182).*

531. **(A)**   Addison's disease is a type of hypoadrenocorticism which results from the destruction of the adrenal cortex. The manifestations of this disease are related to decreased levels in the hormones aldosterone and cortisol. Affected patients may present with hypotension, muscle fatigue, and weight loss. Decreased cortisol levels predispose the patient to hypoglycemia. Decreased mineralocorticoid levels lead to hyperkalemia and hyponatremia. These patients are at risk for circulatory collapse from any number of physiologically stressful events *(Stoelting: Anesthesia and Co-existing Disease, ed 3, p 361).*

532. **(E)**   Thyroid storm is a potentially life-threatening exacerbation of hyperthyroidism caused by the acute release of excessive amounts of thyroid hormones in to the circulation. All of the drugs listed should be used to treat specific manifestations of thyroid storm. Sodium iodide acutely reduces the release of physiologically active hormones from the thyroid gland *(Stoelting: Anesthesia and Co-existing Disease, ed 3, p 349).*

533. **(E)**   Mannitol and furosemide promote diuresis. Fresh-frozen plasma contains haptoglobin, which binds to free hemoglobin and reduces the amount of the hemoglobin excreted by the kidneys. Alkalinization of the urine promotes renal excretion of hemoglobin *(Davison: Clinical Anesthesia Procedures of the Massachusetts General Hospital, ed 4, p 329).*

534. **(E)**   Retinopathy of prematurity is a hazard associated with O_2 administration to neonates, particularly those with a birth weight < 1,500 g and a gestational age < 44 weeks. CO_2 retention is a hazard in patients with chronic obstructive lung disease. Bronchopulmonary dysplasia is a disorder which afflicts infants who have required mechanical ventilation at birth to treat respiratory distress syndrome. Adsorption atelectasis is a potential hazard of oxygen administration in any patient receiving concentrations > 50%. It results from rapid uptake of oxygen greater than the delivery of oxygen by ventilation. Normally, the presence of nitrogen serves as an internal splint protecting the alveoli from collapse *(Stoelting: Basics of Anesthesia, ed 3, pp 388-389).*

535. **(B)**   Intrathecal opiates bind to receptors in the substantia gelatinosa of the spinal cord producing analgesia. For example, a single dose of morphine (0.5 to 1 mg) injected intrathecally into an adult may produce analgesia for up to 20 hours. Unlike local anesthetics, intrathecal opiates do not produce a sympathectomy and are therefore not associated with orthostatic hypotension. Analgesia produced by intrathecal opiates is specific for visceral rather than somatic pain. The

more lipid-soluble opiates such as fentanyl and meperidine have a decreased incidence of delayed respiratory depression compared with morphine *(Stoelting: Pharmacology & Physiology, ed 2, p 73)*.

536. **(B)** Although renal function declines with increasing age, serum creatinine does not change because there is also a decrease in muscle mass. Hepatic production of albumin is decreased resulting in a decreased serum albumin concentration which may have an impact on the plasma protein binding of some drugs. Older adults who maintain an active lifestyle and remain physically fit are likely to have a normal cardiac output *(Stoelting: Basics of Anesthesia, ed 3, pp 396-397)*.

537. **(E)** The decision to stop mechanical support of the lungs is based on a variety of factors which can be measured. Guidelines which suggest that cessation of mechanical inflation of the lungs is likely to be successful include a vital capacity > 15 mL/kg, arterial P_aO_2 > 60 mm Hg (F_IO_2 below 0.5), A-a gradient < 350 mm Hg (F_IO_2 = 1.0), arterial pH > 7.3, P_aCO_2 < 50 mm Hg, dead space/tidal volume ratio < 0.6, and a maximum inspiratory pressure > -20 cm H_2O. In addition to these, the patient should be hemodynamically stable, conscious and oriented, and in good nutritional status *(Stoelting: Basics of Anesthesia, ed 3, p 463)*.

538. **(D)** Drugs and events that increase cardiac contractility should be avoided in patients with asymmetric septal hypertrophy because they increase the obstruction to left ventricular outflow. Tachycardia, afterload reduction, and digitalis should be avoided. Increasing preload is of benefit *(Stoelting: Anesthesia and Co-existing Disease, ed 3, p 99)*.

539. **(B)** Radiographic changes consistent with chronic obstructive pulmonary disease include decreased radiolucency because of decreased pulmonary blood flow and hyperinflated lungs with a flattened diaphragm. Heart size is reduced unless pulmonary hypertension has caused right ventricular enlargement. Notching along the lower border of the ribs is seen in patients with coarctation of the aorta *(Stoelting: Anesthesia and Co-existing Disease, ed 3, p 138)*.

540. **(A)** This patient is beginning to show some of the signs of TURP syndrome. There are a number of potential causes of hypokalemia in this patient. Volume overload by virtue of dilution is capable of reducing the plasma potassium concentration. Use of ß$_2$-stimulating drugs also results in reduction of the serum potassium concentration by driving potassium intracellularly. Lastly, hyperventilation leads to respiratory alkalosis. This too will cause the intracellular migration of potassium and result in an overall decreased serum concentration. Aminophylline has no effect on serum potassium concentration *(Barash: Clinical Anesthesia, ed 2, p 221; Stoelting: Pharmacology and Physiology, ed 2, pp 308-309)*.

541. **(D)** Short-term abstinence from cigarette smoking results in restoration of the P_{50} to its normal value of 26 mm Hg. Other benefits require longer periods of abstinence (i.e., weeks) *(Stoelting: Anesthesia and Co-existing Disease, ed 3, pp 140-141)*.

542. **(C)** Succinylcholine should be avoided in patients with multiple sclerosis because of the significant risk of hyperkalemia. Although the mechanism is not known, spinal anesthesia has been implicated in postoperative exacerbations of multiple sclerosis. Lumbar epidural anesthesia can be used safely in these patients *(Stoelting: Anesthesia and Co-existing Disease, ed 3, p 217)*.

543. **(A)** Succinylcholine increases intraocular pressure, which peaks 2 to 4 minutes after administration. Scopolamine produces mydriasis and thus should be avoided in these patients. Hypercarbia and increased CVP also increase intraocular pressure *(Miller: Anesthesia, ed 4, pp 2177-2178).*

544. **(B)** Patients with hypothyroidism are at increased risk for congestive heart failure during general anesthesia. Impaired renal excretion of free water can lead to edema and hyponatremia. Thus, 5% dextrose in water is a poor choice for fluid maintenance during surgery. Thyroid function has no effect on anesthetic requirement *(Stoelting: Anesthesia and Co-existing Disease, ed 3, pp 352-354).*

545. **(A)** Hepatic perfusion pressure is equal to hepatic vein pressure minus portal pressure or hepatic vein pressure minus mean hepatic artery pressure. Any factor that raises hepatic vein pressure (e.g., positive pressure) or lowers mean arterial pressure (e.g., spinal or general anesthesia) will lower perfusion pressure and hepatic flow. Hyperventilation lowers splanchnic vascular resistance and improves hepatic flow *(Stoelting: Anesthesia and Co-existing Disease, ed 3, p 253).*

546. **(A)** Severe autonomic neuropathy can affect the autonomic nervous system to such an extent that atropine and propranolol would have little effect (since there would be nothing to block). After heart transplantation, the new heart (donor heart) is denervated and will not respond to autonomic nervous system blocking drugs. Brain death is associated with absence of autonomic function by definition. A high spinal would be associated with total sympathectomy and propranolol would have no effect on heart rate, but the vagus nerve would be unaffected *(Stoelting: Anesthesia and Co-existing Disease, ed 3, pp 342-343; Miller: Anesthesia, ed 4, pp 568-570 & 1487; Rogers: Principles and Practice of Anesthesiology, p 1477; Kaplan: Cardiac Anesthesia, ed 3, p 1188).*

547. **(E)** Drugs considered unsafe for patients susceptible to malignant hyperthermia include all the volatile anesthetics and the depolarizing muscle relaxants, succinylcholine and decamethonium. All local anesthetics (both amide and ester), N_2O, opiates, barbiturates, and the nondepolarizing muscle relaxants except curare are unquestionably safe (i.e., nontriggering) in patients susceptible to malignant hyperthermia. Curare, because it is a weak depolarizer, is controversial and is probably best avoided in these patients in view of the numerous other nondepolarizing muscle relaxants available *(Barash: Clinical Anesthesia, ed 2, pp 592-593; Miller: Anesthesia, ed 4, pp 1084-85).*

548. **(E)** Metabolic derangements associated with acute diabetic ketoacidosis include hyperglycemia and glycosuria leading to dehydration and loss of Na^+, K^+, and Cl^- in the urine. Therapy consists of rehydration with normal saline, replacement of K^+, and treatment of acidosis with HCO_3^-. Even a small dose of insulin will stop production of ketoacids *(Stoelting: Anesthesia and Co-existing Disease, ed 3, p 341).*

549. **(E)** Rheumatoid arthritis is a systemic disease which affects many organs. In addition to the items listed in this question, other organ involvement may include pericardial effusion, myocarditis, conduction disturbances, restrictive lung disease, cervical nerve root compression, and mononeuritis multiplex *(Stoelting: Anesthesia and Co-existing Disease, ed 3, pp 446-448).*

550. **(D)** The two most important compensatory mechanisms for chronic anemia are 1) a rightward shift in the oxyhemoglobin dissociation curve and 2) an increase in cardiac output. When elective surgery is performed in the presence of chronic anemia, steps should be taken to minimize factors that could interfere with adequate tissue O_2 delivery. For example, leftward shifts in the oxyhemoglobin dissociation curve, as may occur during hyperventilation of the lungs (which causes respiratory alkalosis) or hypothermia, can reduce tissue O_2 delivery. A leftward shift in the oxyhemoglobin dissociation curve impairs the release of O_2 from hemoglobin to tissues. Shivering or hyperthermia should be avoided in patients with chronic anemia, since these can greatly increase total body O_2 requirement. An interesting observation is that volatile anesthetics may be less soluble in blood deficient in lipid-rich erythrocytes. Consequently, the rate of increase in the arterial anesthetic partial pressure may be accelerated in anemic patients *(Stoelting: Anesthesia and Co-existing Disease, ed 3, pp 393-395)*.

551. **(E)** Successful treatment of malignant hyperthermia depends on early recognition of the syndrome and institution of a preplanned therapeutic regimen. Although there are a number of symptomatic therapies which should be implemented to maintain renal function and correct the metabolic derangements (e.g., hyperthermia, acidosis, and arterial hypoxemia), the most effective treatment for malignant hyperthermia is administration of dantrolene 1 to 2 mg/kg IV. This dose should be repeated every 5 to 10 minutes to a maximum dose of 10 mg/kg. Dantrolene should be continued in the postoperative period to prevent possible recurrence of malignant hyperthermia. Although the site of action of dantrolene is not clear, it is thought to inhibit excitation/contraction of skeletal muscle by reducing calcium release from the sarcoplasmic reticulum. Symptomatic treatments for malignant hyperthermia include termination of the volatile anesthetic and surgical procedure, hyperventilation of the patient's lungs with 100% O_2, and active cooling of the patient. Other symptomatic therapies should include hydration with a balanced salt solution and administration of osmotic or loop diuretics to maintain urine output at 1 to 2 mL/kg/hour, administration of HCO_3^- to correct metabolic acidosis, and administration of antidysrhythmic agents, such as procainamide, for the treatment of ventricular dysrhythmias *(Stoelting: Anesthesia and Co-existing Disease, ed 3, pp 611-613)*.

552. **(D)** The physiologic response to drugs is altered significantly by burn injuries. In the initial period after a burn the patient is hypovolemic from fluid loss and third spacing. Additionally, decreased myocardial function and release of vasoactive substances results to decreased tissue perfusion to most organs with sparing of the brain and the heart. For these reasons, administration of drugs by any route other than intravenously may result in a decreased onset of action. At approximately 48 hours post-burn after fluid resuscitation, the hypermetabolic phase begins. This period is heralded by an increase in glucose utilization and oxygen consumption. In the post-burn period, plasma albumen concentrations are decreased whereas the plasma concentration of alpha-1 glycoprotein is increased. Accordingly, drugs bound to albumen such as benzodiazepines (e.g., midazolam) and anticonvulsants will have an increased free fraction. On the other hand, drugs bound to alpha-1 acid glycoprotein such as tricyclic antidepressants and muscle relaxants will have a decreased free fraction. An additional reason for the increased requirement for muscle relaxants is the extrajunctional proliferation of cholinergic receptors on the muscles. The requirement for opiates in burn patients may also be increased. In children, it has been observed that the thiopental requirements may be increased for up to a year after the burn injury *(Stoelting: Anesthesia and Co-existing Disease, ed 3, p 624)*.

553. **(A)** Calcium levels greater than 16 mg/dl may be life-threatening and are therefore a medical emergency. Treatment for hypercalcemia includes saline diuresis with furosemide, not thiazides, because the latter may actually increase the plasma calcium concentrations. Other therapy may include salmon calcitonin 4 IU/kg SQ every 12 hours, mithramycin, and corticosteroids. *(Stoelting: Anesthesia and Co-Existing Disease, ed 3, p 356; Rogers: Principles and Practice of Anesthesiology, p 285).*

554. **(E)** The history described in this question is consistent with Reye's syndrome. Reye's syndrome is characterized by fatty infiltration of viscera (particularly the liver), cerebral edema, and intracranial hypertension, which may result in brain infarction and herniation, and death. Reye's syndrome usually begins with symptoms consistent with an upper respiratory tract viral illness. These symptoms then give way to vomiting and other signs and symptoms associated with intracranial hypertension. Interestingly, there appears to be an association between the use of salicylates during the prodromal respiratory viral illness and the development of Reye's syndrome. Treatment for Reye's syndrome is directed primarily toward reversing associated metabolic derangements (which results from hepatic failure), monitoring and reducing intracranial pressure (e.g., osmotic diuretics, hyperventilation), and nutritional support until natural resolution of the disease process occurs *(Stoelting: Anesthesia and Co-existing Disease, ed 3, pp 603-604).*

555. **(D)** 556. **(C)** 557. **(D)** 558. **(C)** 559. **(C)** 560. **(A)** Pulmonary function tests can be used to classify patients with chronic pulmonary disease into those with obstructive airway diseases and those with restrictive pulmonary diseases. Bronchial asthma, pulmonary emphysema, and chronic bronchitis are examples of obstructive airway disease. In the presence of obstructive airway disease, the FEV_1 is < 80% of the FVC, and the total lung capacity and functional residual capacity are increased; in the presence of restrictive pulmonary disease, the FEV_1 is normal or > 80% of the FVC, and the total lung capacity, functional residual capacity, and total pulmonary compliance are reduced. In patients with pulmonary emphysema, the lung compliance is increased because the elastic recoil of the lungs is decreased *(Stoelting: Basics of Anesthesia, ed 3, pp 278-280).*

561. **(A)** 562. **(B)** 563. **(C)** 564. **(D)** Injury to peripheral nerves results primarily from stretching or compression of the nerves, which ultimately leads to ischemia of the intraneural vasa nervosum. Peripheral nerve injuries in the lower extremity most often occur when patients are placed improperly into the lithotomy position. Proper padding between the metal leg braces and positioning of the legs will limit the occurrence of these injuries. The sciatic nerve provides motor function for all the skeletal muscles below the knees, and sensory innervation for the lateral half of the leg and most of the foot. The common peroneal nerve, which is a branch of the sciatic nerve, provides motor function to the skeletal muscles that dorsiflex and evert the foot, and extend the toes. Injury to the femoral nerve will manifest in paresis of the quadriceps femoris muscle. The inability to adduct the leg and thigh are clinical manifestations consistent with damage to the obturator nerve *(Stoelting: Basics of Anesthesia, ed 3, pp 198-199).*

565. **(D)** 566. **(C)** The likelihood for reinfarction during the perioperative period, if the operation is carried out < 3 months after the acute infarction, is 37%. If the time interval is 3 to 6 months after the acute infarction, the chance of reinfarction is 16% *(Stoelting: Anesthesia and Co-existing Disease, ed 3, pp 4-5).*

Pediatric Physiology and Anesthesia

DIRECTIONS (Questions 567 through 604): Each of the questions or incomplete statements in this section is followed by answers or by completions of the statement, respectively. Select the ONE BEST answer or completion for each item.

567. A 6-year-old child who has sustained a severe thermal injury to the face, upper extremities, and chest is brought to the emergency room. On examination, the child has singed nasal hairs and soot in the oropharynx, is hoarse, has inspiratory and expiratory stridor, and is tachypneic. Which of the following would be the most appropriate management of this child's respiratory condition?

    A. O_2 supplementation with a nasal cannula
    B. Nasotracheal suction to remove debris in the upper airway
    C. Administer 100% O_2 by closed face mask
    D. Immediate direct laryngoscopy and tracheal intubation
    E. Emergency cricothyrotomy

568. In the newborn the cricoid cartilage is at which level relative to the cervical spine?

    A. C-3
    B. C-4
    C. C-5
    D. C-6
    E. C-7

569. A 5-month-old infant is scheduled for operative reduction of a right inguinal hernia. Spinal anesthesia is performed. The first sign of a high spinal in this patient would be

    A. Hypotension
    B. Tachycardia
    C. Hypoxia
    D. Bradycardia
    E. Asystole

570. What percent of an infant's total body weight consists of water?

    A. 20%
    B. 40%
    C. 60%
    D. 75%
    E. 90%

571. What is the maximum F_IO_2 that can be administered to the mother without increasing the risk of retinopathy of prematurity in utero?

    A. 0.35
    B. 0.50
    C. 0.65
    D. 0.80
    E. 1.0

572. Which of the following patients is **LEAST** likely to develop retinopathy of prematurity?

    A. A term infant, 51 weeks postconceptual age, exposed to an F_IO_2 of 60% for 4 hours
    B. A premature infant 29 weeks postconceptual age exposed to a P_aO_2 of 150 mm Hg for 1 hour
    C. A premature infant 28 weeks postconceptual age never exposed to supplemental oxygen
    D. An infant with tetralogy of Fallot 34 weeks postconceptual age with a P_aO_2 50 mm Hg receiving an F_IO_2 of 50% by endotracheal tube
    E. A term infant receiving 100% oxygen for 6 hours after birth

573. A 5-week-old male infant is brought to the emergency room with projectile vomiting. At the time of admission the patient is lethargic with a respiratory rate of 12/minute and has had no urine output in the preceding 3 hours. A diagnosis of pyloric stenosis is made and the patient is brought to the operating room for pyloromyotomy. The most appropriate anesthetic management would be

    A. Induction with IM ketamine, glycopyrrolate, and succinylcholine with cricoid pressure followed by immediate intubation
    B. Inhalation induction with halothane with cricoid pressure
    C. Awake intubation
    D. Awake saphenous IV followed by rapid sequence induction with ketamine, atropine, and succinylcholine
    E. Postpone surgery

574. Which of the following is the most common type of tracheoesophageal fistula?

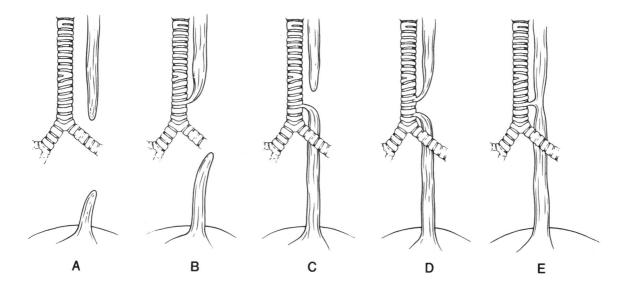

A   B   C   D   E

575. A 4-year-old boy is scheduled for completion of a hypospadias repair. The child has a history of a viral illness with a cough 2 weeks prior to surgery which has resolved. Anesthesia is induced with halothane and nitrous oxide. During induction the patient's rhythm changes from normal sinus rhythm to ventricular tachycardia. No pulse is palpable. The most likely explanation for this patient's heart rhythm is

   A. Undiagnosed viral myocarditis
   B. Hypoxia
   C. Halothane irritability
   D. Hyperkalemia
   E. Undiagnosed Wolff-Parkinson-White syndrome

576. Preterm neonates are at an increased risk for retinopathy of prematurity until what postconceptual age?

   A. 36 weeks
   B. 38 weeks
   C. 42 weeks
   D. 44 weeks
   E. 60 weeks

577. Cuffed endotracheal tubes are not indicated in children younger than

   A. 3 years of age
   B. 5 years of age
   C. 10 years of age
   D. 12 years of age
   E. 15 years of age

578. A 4-year-old otherwise healthy male patient is undergoing elective tonsillectomy. Prior to induction of general anesthesia the patient is breathing at a rate of 20. An inhalation induction is begun with halothane and nitrous oxide and 60 seconds later the patient is noted to breathe at 40/minute. This rapid respiratory rate most likely represents

   A. Hypoxia
   B. Hypercarbia
   C. The excitement stage of anesthesia
   D. Malignant hyperthermia
   E. Pulmonary embolism

579. A healthy 1-month-old neonate is anesthetized for an inguinal hernia repair. An inhalation induction with halothane is carried out and the patient is intubated. Prior to making the surgical incision, the blood pressure is noted to be 60 mm Hg systolic. Heart rate is 120 beats/minute. The most appropriate intervention for this patient's blood pressure would be

   A. Administration of ephedrine
   B. Administration of phenylephrine
   C. 50 cc fluid bolus
   D. Administration of epinephrine
   E. None of the above

580. A 5-year-old male is anesthetized for elective repair of an umbilical hernia. General anesthesia is induced and maintained with halothane and nitrous oxide via an anesthesia mask. At the conclusion of the operation the patient is taken to the recovery room and subsequently discharged to the outpatient ward. Prior to discharge, the patient's urine is noted to be dark brown. The most appropriate action at this time would be

A. Discharge the patient with instructions to return if urine color does not normalize
B. Discharge the patient in 3 hours if no other signs or symptoms are manifested
C. Obtain a serum creatinine and BUN and discharge the patient if these are normal
D. Admit the patient to rule out acute tubular necrosis
E. Work patient up for malignant hyperthermia

581. At what inspiratory pressure should an uncuffed endotracheal tube leak in an infant?

A. Less than 20 cm H_2O
B. 20 to 30 cm H_2O
C. 30 to 40 cm H_2O
D. 40 to 50 cm H_2O
E. No leak necessary

582. A premature newborn delivered at 32 weeks gestation is brought to the operating room for repair of a left-sided congenital diaphragmatic hernia. After awake tracheal intubation, general anesthesia is maintained with halothane, O_2, and fentanyl. Shortly thereafter the anesthesiologist notes difficulty with ventilation. The S_aO_2 subsequently falls to 65% and the heart rate decreases to 50 beats/min. What would be the most appropriate step to take at this time?

A. Pull the endotracheal tube from the right mainstem bronchus
B. Ventilate with PEEP and administer furosemide
C. Pass an oral gastric tube to decompress the stomach
D. Place a chest tube on the right side
E. Reintubate the patient

583. Symptoms of infantile pyloric stenosis occur most frequently between the ages of

A. 1 and 2 weeks
B. 2 and 6 weeks
C. 6 and 12 weeks
D. 3 and 6 months
E. 6 and 12 months

584. In a 12-year-old child, the length of an oral endotracheal tube (from the lips to the mid trachea) should be

A. 12 cm
B. 14 cm
C. 16 cm
D. 18 cm
E. 20 cm

585. In which of the following conditions would a preoperative evaluation of the heart with echocardiogram be indicated prior to anesthesia and surgery?

    A. Necrotizing enterocolitis
    B. Pyloric stenosis
    C. Gastroschisis
    D. Imperforate anus
    E. Hypospadias

586. A 14-day-old otherwise healthy neonate is transported to the operating room well hydrated for surgery for a bowel obstruction. A rapid sequence induction is planned. Compared with the adult dose, the dose of succinylcholine administered to this patient should be

    A. Diminished because of the immature nervous system
    B. The same as the adult dose
    C. Increased because of increased acetylcholine receptors
    D. Decreased because of decreased acetylcholine receptors
    E. Increased because of a greater volume of distribution

587. The most common cause of gastrointestinal obstruction in children is

    A. Intussusception
    B. Infantile pyloric stenosis
    C. Duodenal atresia
    D. Congenital aganglionic megacolon
    E. Imperforate anus

588. A 10-week-old infant born at 31 weeks' gestation is anesthetized for repair of an inguinal hernia. General anesthesia is induced by mask with halothane, an endotracheal tube is placed, and anesthesia is maintained with isoflurane, O_2, and N_2O. At the end of the procedure the endotracheal tube is removed and the patient is transported to the recovery room. What is the best postoperative management of this patient?

    A. Ilioinguinal-iliohypogastric nerve block and discharge home with instruction to parents
    B. Caudal block with 0.25% bupivacaine, 1 mL/kg, and admit to a pediatric ward for overnight observation
    C. Caudal block with 0.25% bupivacaine, 2 mL/kg, and admit to a pediatric ward for overnight observation
    D. Oral pain medication and discharge home with instructions to the parent
    E. Fentanyl, 1 cc IV, and admit to a pediatric ward for overnight observation

589. A 6-year-old 20-kg girl develops ventricular fibrillation after induction with halothane for tonsillectomy. An endotracheal tube is placed immediately and position is confirmed. The defibrillator should be charged to what energy level for the initial shock?

    A. 40 joules
    B. 60 joules
    C. 80 joules
    D. 100 joules
    E. 150 joules

590. The spinal cord of neonates extends to the

    A. T12/L1 vertebra
    B. L2 vertebra
    C. L3 vertebra
    D. L5 vertebra
    E. S1 vertebra

591. The most common initial symptom of esophageal atresia and tracheoesophageal fistula is

    A. Respiratory distress at delivery
    B. Failure to thrive
    C. Hypoxia
    D. Respiratory distress during feeding
    E. Projectile vomiting

592. A 3-hour-old preterm newborn with microcephaly is scheduled for surgical repair of an omphalocele. Physical examination reveals macroglossia but no other anomalies are found. Which of the following is likely to occur in this patient?

    A. Hypokalemia
    B. Hyperkalemia
    C. Metabolic acidosis
    D. Hypoxemia
    E. Hypoglycemia

593. Which of the following is the **LEAST** appropriate technique for induction of general anesthesia in a newborn for surgical repair of tracheoesophageal fistula?

    A. Awake tracheal intubation
    B. Inhalation induction and tracheal intubation
    C. Inhalation induction using mask-and-bag positive-pressure ventilation and tracheal intubation
    D. Rapid intravenous induction and tracheal intubation
    E. Intramuscular induction with high-dose ketamine and tracheal intubation

594. Each of the following statements concerning side effects of succinylcholine when used to paralyze neonates is true **EXCEPT**

    A. It seldom causes muscle fasciculation
    B. It can cause bradycardia
    C. Dysrhythmias frequently occur following intramuscular injections
    D. It can cause myoglobinuria
    E. It can cause myalgias

595. The predicted blood volume in a 4-kg neonate is

    A. 190 mL
    B. 280 mL
    C. 320 mL
    D. 420 mL
    E. 500 mL

596.   The pulmonary vascular resistance in newborns decreases to that of adults by

    A.   1 week of age
    B.   1 month of age
    C.   1 year of age
    D.   3 years of age
    E.   5 years of age

597.   A 10-month-old infant is undergoing elective repair of a left testicular hydrocele under general anesthesia with isoflurane, N_2O, and fentanyl. All of following are effective means of preventing hypothermia in this patient **EXCEPT**

    A.   Placement of an infrared heater over the operating table and prewarming the operating room
    B.   Covering the operating room table with a heating blanket
    C.   Wrapping the extremities with sheet wadding and covering the head with a cloth cap
    D.   Ventilating the patient with a Mapleson D circuit at low gas flows
    E.   Warming and humidifying the inspired anesthetic gases

598.   Central postoperative depression of ventilation in a full-term neonate is most likely to occur after surgery for which of the following?

    A.   Gastroschisis
    B.   Omphalocele
    C.   Tracheoesophageal fistula
    D.   Diaphragmatic hernia
    E.   Pyloric stenosis

599.   A premature male neonate born at 32 weeks' gestation is scheduled to undergo emergency repair of a left-sided diaphragmatic hernia. Which of the following vessels could be cannulated for preductal arterial blood sampling?

    A.   Femoral artery
    B.   Umbilical artery
    C.   Dorsalis pedis artery
    D.   Right radial artery
    E.   Left radial artery

600.   In which of the following patients would the minimum alveolar concentration for halothane be the greatest?

    A.   A premature infant-30 weeks postconceptual age
    B.   Full-term neonate
    C.   3-month-old infant
    D.   19-year-old male body builder
    E.   35-year-old woman with hyperthyroidism

601. A 40-kg, 10-year-old child sustains a thermal injury to his legs, buttocks, and back. The estimated area involved is 50%. How much fluid should be administered during the first 24 hours?

    A. 2.5 L
    B. 4.0 L
    C. 5.5 L
    D. 8.0 L
    E. 10.0 L

602. An otherwise healthy 3-month-old black female infant with a hemoglobin of 19 mg/dL at birth presents for elective repair of an inguinal hernia. Her preoperative hemoglobin is 10 mg/dL. Her father has a history of polycystic kidney disease. The most likely explanation for this patient's anemia is

    A. Sickle cell trait
    B. Sickle cell anemia
    C. Iron deficiency
    D. Undiagnosed polycystic kidney disease
    E. It is a normal finding

603. The anesthesiologist is called to the emergency room by the pediatrician to help manage a 3-year-old boy with a high fever and upper airway obstruction. His mother states that earlier that afternoon he complained of a sore throat and hoarseness. The patient is sitting erect and leaning forward, has inspiratory stridor, tachypnea, and sternal retractions, and is drooling. Which of the following is the most appropriate management of airway obstruction in this patient?

    A. Aerosolized racemic epinephrine
    B. Awake tracheal intubation in the emergency room
    C. Transfer to the operating room and awake tracheal intubation
    D. Transfer to the operating room, inhalation induction, and tracheal intubation
    E. Transfer to the operating room, inhalation induction, paralysis with succinylcholine, and tracheal intubation

604. A 2-year-old child with cerebral palsy with known gastroesophageal reflux is scheduled to undergo iliopsoas release under general anesthesia. Which of the following would be the most appropriate technique for inducing general anesthesia in this patient?

    A. Inhalation induction with halothane followed by mask anesthesia with cricoid pressure
    B. Inhalation induction with halothane followed by tracheal intubation
    C. Intravenous induction with thiopental followed by laryngeal mask airway
    D. Intravenous induction with thiopental followed by tracheal intubation
    E. Rapid-sequence induction with thiopental and succinylcholine followed by tracheal intubation

605. A 7-week-old male infant is admitted to the peds ICU with a bowel obstruction. His laboratory values are sodium, 120 mEq/L; chloride, 85 mEq/L; glucose, 85 mg/dL; and potassium, 2.0 mEq/L. Respiratory rate is 10/minute and urine output according to the patient's mother has been 0 for the last four hours. The most appropriate fluid for resuscitation of this patient would be

   A. D5W
   B. D5W with 0.45 sodium chloride and 20 mEq/L potassium chloride
   C. 0.45% sodium chloride
   D. 0.9% sodium chloride with 30 mEq/L potassium chloride
   E. 0.9% sodium chloride

606. An 8-hour-old 2,200 gram neonate, 30 weeks postgestational age, is noted in the ICU to begin making twitching movements. Blood pressure is 45 mm Hg systolic, blood glucose 50 mg/dL, and urine output 10 cc/hr. An O_2 sat on pulse oximeter is 88%. The most appropriate course of action to take at this point would be

   A. Administer calcium gluconate 250 mg (2.5 cc of 10% solution)
   B. Glucose 10 mg IV over 5 minutes (2 cc of D5W)
   C. Hyperventilate with 100% O_2
   D. Administer a 20 cc bolus of 5% albumen
   E. Begin a dopamine infusion

607. EMLA (Eutectic Mixture of Local Anesthetics) creme is a mixture of which local anesthetics?

   A. Lidocaine and prilocaine
   B. Lidocaine and benzocaine
   C. Prilocaine and benzocaine
   D. Ropivacaine and benzocaine
   E. Prilocaine, benzocaine, lidocaine

DIRECTIONS (Questions 608 through 639): For each of the items in this section, ONE or MORE of the numbered options is correct. Select the answer:

Select A if options *1, 2 and 3* are correct,
Select B if options *1 and 3* are correct,
Select C if options *2 and 4* are correct,
Select D if only option *4* is correct,
Select E if *all* options are correct.

608. Advantages of catheterization of the umbilical artery versus the umbilical vein in a newborn include

   1. It allows assessment of oxygenation
   2. Hepatic damage from hypertonic infusion is avoided
   3. It permits assessment of systemic blood pressure
   4. It is easier to cannulate

Select A if options *1, 2 and 3* are correct,
Select B if options *1 and 3* are correct,
Select C if options *2 and 4* are correct,
Select D if only option *4* is correct,
Select E if *all* options are correct.

609. True statements concerning thermoregulation in neonates include which of the following?

    1. A significant proportion of their heat loss can be accounted for by their small surface-to-volume ratio
    2. Heat loss through conduction can be reduced by humidification of inspired gases
    3. They compensate for hypothermia by shivering
    4. The principal method of heat production is metabolism of brown fat

610. Normal values for a healthy 6-month-old, 7-kg infant include

    1. Hemoglobin 17 gm/dL
    2. Heart rate 72 beats/min
    3. Respiratory rate 20 breaths/min
    4. O_2 consumption at rest 35 mL/min

611. A 5-year-old child undergoing strabismus surgery under general anesthesia suddenly develops sinus bradycardia and intermittent ventricular escape beats, but is hemodynamically stable. Which therapy is appropriate for treating this dysrhythmia?

    1. Administer atropine
    2. Infiltrate the recti with lidocaine
    3. Ask the surgeon to stop pressing on the eye
    4. Turn off the volatile anesthetic

612. Which of the following respiratory indices is decreased in neonates compared to adults?

    1. Tidal volume
    2. Arterial pH
    3. O_2 consumption
    4. Functional residual capacity

613. A 14-year-old girl with neurofibromatosis is anesthetized for resection of an acoustic neuroma. Which of the following may potentially complicate the anesthetic management of this patient?

    1. The presence of a pheochromocytoma
    2. Upper airway obstruction from a laryngeal neurofibroma
    3. Intracranial hypertension
    4. Increased risk for malignant hyperthermia

Select A if options *1, 2 and 3* are correct,
Select B if options *1 and 3* are correct,
Select C if options *2 and 4* are correct,
Select D if only option *4* is correct,
Select E if *all* options are correct.

614. Retinopathy of prematurity

    1. Occurs only after exposure to high concentrations of O_2 for 12 or more hours
    2. Cannot occur in patients who have never received supplemental O_2
    3. Is caused by obliteration of immature retinal arteries
    4. Is most commonly seen in neonates < 44 weeks postconceptual age

615. Indices of renal function that are decreased in healthy infants compared with adults include?

    1. Glomerular filtration rate
    2. Ability to concentrate urine
    3. Urea clearance
    4. Reabsorption of HCO_3^-

616. The precipitous decrease in pulmonary vascular resistance that occurs in newborns immediately following birth result from which of the following?

    1. Expansion of the lungs during inspiration
    2. Decreased arterial pH
    3. Improved alveolar oxygenation
    4. Closure of the foramen ovale

617. Blood gas samples from an umbilical venous catheter placed into a 32-week gestational age newborn breathing room air reveal a PO_2 of 60 mm Hg. Possible explanations for this value include

    1. The tip of the catheter is in the left ventricle
    2. The catheter has been inadvertently placed into the umbilical artery
    3. The tip of the catheter is in the left atrium
    4. It is a normal umbilical venous blood gas value in a newborn

618. Variables that are greater in healthy full-term neonates than in adults (per kilogram body weight) include

    1. Functional residual capacity
    2. Blood volume (per kilogram)
    3. Tidal volume
    4. Heart rate

619. Signs and symptoms consistent with acute epiglottis include

    1. Gradual onset
    2. Drooling
    3. Age < 2 years
    4. Leaning forward

Select A if options *1, 2 and 3* are correct,
Select B if options *1 and 3* are correct,
Select C if options *2 and 4* are correct,
Select D if only option *4* is correct,
Select E if *all* options are correct.

620. Correct techniques for resuscitation of a 6-month-old include

    1. Mouth-to-mouth and nose ventilation
    2. Chest compressions with 2 fingers on the sternum
    3. Sternal compression rate of at least 100/minute
    4. Blind finger sweep for aspirated foreign body is patient is unconscious

621. True statements concerning metabolism in infants compared with that in adults include which of the following?

    1. A smaller percentage of the cardiac output is distributed to the vessel-rich tissue group
    2. A greater percentage of total body water is extracellular
    3. Infants are less sensitive to thiopental
    4. By 1 year of age the glomerular filtration rate (per square meter of body surface area) is equal to that of an adult

622. True statements concerning the anatomy of the infant airway compared with the adult airway include which of the following?

    1. The cricoid cartilage is the narrowest part of the larynx in infants, whereas the vocal cords are the narrowest part of the larynx in adults
    2. The epiglottis is stiffer in infants than in adults
    3. The glottic opening is more anterior in infants than in adults
    4. The cricoid ring is in a more horizontal position within the larynx in infants than in adults

623. A 4-week-old infant with infantile pyloric stenosis is scheduled to undergo general anesthesia for pyloroplasty. **Initial** steps to correct the fluid and electrolyte abnormalities commonly associated with this condition should include

    1. Intravenous infusion of sodium bicarbonate
    2. Intravenous infusion of potassium chloride
    3. Hydration with lactated ringers solution
    4. Hydration with normal saline

624. Anomalies and features associated with Down's syndrome include

    1. Endocardial cushion defect
    2. Thyroid hypofunction
    3. Large tongue
    4. Atlanto-occipital instability

Select A if options *1, 2 and 3* are correct,
Select B if options *1 and 3* are correct,
Select C if options *2 and 4* are correct,
Select D if only option *4* is correct,
Select E if *all* options are correct.

625. Congenital syndromes frequently associated with cardiac abnormalities include

   1. Tracheoesophageal fistula
   2. Meningomyelocele
   3. Omphalocele
   4. Gastroschisis

626. Appropriate management of a neonate born with congenital diaphragmatic hernia should include

   1. Expansion of the hypoplastic lung with positive pressure ventilation
   2. Insertion of an orogastric tube
   3. Ventilation of the lungs with a bag and mask to prevent hypoxia
   4. Evaluation for the presence of associated congenital anomalies

627. Which of the following should be avoided in the anesthetic management of neonates undergoing surgical correction of a congenital diaphragmatic hernia?

   1. N_2O
   2. Cannulation of the right radial artery (vs left)
   3. Ketamine
   4. Hyperventilation

628. Which of the following resuscitation techniques is (are) appropriate for a 6-month-old who is pulled pulseless out of a swimming pool?

   1. Chest compressions should be carried out 80-100 per minute
   2. Ventilation should be mouth-to-mouth and nose
   3. Restoration of circulation may be best determined through palpation of the carotid pulse
   4. Sternal compression depth should be 0.5-1.0 inches

629. Klippel-Feil syndrome is associated with

   1. Short neck
   2. Micrognathia
   3. Congenital heart abnormalities
   4. Scoliosis

Select A if options *1, 2 and 3* are correct,
Select B if options *1 and 3* are correct,
Select C if options *2 and 4* are correct,
Select D if only option *4* is correct,
Select E if *all* options are correct.

630. A 2-month-old, 9-kg infant is undergoing general anesthesia for an elective urologic procedure. The patient is breathing spontaneously through a Mapleson D breathing circuit. Which of the following maneuvers would decrease rebreathing through this circuit?

    1. Decrease the I:E ratio
    2. Decrease the tidal volume
    3. Decrease the respiratory rate
    4. Decrease the fresh-gas inflow rate

631. A 16-week-old male infant born at 29 weeks gestation is scheduled for elective repair of a left inguinal hernia. The patient is induced with halothane and nitrous oxide. An intravenous cannula is placed, and the patient is intubated uneventfully. Which of the following statements concerning the anesthetic care of this patient is (are) true?

    1. The patient should be NPO for 6 hours prior to induction
    2. The patient is at high risk for retinopathy of prematurity
    3. Fluid deficits should be replaced with a 0.45 saline and 10% dextrose solution
    4. The patient is at risk for apnea and bradycardia postoperatively

632. Hemolytic disease of the newborn (Rh incompatibility)

    1. Has a higher incidence when the fetus and mother are both Rh- and ABO-incompatible
    2. Can only be diagnosed at birth by the presence of jaundice
    3. Occurs when maternal erythrocytes cross the placenta
    4. Can lead to high-output cardiac failure in utero

633. Variables which are doubled in infants compared with adults include

    1. CO_2 production/kg
    2. Heart rate
    3. O_2 consumption/kg
    4. Tidal volume/kg

634. In the infant hypothermia can be manifested as

    1. Metabolic acidosis
    2. Bradycardia
    3. Hypoglycemia
    4. Respiratory depression

Select A if options *1, 2 and 3* are correct,
Select B if options *1 and 3* are correct,
Select C if options *2 and 4* are correct,
Select D if only option *4* is correct,
Select E if *all* options are correct.

635. Necrotizing enterocolitis is

1. A potential complication of umbilical artery catheterization
2. Caused by intestinal mucosal injury from ischemia
3. Commonly associated with prenatal asphyxia and postnatal respiratory complications
4. A surgical emergency

636. Midazolam premedication may be administered to pediatric patient via the following route(s)

1. Nasally
2. Orally
3. Sublingually
4. Rectally

637. True statements regarding anesthetic concerns for strabismus surgery include

1. There is a very high incidence of postoperative nausea and vomiting
2. The oculocardiac reflex can be prevented by a retrobulbar block
3. Succinylcholine may interfere with the forced duction test
4. Patients with strabismus are at increased risk for malignant hyperthermia

638. A 5-year-old girl with hemolytic-uremic syndrome is brought to the operating room for placement of a dialysis catheter. Anesthetic management issues typical for this disease include

1. Thrombocytopenia
2. Increased intracranial pressure
3. Anemia
4. Glucose intolerance

639. A 3-year-old child status post resection of Wilm's tumor at age 2 is receiving doxorubicin (adriamycin) and cyclophosphamide for metastatic disease. The patient is scheduled for placement of a Hickman catheter for continued chemotherapy. Anesthetic concerns related to this patient's chemotherapeutic treatment include

1. Thrombocytopenia
2. Inhibition of plasma cholinesterase
3. Cardiac depression
4. Pulmonary fibrosis

PEDIATRIC PHYSIOLOGY AND ANESTHESIA ANSWERS, REFERENCES, AND EXPLANATIONS

567. **(D)** Thermal injuries of the upper airways can cause severe edema, resulting in hoarseness, stridor, and respiratory distress. Swelling of the supraglottic tissues can result in complete upper airway obstruction, even hours after the original thermal injury. Therefore, the airway should be secured immediately in patients with thermal injuries of the upper airway before respiratory decompensation occurs. Nasotracheal tubes are preferred over orotracheal tubes, as they are more easily secured *(Stoelting: Anesthesia and Co-existing Disease, ed 3, pp 620-621).*

568. **(B)** The anatomy of the oropharynx and larynx of the infant is different from that of the adult in many aspects. These differences may make it more difficult for a successful direct laryngoscopy and tracheal intubation. Infants have larger arytenoids and tongue, and the lower border of the larynx (the cricoid cartilage) is positioned more cephalad at the lower border of the C4 vertebra. Additionally, the epiglottis of the infant is relatively larger and stiffer compared to the adult *(Rogers: Principles and Practice of Anesthesiology, pp 1020-1021).*

569. **(C)** Spinal anesthesia can be administered safely to children of all ages. The anatomy of the spinal cord and dural sac is different from the adult. The spinal cord and dural sac extend farther down the vertebral canal in small children such that the tip of the spinal cord at birth is at the level of L2 or L3, and will ascend with the dural sac to reach its permanent position at the L1 interspace by one year of age. The complications associated with subarachnoid block are different from those of adults. Respiratory depression with hypoxia will likely be the initial symptom associated with a high spinal anesthetic in infants *(Berry: Anesthetic Management of Difficult and Routine Pediatric Patients, ed 2, p 328).*

570. **(D)** An infant's total body weight consists of approximately 75% water. Fifty-five percent of a male adult's weight and 45% of female adult's weight consists of water *(Miller: Anesthesia, ed 4, pp 1595, 1596).*

571. **(E)** The fetal P_aO_2 does not increase above 45 mm Hg when O_2 is administered to the mother because of the high O_2 consumption of the placenta and uneven distribution of the maternal and fetal blood flow in the placenta. For these reasons, the F_IO_2 administered to the mother is not a factor in the etiology of retinopathy of prematurity in utero *(Stoelting: Basics of Anesthesia, ed 3, p 374).*

572. **(A)** Retinopathy of prematurity (retrolental fibroplasia) typically occurs in newborns who are born at less than 35 weeks gestational age. Additionally, the risk of retinopathy is inversely related to birth weight, with significant risk occurring in infants weighing less than 1.5-2.0 kg. The risk is negligible after 44 weeks postconception. The mechanism for retrolental fibroplasia is related to the complicated process of retinal development and maturation. Under normal circumstances, retinal vasculature develops from the optic disk toward the periphery of the retina. This process is typically complete by 40 weeks gestation. Hyperoxia causes constriction of the retinal arterioles, causing swelling and degeneration of the endothelium, disrupting normal retinal develop-

ment. Vascularization of the retina resumes in an abnormal fashion when normoxic conditions returned, resulting in neovascularization and scarring of the retina. In the worst case scenario, this process can lead to retinal detachment and blindness. Consequently, hyperoxia should be avoided when anesthetizing preterm infants. Exposure of preterm infants to $P_aO_2 > 80$ mmHg for prolonged periods may be associated with increased incidence and severity of retinopathy. To reduce this risk, it is recommended that the P_aO_2 be maintained between 60-80 mm Hg during anesthesia. On the other hand, one must never compromise O_2 delivery to the neonates brain to protect the eyes *(Gregory: Pediatric Anesthesia, ed 3, pp 358-359)*.

573. **(E)** This patient has signs consistent with severe dehydration and needs resuscitation with fluid and electrolytes prior to surgery. Surgery should be delayed until there is thorough evaluation and treatment of the fluid and electrolyte imbalances. Patients with pyloric stenosis and vomiting can become alkalotic, with hypokalemia, hypochloremia, and dehydration. Fluid resuscitation should be initiated with a balanced salt solution that does not contain potassium until the patient voids. Potassium can then be safely added to the intravenous fluids. Once there has been adequate hydration and correction of the electrolyte and acid-base abnormalities, the patient could then undergo surgery. Several days may be required to restore normal fluid and electrolyte balance *(Gregory: Pediatric Anesthesia, ed 3, p 562)*.

574. **(C)** Tracheoesophageal fistulas result from failure of the esophagus and the trachea to completely separate during their development, leaving a communication between the two structures. This lesion occurs with an incidence of approximately 1 in 4,000 live births. The most common type of tracheoesophageal fistula is esophageal atresia, with the lower segment of the esophagus communicating with the back of the trachea. This type of lesion occurs in more than 90% of all tracheoesophageal fistulas *(Gregory: Pediatric Anesthesia, ed 3, pp 438, 439)*.

575. **(C)** Volatile anesthetics, particularly halothane, can have significant adverse effects on cardiac heart rate and rhythm. Halothane may cause direct depression of the S-A node and has been shown to increase the refractory period of the A-V conduction system. Both brady- and tachydysrhythmias have been reported during inhalation induction of anesthesia with halothane. These include sinus bradycardia, nodal or junctional rhythms, and ventricular dysrhythmias. Whereas cardiac dysrhythmias following inhalation induction with halothane are common, they are usually benign and do not represent a disease state. Cardiac dysrhythmias induced by halothane, however, may be exacerbated by hypoxia, hypercarbia, or electrolyte abnormalities. Halothane "sensitizes" the myocardium to catecholamines, particularly in the presence of acute hypercarbia and acidosis. Under these conditions, ventricular rhythms such as bigeminy, multifocal ventricular ectopic beats, and even ventricular tachycardia may occur *(Wood: Drugs and Anesthesia: Pharmacology for Anesthesiologists, ed 2, pp 240-241)*.

576. **(D)** Retinopathy of prematurity occurs most commonly in association with premature newborns who have received O_2 therapy for respiratory distress syndrome. Neonates should be considered at risk for retinopathy of prematurity until 44 weeks postconceptional age, because a significant number of full-term newborns will have immature retinal vasculature *(Miller: Anesthesia, ed 4, p 614; Motoyama: Smith's Anesthesia for Infants and Children, ed 2, p 430)*.

577. **(C)** In general, cuffed endotracheal tubes are not indicated for patients younger than 10 years of age. The external diameter of uncuffed endotracheal tubes should be small enough to allow a

small gas leak around the tube at peak inflation pressures of 20 to 30 cm H_2O *(Miller: Anesthesia, ed 4, p 2112)*.

578. **(C)** In contrast to intravenous induction, patients who undergo induction of anesthesia by inhalation of a volatile anesthetic passes through various stages of depth. These stages can be monitored by observation of the pupils, muscle activity, tearing, respiratory patterns, and muscle relaxation. The earliest or "lightest" stage of anesthesia is associated with sensory and mental depression. Patients in this stage open their eyes to command, tolerate mild painful stimuli, such as superficial debridement, have normal respiratory patterns, and maintain intact airway reflexes. The second stage of anesthesia is marked by excitement, which is associated with muscle movement, heightened laryngeal reflexes, disconjugate pupils, tachycardia, hypertension, and hyperventilation. The third stage of anesthesia, which is the level associated with the minimum alveolar concentration (MAC), is notable by the absence of movement (in 50% of patients) in response to a surgical incision. As anesthesia with inhaled anesthetics is deepened beyond the MAC, significant respiratory, cardiovascular, and CNS depression occurs *(Barash: Clinical Anesthesia, ed 2, p 453)*.

579. **(E)** The hemodynamic indices described in this question are normal for healthy 1-month-old neonates *(Stoelting: Basics of Anesthesia, ed 3, p 382)*.

580. **(E)** The presence of dark brown urine may be caused by myoglobin, a possible sign of undiagnosed malignant hyperthermia. Accordingly, this patient should be evaluated for malignant hyperthermia. Arterial blood gas analysis should be performed to assess the patient's metabolic status, which would include acidosis, a base deficit, and an increase in P_aCO_2 if MH has been triggered. If a metabolic acidosis or a mixed acidosis is present despite adequate ventilation, it should be presumed that the patient has malignant hyperthermia and therapy should be initiated *(Berry: Anesthetic Management of Difficult and Routine Pediatric Patients, ed 2, p 391)*.

581. **(B)** In infants and young children, there should be a small air leak around the endotracheal tube at peak inflation pressures of approximately 20 to 30 cm H_2O. An air leak within this pressure range reduces the incidence of postextubation complications, such as subglottic edema *(Berry: Anesthetic Management of Difficult and Routine Pediatric Patients, ed 2, p 420)*.

582. **(D)** A congenital diaphragmatic hernia is the herniation of abdominal viscera into the chest cavity through a defect in the diaphragm and occurs in approximately 1 in every 5,000 live births. Approximately 75% to 85% of congenital diaphragmatic hernias occur through a posterolateral defect in the left side of the diaphragm at the foramen of Bochdalek. A tension pneumothorax is a potential complication of positive-pressure ventilation in neonates with congenital diaphragmatic hernias. If a patient experiences sudden O_2-desaturation during positive-pressure ventilation, a tension pneumothorax should be suspected and if confirmed, a chest tube should be placed on the side contralateral to the congenital diaphragmatic hernia *(Barash: Clinical Anesthesia, ed 2, p 1322)*.

583. **(B)** Infantile pyloric stenosis is one of the most common surgical diseases of neonates and infants. Symptoms can appear as early as the second week of life but usually before the sixth week of life *(Miller: Anesthesia, ed 4, p 2118)*.

584. **(D)** The depth of insertion of an oral endotracheal tube from the lips to the mid-trachea is approximately 7 cm for 1 kg neonates and is an additional centimeter for each kilogram increase in body weight to a maximum depth of 10 cm for full-term neonates. A convenient formula for estimating the appropriate depth of insertion of an oral endotracheal tube (in cm) for infants and children is as follows:

$$12 + \frac{age\ (years)}{2} = tube\ length$$

(Barash: Clinical Anesthesia, ed. 2, p 690).

585. **(D)** The preanesthetic assessment of neonates with imperforate anus or omphalocele should include an assessment for abnormalities not involving the gastrointestinal tract. The diagnosis of gastrointestinal abnormalities is often made by antenatal examination. For example, omphalocele is associated with a greater than 70 percent incidence of other congenital anomalies, including cardiac anomalies, trisomy 21, and Beckwith's syndrome. Conversely, gastroschisis is rarely associated with other congenital anomalies *(Gregory: Pediatric Anesthesia, ed 3, pp 558-563 & 594; Stoelting: Anesthesia and Co-existing Disease, ed 3, p 596; Rogers: Principles and Practice of Anesthesiology, p 2148).*

586. **(E)** Neonates and infants require more succinylcholine per body weight than do older children and adults to produce neuromuscular blockade, because the extracellular fluid volume is much greater in neonates and infants. Since the volume of distribution of succinylcholine is greater, the recommended dose of succinylcholine in neonates and infants to provide optimal conditions for tracheal intubation is 2 mg/kg compared to 1 mg/kg for adults *(Stoelting: Anesthesia and Co-existing Disease, ed 3, p 586).*

587. **(B)** Pyloric stenosis occurs in approximately 1 in every 500 to 750 live births, making it the most common cause of gastrointestinal obstruction in pediatric patients. Pyloric stenosis occurs as frequently in preterm as in term neonates and there is a predilection for male infants. Persistent vomiting usually manifests itself between the second and sixth week(s) of age and can result in dehydration, hypokalemia, hypochloremia, and metabolic alkalosis *(Gregory: Pediatric Anesthesia, ed 3, p 562).*

588. **(B)** Apnea spells are defined as cessation of breathing for at least 20 seconds which result in cyanosis. Infants who are born prematurely and who are still younger than 60 weeks postconceptual age are at risk for apnea and bradycardia following general anesthesia. These patients should not undergo outpatient surgery because volatile and intravenous anesthetic agents affect control of breathing, but should be admitted to the hospital and monitored for apnea spells for 12 to 18 hours after surgery *(Barash: Clinical Anesthesia, ed 2, pp 1328, 1343, 1565; Motoyama: Smith's Anesthesia for Infants and Children, ed 2, pp 324, 325).*

589. **(A)** The treatment for documented ventricular fibrillation or pulseless ventricular tachycardia is electrical defibrillation. The initial defibrillation should be 2 joules/kg, increasing to 4 joules/kg for a second or third shock. The maximum defibrillation charge should be 6 joules/kg *(Gregory: Pediatric Anesthesia, ed 3, p 841).*

590. **(C)**

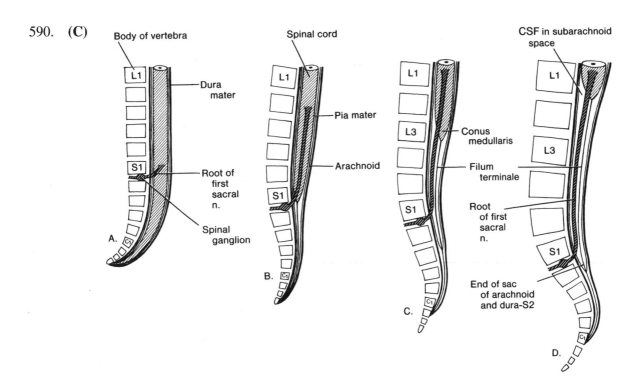

The position of the inferior end of the spinal cord in relation to the vertebral column and meninges at various stages of development. (A) Eight weeks; (B) 24 weeks; (C) newborn; (D) 8-year-old child and adult.

The spinal cord of neonates can extend as far down as L-3. Therefore, lumbar puncture should be performed in these patients no higher than the L-4 to L-5 interspace *(Gregory: Pediatric Anesthesia, ed 3, p 379).*

591. **(D)** Esophageal atresia and tracheoesophageal fistula is frequently suspected soon after birth when an oral suction catheter cannot be introduced into the stomach or when the patient has excessive salivation, drooling, and coughing that is exacerbated during feeding. These patients should be placed in the head-up position and the blind upper pouch of the esophagus should be decompressed with a suction tube immediately after the diagnosis is made to reduce pulmonary aspiration of secretions *(Gregory: Pediatric Anesthesia, ed 3, pp 438-439).*

592. **(E)** Beckwith-Weidemann syndrome is characterized by omphalocele, organomegaly, congenital heart disease, macroglossia, and hypoglycemia. These patients can be very difficult to intubate because they have significant macroglossia *(Stoelting: Anesthesia and Co-existing Disease, ed 3, pp 595, 596; Berry: Anesthetic Management of Difficult and Routine Pediatric Patients, ed 2, p 152).*

593. **(C)** Anesthesia for patients with esophageal atresia and tracheoesophageal fistula can be safely induced with either an intravenous or volatile anesthetic. However, mask-and-bag ventilation will force gas into the stomach, potentially making ventilation of the lungs difficult; thus it should be avoided. A frequently used technique to facilitate correct placement of the endotra-

cheal tube is to advance the tube into a bronchus, then while listening over the stomach, slowly withdraw the tube until sounds are heard over the stomach. Then advance the tube until these sounds become diminished *(Miller: Anesthesia, ed 4, p 2119)*.

594. **(C)** Unlike adults, neonates and infants seldom have muscle fasciculations to succinylcholine. The most frequently encountered side effect associated with succinylcholine in neonates and infants is bradycardia, especially when given intravenously. The incidence of bradydysrhythmias is significantly decreased when the succinylcholine is administered intramuscularly. Other side effects include myoglobinuria, myalgias, and sore throat *(Gregory: Pediatric Anesthesia, ed 3, p 28; Berry: Anesthetic Management of Difficult and Routine Pediatric Patients, ed 2, pp 68-69)*.

595. **(C)** The blood volume of healthy, full-term neonates is approximately 80 mL/kg. Because this patient weighs 4 kg, the predicted blood volume is 320 mL *(Gregory: Pediatric Anesthesia, ed 3, p 807)*.

596. **(C)** In the fetus, pulmonary vascular resistance is extremely high. Most of the right ventricular output bypasses the lungs and flows into the descending aorta through the ductus arteriosus. With the onset of ventilation at birth, an increase in P_aO_2 causes a precipitous decrease in pulmonary vascular resistance enabling blood to flow through the lungs. Pulmonary vascular resistance continues to decrease after birth, approaching the adult level within the first year of life *(Motoyama: Smith's Anesthesia for Infants and Children, ed 2, p 45)*.

597. **(D)** A comprehensive understanding of thermoregulation and meticulous attention to details during the anesthetic care of infants are necessary to minimize intraoperative heat loss. In anesthetized infants, the majority of heat loss occurs through the transfer of heat from the patient to the environment. For this reason, placement of an infrared heater over the operating room table and pre-warming the operating room atmosphere are the most effective means of preventing hypothermia in these patients. Covering the operating room table with a heating blanket, ventilating the patient with warm, humidified anesthetic gases, wrapping the extremities of the patient with sheet wadding, and covering the patient's head with a cloth or plastic cap are also effective means of reducing heat loss and preventing hypothermia. A Mapleson D breathing circuit is not a circle system and does not preserve heat or moisture. Low flows with Mapleson circuits may result in respiratory acidosis because of rebreathing *(Miller: Anesthesia, ed 4, pp 1373-1375; Motoyama: Smith's Anesthesia for Infants and Children, ed 2, pp 152 & 155)*.

598. **(E)** Patients with pyloric stenosis often have protracted vomiting, which can lead to dehydration, hypokalemia, hypochloremia, hyponatremia, and a metabolic alkalosis. If dehydration is severe, hypoperfusion can occur, which can manifest itself as metabolic acidosis. Postoperative ventilatory depression frequently occurs in these patients which is thought to be related to hyperventilation and cerebral spinal fluid alkalosis. Thus, before the endotracheal tube is removed, these patients should be alert and awake with a normal rate and pattern of respiration *(Stoelting: Anesthesia and Co-existing Disease, ed 3, p 597)*.

599. **(D)** In addition to routine monitors, newborns with persistent fetal circulation should have a pre-ductal (ductus arteriosus) artery cannulated for monitoring of arterial blood pressure and gases and pH. The right radial or temporal arteries arise from vessels that originate from the aorta

proximal to the ductus arteriosus *(Stoelting: Anesthesia and Co-existing Disease, ed 3, pp 592, 593)*.

600. **(C)** The minimum alveolar concentration for volatile anesthetics is greatest at 3 months of age. The minimum alveolar concentrations is least in preterm neonates. This is thought to be related to the immaturity of the central nervous system and to elevated levels of progesterone and ß-endorphins. After 3 months of age, the minimum alveolar concentrations of volatile anesthetics steadily declines with aging except for a slight increase at puberty *(Stoelting: Anesthesia and Co-existing Disease, ed 3, pp 584-585)*.

601. **(D)** Intravascular fluid-volume deficits in patients with burn injuries are roughly proportional to the extent and depth of the burn. For reasons that are unclear, the vascular compartment, particularly in the area of the burn, becomes hyperpermeable to plasma proteins, such as fibrinogen and albumin. These proteins subsequently exert an osmotic pressure gradient that favors the translocation of intravascular fluid into the extravascular third space. Therefore, during this period (approximately 24 hours), administration of colloid solutions would be of no benefit to the patient and may exacerbate third-space translocation of fluids. As a rule of thumb, an estimated 4 mL/kg of fluid is lost for each percent of body surface area burned. Approximately two-thirds of this fluid should be replaced with isotonic crystalloid solutions during the first 8 hours following the injury *(Stoelting: Anesthesia and Co-existing Disease, ed 3, pp 620, 621)*.

602. **(E)** The most likely explanation for anemia in this patient is that this is a normal physiologic finding. At birth, a full-term infant has a hemoglobin of approximately 19 g/dl. A physiologic anemia occurs by 2-3 months of age resulting in hemoglobin concentrations of approximately 10 g/dl. After 3 months, there is a progressive increase in hemoglobin concentration, which reaches levels similar to that of adults by 6-9 months of age *(Stoelting: Anesthesia and Co-existing Disease, ed 3, p 583)*.

603. **(D)** This history is consistent with acute epiglottitis, which is a life-threatening acute bacterial infection involving the epiglottis and other supraglottic structures. When acute epiglottitis is suspected, the anesthesiologist and otolaryngologist should be notified and the patient should immediately be transferred to the operating room before complete upper airway obstruction ensues. In the operating room, anesthesia should be induced with halothane and O_2 with the child in a sitting position. Halothane is less likely to induce laryngospasm than is enflurane or isoflurane. Intravenous access should be established as soon as the child is deeply anesthetized. Atropine should be administered to block vagally-mediated bradycardia induced by direct laryngoscopy. Muscle relaxants are contraindicated since they can cause complete obstruction of the upper airway in these patients. The trachea should then be intubated under direct laryngoscopy when the depth of anesthesia is sufficient to blunt laryngeal reflexes *(Gregory: Pediatric Anesthesia, ed 3, p 672)*.

604. **(E)** Cerebral palsy is a group of nonspecific neurologic disorders characterized by central motor deficits resulting from various etiologic factors including genetic abnormalities, such as congenital cerebrovascular malformations, metabolic defects, such as kernicterus and hypoglycemia, injury to the brain, intrauterine and neonatal infections, and a variety of anatomic disorders which cause localized or diffuse atrophy of the cerebral cortex, basal ganglia, and subcortical white matter. Clinical manifestations of cerebral palsy can include skeletal muscle

spasticity, cerebellar ataxia, seizure disorders, varying degrees of mental retardation and speech deficits, and extrapyramidal symptoms such as skeletal muscle rigidity, choreoathetosis, and dyskinesia. In addition, gastroesophageal reflux is common in children with cerebral palsy. For this reason, induction of general anesthesia in these patients should include a rapid-sequence intravenous induction followed by immediate tracheal intubation. Even though these patients have skeletal muscle spasticity, there have been no reports of succinylcholine-induced hyperkalemia *(Stoelting: Anesthesia and Co-existing Disease, ed 3, p 599)*.

605. **(E)**   The symptoms described in this patient are consistent with severe dehydration. Thus, the vascular volume should be expanded initially with a balanced salt solution or a colloid solution until the patient voids. When the urine output increases, potassium can be added to the intravenous fluids *(Gregory: Pediatric Anesthesia, ed 3, p 563)*.

606. **(A)**   Preterm infants have very limited calcium reserves and are very susceptible to hypocalcemia. Hypocalcemia manifests itself in a number of nonspecific ways, including irritability, twitching, hypotension, and seizure. Some of the signs of hypoglycemia are similar to those of hypocalcemia and include seizure, irritability, hypotension, and sometimes bradycardia and apnea. In the patient described in this question, the glucose has already been measured at 50 mg/dl, which is acceptable for a preterm infant. An O_2 saturation of 88 is also acceptable since the patient is at risk for retinopathy of prematurity. Hyperventilation would cause alkalosis, which would decrease the unbound fraction of calcium making the patient more susceptible to seizures. Furthermore, calcium binds to albumin and this would further reduce the free calcium. Because the urine output is more than adequate, it is unlikely that the patient needs a fluid bolus to correct hypotension *(Stoelting: Anesthesia and Co-existing Disease, ed 3, p 590; Gregory: Pediatric Anesthesia, ed 3, pp 99 & 358)*.

607. **(A)**   EMLA is a eutectic mixture of lidocaine and prilocaine. Recent studies have shown that when 5% EMLA cream is applied for 45 minutes or more, there is significantly less pain associated with venipuncture in children age 1-5 years. In most studies, the plasma concentrations methemoglobin were well below toxic levels, with 2 percent of total hemoglobin the highest individual concentrations reported. However, EMLA cream should be used with caution in infants and small children receiving other drugs that may potentially produce methemoglobin to avoid the risk of clinically significant methemoglobinemia *(Gregory: Pediatric Anesthesia, ed 3, pp 311-312)*.

608. **(A)**   Although the umbilical vein is larger and easier to cannulate than the artery, using this vessel will not allow for adequate assessment of oxygenation or systemic blood pressure. Additionally, administration of drugs or hypertonic solutions into the umbilical vein may be hazardous, since the catheter can become wedged in a venous radical of the liver or enter the portal veins thereby causing hepatic injury or portal vein thrombosis. If a catheter is inserted into the umbilical vein, the catheter tip must be advanced through the ductus venosus into the inferior vena cava near the right atrium and should be checked by x-ray. Careful placement of an umbilical artery catheter is equally important. The tip of the umbilical artery catheter should be placed just above the bifurcation of the aorta and below the celiac, renal, and mesenteric arteries. Dislocation may be hazardous because improper placement may be associated with thrombosis or embolism in these major aortic vessels *(Shnider: Anesthesia for Obstetrics, ed 3, p 702)*.

609. **(D)** Because of the large surface-to-volume ratio, thin layer of insulating subcutaneous fat, and limited ability to compensate for cold stress, neonates and infants are at greater risk for intraoperative hypothermia than are adults. Infants less than 3 months of age do not produce heat by shivering, thus metabolism of brown fat is the principle method of thermogenesis *(Miller: Anesthesia, ed 4, p 2102)*.

610. **(D)** In a 6-month-old infant, a normal hemoglobin value is approximately 11 gm/dL, a normal heart rate is about 120 beats/min, and a normal respiratory rate is about 30 breaths/min. O_2 consumption in infants is 5 to 6 mL/kg/min, approximately two times that of adults *(Stoelting: Basics of Anesthesia, ed 3, p 382)*.

611. **(A)** The initial treatment of bradycardia and hypotension in patients undergoing surgical correction of strabismus is to stop the stimulus. Subsequently, the depth of anesthesia can be increased and the adequacy of ventilation should be assessed (as hypercarbia decreases the threshold to elicit the oculocardiac reflex). Infiltrating lidocaine locally into the recti muscles may also be effective in preventing and treating the oculocardiac reflex. Atropine can be administered if the bradydysrhythmia persists. Retrobulbar block will block the oculocardiac reflex, but it is associated with other potentially dangerous complications, and should only be performed if the aforementioned steps have been unsuccessful *(Miller: Anesthesia, ed 4, pp 1281-1282)*.

612. **(C)** There is no difference in tidal volume between neonates and adults. Neonates are more susceptible to atelectasis than are adults because of their high O_2 consumption and reduced chest-wall compliance and functional residual capacity. Consequently, they are at an increased risk for hypoxia during general anesthesia and pulmonary complications in the perioperative period. Neonates have difficulty in reabsorbing HCO_3^- from their urine, which results in a persistent mild metabolic acidosis. When protein is added to their diets, renal excretion of H^+ and ammonia increases which lowers the urine pH and corrects the metabolic acidosis *(Stoelting: Anesthesia and Co-existing Disease, ed 3, p 580)*.

Mean Pulmonary Function Values

	Neonate (3 kg)	Adult (70 kg)
Oxygen consumption (ml $\cdot$ kg^{-1} $\cdot$ min^{-1})	6.4	3.5
Alveolar ventilation (ml $\cdot$ kg^{-1} $\cdot$ min^{-1})	130	60
Carbon dioxide production (ml $\cdot$ kg^{-1} $\cdot$ min^{-1})	6	3
Tidal volume (ml $\cdot$ kg^{-1})	6	6
Breathing frequency (min)	35	15
Vital capacity (ml $\cdot$ kg^{-1})	35	70
Functional residual capacity (ml $\cdot$ kg^{-1})	30	35
Tracheal length (cm)	5.5	12
P_aO_2 (F_1O_2 0.21, mm Hg)	65-85	85-95
P_aCO_2 (mm Hg)	30-36	36-44
pH	7.34-7.40	7.36-7.44

From: Stoelting RK, Dierdorf SF (eds): Anesthesia and Co-Existing Disease, ed 3. New York, Churchill Livingstone, Inc., 1993, p 580. Used with permission.

613. **(A)**   Neurofibromatosis (von Recklinghausen's disease) is an autosomal dominant genetic disorder characterized by multiple neurofibromas involving the skin and peripheral and central nervous systems. The clinical features of this disease are diverse and always progress with time. The anesthetic management of patients with neurofibromatosis can be complicated by the associated clinical features of this disease. For example, a pheochromocytoma may be present in approximately 1% of patients. If this is unrecognized, severe hypertension can occur during anesthesia. Signs and symptoms of intracranial hypertension may reflect the presence of an expanding intracranial tumor. If intracranial pressure is elevated, efforts to reduce intracranial pressure should be initiated. Finally, compromise of the upper airway may occur when neurofibromas develop in the cervical or mediastinal regions. There is no evidence that these patients are at increased risk for malignant hyperthermia *(Stoelting: Anesthesia and Co-existing Disease, ed 3, pp 244-245).*

614. **(D)**   Retinopathy of prematurity is an abnormal proliferation of immature retinal vessels, which usually occurs after exposure to hyperoxia. The most significant risk factor for retinopathy of prematurity is prematurity, the risk being inversely related to birth weight, with significant risk occurring in infants weighing < 1,500 grams. The risk of retinopathy of prematurity is increased when the F_IO_2 is sufficient to cause a retinal artery $P_aO_2 > 80$ to 90 mm Hg for prolonged periods in neonates younger than 44 weeks postconceptual age. However, it is possible to develop retinopathy of prematurity with exposures as short as 1-2 hours to a P_aO_2 of 150 mm Hg. Likewise, it is possible to develop ROP in patients who have never received supplemental oxygen and even those who have cyanotic heart disease. Retinopathy of prematurity is clearly a multifactorial disease which cannot be explained simply by exposure to high concentrations of oxygen *(Gregory: Pediatric Anesthesia, ed 3, pp 358-359).*

615. **(E)**   Although nephrogenesis is complete by 36 weeks of gestation, many aspects of renal function are not fully developed at birth. Neonates and infants are unable to concentrate urine as well as adults until 6 months to 12 months of age. Furthermore, glomerular filtration rate, reabsorption of sodium or HCO_3^- by the proximal and distal renal tubule cells, and secretion of H^+ do not reach adult values until 1 to 2 years of age. The clinical implication of these differences is that these patients are less able to compensate for extremes of fluid and electrolyte balance. Specifically, neonates and infants excrete volume loads more slowly than do adults and therefore are more susceptible to fluid overload *(Stoelting: Basics of Anesthesia, ed 3, p 382).*

616. **(B)**   Improved oxygenation of the lung parenchyma, lung expansion during inspiration, and a rise in arterial pH are all factors responsible for the precipitous drop in pulmonary vascular resistance in newborns at birth. Closure of the foramen ovale is caused by an increase in left atrial pressure and does not influence the change in pulmonary vascular resistance at birth under normal circumstances *(Miller: Anesthesia, ed 4, p 2098).*

617. **(A)**   Once an umbilical venous catheter has been placed, the PO_2 of the blood should be measured. If the PO_2 is greater than 40 mm Hg, it is likely that the catheter tip is located in the left atrium or left ventricle, and should be withdrawn into the right atrium or inferior vena cava *(Miller: Anesthesia, ed 4, p 2088).*

618. **(C)**   The blood volume in neonates is about 85 mL/kg, and the blood volume in adults is about 65 mL/kg. Tidal volume is the same in infants and adults (6 mL/kg). The functional residual

capacity is about 25 mL/kg in infants versus 40 mL/kg in adults *(Stoelting: Basics of Anesthesia, ed 3, p 382)*.

619. **(C)**   Patients with acute epiglottitis are usually 2 to 6 years of age. These patients usually present with difficulty swallowing, high fever, and inspiratory stridor. Other signs and symptoms include drooling, lethargy, cyanosis, tachypnea, and a propensity to sitting up and leaning forward. The onset of signs and symptoms of acute epiglottitis is typically rapid, within a 24-hour period. Acute epiglottitis accounts for approximately 5% of children with stridor and the most common etiologic agent is a bacterial infection with Hemophilus Influenzae. Total upper airway obstruction can occur in these children at any time because of the rapid progression of the disease. For this reason, attempts to visualize the epiglottis should not be undertaken until the patient is in the operating room and appropriate preparations are completed for direct laryngoscopy and tracheal intubation, and possible emergency tracheostomy. The definitive treatment of acute epiglottitis includes appropriate antibiotic therapy and a secured airway *(Stoelting: Anesthesia and Co-existing Disease, ed 3, pp 607, 608)*.

620. **(B)**   The technique for cardiopulmonary resuscitation of infants and children is different from that of adults. For adults, sternal compression should be accomplished with the heel of the hand on the lower one-third of the sternum at a depth of 4-5 cm and a compression rate of 80-100/min. For infants, sternal compression should be accomplished by encircling the chest with both hands and depressing the midsternum with the thumbs at a depth of 1-2½ cm and a rate no less than 100/min. A finger sweep of the mouth should only be performed in infants when foreign object is visible to reduce the likelihood of impacting the foreign object into the airway *(Stoelting: Basics of Anesthesia, ed 3, p 480)*.

621. **(C)**   A number of physiologic differences between pediatric and adult patients have important implications concerning anesthetic management. For example, a greater percentage of the cardiac output is distributed to the vessel-rich tissue group in infants compared to adults. This physiologic difference, along with differences in body water composition, alveolar ventilation, blood solubility of volatile anesthetics, and functional residual capacity, is an important factor in producing a more rapid induction of general anesthesia in infants and small children compared to adults. Neonates are more sensitive to central-acting hypnotic sedatives such as thiopental, narcotics, and benzodiazepines because of an immature blood-brain barrier. The glomerular filtration rate in healthy full-term neonates is approximately one-fifth to one-tenth that of adults. This decrease in renal function can delay excretion of drugs that are dependent on renal clearance for elimination *(Stoelting: Basics of Anesthesia, ed 3, pp 382, 383)*.

622. **(A)**   The cricoid ring of the adult is in a horizontal (not diagonal) position within the larynx, making the vocal cords the narrowest portion of the upper airway *(Miller: Anesthesia, ed 4, p 2100 & 2101)*.

623. **(D)**   Fluid and electrolyte abnormalities commonly associated with infantile pyloric stenosis include hyponatremia, hypokalemia, hypochloremia, and hypovolemia. These abnormalities must be corrected before surgery. Severe dehydration is not uncommon in these patients; accordingly, correction of hypokalemia with potassium chloride should be delayed until the patient has been adequately hydrated with normal saline and urine output is normal. As a result of the vomiting, the kidneys secrete potassium instead of hydrogen ions (which are lost through vomiting) in an

attempt to maintain a normal arterial pH. Once hypokalemia occurs, the kidneys can no longer secrete potassium and metabolic alkalosis occurs. Correction of hypokalemia is necessary for correction of the metabolic alkalosis *(Gregory: Pediatric Anesthesia, ed 3, pp 562-563).*

624. **(E)** Down's syndrome (trisomy 21) occurs in approximately 0.2% of live births. There is a direct correlation between the incidence of Down's syndrome and maternal age. The risk of Down's syndrome is approximately 1 in 2,000 live births for 20-year-old mothers whereas the incidence increases to approximately 1 in 40 live births for mothers over the age of 45. The most important considerations for the anesthetic management of these patients is the diagnosis of the associated congenital abnormalities, in particular endocardial cushion defects, and adequate management of the airway. Patients with Down's syndrome have a short neck, small mouth, narrow nasopharynx, and large tongue. Despite these abnormalities, tracheal intubation is usually not difficult in the hands of an experienced anesthesiologist. Asymptomatic dislocation of the atlas on the axis is present in approximately 20% of these patients and should be diagnosed by lateral neck x-ray prior to surgery. If present, the neck should not be extended during direct laryngoscopy for tracheal intubation *(Miller: Anesthesia, ed 4, pp 968, 969).*

625. **(B)** Congenital cardiac abnormalities frequently occur in association with esophageal atresia and tracheoesophageal fistula, and with omphalocele. Gastroschisis is the external herniation of abdominal viscera through a defect in the anterior abdominal wall, lateral to the umbilical cord. In contrast to omphalocele, the herniated abdominal viscera is not covered by a sac. Gastroschisis is rarely associated with other congenital anomalies *(Barash: Clinical Anesthesia, ed 2, pp 1322-1326).*

626. **(C)** Following repair of a congenital diaphragmatic hernia, the hypoplastic lung should **NOT** be expanded. Attempts to do so may cause a pneumothorax. Airway pressures should be monitored during mechanical ventilation and should be maintained below 25 to 30 cm H_2O. Ventilation of the lungs with a bag and mask can cause gastric and intestinal distension, which can further impair respiration and worsen pulmonary gas exchange. In addition, the abdominal cavity is usually underdeveloped. Thus, the surgical abdominal closure can be tight, which can cause a cephalad displacement of the diaphragm, a reduced functional residual capacity, and hypoventilation *(Gregory: Pediatric Anesthesia, ed 3, pp 432-435).*

627. **(B)** N_2O should not be used in patients with a congenital diaphragmatic hernia because it causes gastric and intestinal distension, which can compromise ventilation. Furthermore, it may increase pulmonary artery pressure. A right radial artery catheter is preferable over a left because it allows preductal blood sampling. These patients usually have persistent fetal circulation (a right-to-left intracardiac shunt), which can lead to profound hypoxia. Hyperventilation of the lungs will cause alkalosis which will reduce pulmonary vascular resistance and improve oxygenation. Ketamine, and other anesthetics and anesthetic adjuvants that increase pulmonary vascular resistance, will increase the right-to-left intracardiac shunt and worsen oxygenation *(Gregory: Pediatric Anesthesia, ed 3, pp 432-435).*

628. **(C)** As previously described in question 620, the technique for cardiopulmonary resuscitation of infants and children is different from that of adults. In contrast to children and adults where the carotid artery should be used to check for a pulse and adequate circulation, in infants, the brachial artery at the mid forearm should be used. Additionally, infants and children are best

ventilated by mouth-to-mouth and nose, instead of simply mouth-to-mouth. The sternol compression rate should be at least 100 per minute *(Stoelting: Basics of Anesthesia, ed 3, p 480)*.

629. **(E)** Klippel-Feil syndrome is characterized by musculoskeletal abnormalities, such as spinal canal stenosis and scoliosis, cervical vertebra fusion, micrognathia, a short neck (which results from reduction in the number of cervical vertebra), and cardiac and genitourinary anomalies. The most important consideration in the anesthetic management of these patients is a possibility of cervical spine instability, which can result in neurologic damage during direct laryngoscopy. Preoperative lateral neck radiographs should be performed to assist in the evaluation of the stability of the cervical spine in these patients *(Stoelting: Anesthesia and Co-existing Disease, ed 3, p 455)*.

630. **(A)** Mapleson circuits are semiopen anesthesia breathing systems that lack unidirectional valves and thus require high fresh-gas inflow rates to prevent rebreathing of exhaled gases. In fact, the fresh-gas inflow rate required to prevent rebreathing of exhaled gases is the limiting factor in the use of these systems. During spontaneous breathing, an increase in fresh-gas inflow rate or a reduction in minute ventilation will decrease rebreathing of exhaled gases. Accordingly, a decrease in the inspiratory time, respiratory rate, or tidal volume, or an increase in the fresh gas inflow rate will decrease rebreathing of exhaled gases *(Miller: Anesthesia, ed 4, p 205)*.

631. **(D)** The patient described in this question is at increased risk of developing postanesthesia apnea and bradycardia. The majority of retrospective and prospective studies investigating this issue have found that infants under 46 weeks postconceptual age are at greatest risk. However, episodes of apnea have been reported in preterm infants up to 60 weeks postconceptual age. Additional risk factors include a history of respiratory distress syndrome, bronchopulmonary dysplasia, neonatal apnea, necrotizing enterocolitis, ongoing apnea at the time of surgery, use of narcotics or long-acting muscle relaxants intraoperatively, and the use of general versus regional anesthesia. Outpatient anesthesia should be considered only for term infants greater than 44 weeks postconceptual age who have had an unremarkable neonatal history and are currently healthy. The premature infant who is less than 60 weeks postconceptual age should be monitored in the hospital the night following surgery. Premature infants less than 44 weeks postconceptual age are susceptible to retinopathy of prematurity, and thus, oxygen saturation should be kept between 93-95 percent in these patients *(Miller: Anesthesia, ed 4, pp 2100, 2109, & 2118)*.

632. **(D)** Erythroblastosis fetalis (hemolytic disease of the newborn) results from intravascular hemolysis of sensitized fetal erythrocytes. Hemolysis of fetal erythrocytes usually occurs when maternal antibodies against fetal erythrocytes cross the placenta. Hemolysis can be detected in utero. Although both Rh and ABO incompatibility can cause this type of hemolytic anemia, severe anemia rarely develops from ABO incompatibility. ABO antibodies are of the immunoglobulin M class, which cannot readily cross the placenta. However, maternal antibodies to Rh antigens can readily cross the placenta and destroy fetal erythrocytes. There is no evidence that incompatibility for both ABO and Rh antigens increases the incidence of erythroblastosis fetalis above the risk from Rh incompatibility alone. The clinical features of erythroblastosis fetalis are related primarily to anemia and hyperbilirubinemia, and in cases of severe anemia, high-output cardiac failure can occur in the fetus in utero *(Frigoletto: Erythroblastosis Fetalis: Identification, Management, and Prevention, pp 321-331)*.

633. **(A)**   Heart rate in the neonate at rest is about 130 beats/min compared to 65 beats/min in the adult. CO_2 production (approximately 6 mL/kg/min) and O_2 consumption (approximately 5-6 mL/kg/min) are roughly double the adult values. Tidal volume is the same for infants and adults (6 mL/kg) *(Stoelting: Basics of Anesthesia, ed 3, p 382)*.

634. **(E)**   In neonates or infants, hypothermia can result in increased total-body O_2 consumption, depression of ventilation, metabolic acidosis, hypoglycemia, and bradycardia. Therefore, monitoring the body temperature and maneuvers to minimize or eliminate significant loss of body heat during anesthesia for neonates and small infants is essential during the perioperative period *(Stoelting: Anesthesia and Co-existing Disease, ed 3, p 587)*.

635. **(A)**   Necrotizing enterocolitis classically occurs in premature infants and in infants with low birth weight, usually following intestinal mucosal injury from ischemia. It is most commonly associated with prenatal asphyxia and respiratory complications in the early postnatal period. Other factors associated with the pathogenesis of necrotizing enterocolitis include a history of umbilical artery catheterization, enteral feeding of small preterm infants, bacterial infection, polycythemia, and gram-negative endotoxemia. Unless there is intestinal necrosis or perforation, medical therapy should be instituted, which should include cessation of enteral feeding, decompression of the stomach, administration of broad-spectrum antibiotics, fluid and electrolyte therapy, parenteral nutrition, and correction of hematologic abnormalities *(Motoyama: Smith's Anesthesia for Infants and Children, ed 2, pp 443-445)*.

636. **(E)**   Midazolam is an excellent choice for premedicating children, since it is water soluble, and has a short ß-elimination half-life (< 2 hours). Midazolam is rapidly absorbed following intramuscular, oral, rectal, nasal, or sublingual administration *(Miller: Anesthesia, ed 4, p 2105)*.

637. **(A)**   Strabismus is misalignment of the visual axis. Infantile strabismus occurs secondary to an innervation abnormality and occurs frequently in patients with central nervous system problems, such as a meningomyelocele, traumatic nerve palsy, or congenital myopathy. Surgical correction of infantile strabismus is most successful when it is done early. The primary anesthetic considerations for these patients include the cardiovascular effects of eye drops, the oculocardiac reflex, and an increased risk for postoperative nausea and vomiting. The use of phenylephrine to produce mydriasis and hemostasis should be minimized to avoid systemic hypertension. Other drugs, such as cyclopentolate, can be used to produce mydriasis without causing hypertension in these patients. In general, approximately 50-80 percent of patients undergoing strabismus surgery will have nausea and vomiting postoperatively. Although the mechanism of this high incidence of vomiting is not known, it is believed to be secondary altered visual perception postoperatively or secondary to an oculoemetic reflex, analogous to the oculocardiac reflex. Administration of droperidol prior to surgery is effective in preventing nausea and vomiting postoperatively. Additionally, avoiding narcotics is commonly recommended. Most recently, propofol has been reported to reduce the incidence of postoperative vomiting in pediatric outpatients having strabismus surgery. Finally, the serotonin antagonist, ondansetron, has been shown to be extremely effective in reducing the incidence of nausea and vomiting in these patients. It was previously held that patients who underwent surgery for strabismus had a higher incidence of malignant hyperthermia. This has since been proven untrue. Some suggest that succinylcholine should be avoided because of its effect on the extraocular muscles, which undergo sustained contracture rather than paralysis after a dose of succinylcholine. It is thought

that this contraction may affect the forced duction test performed by the ophthalmologist at the time of surgery to estimate any restriction in movement of the extraocular muscles *(Gregory: Pediatric Anesthesia, ed 3, pp 684-685).*

638. **(A)** Hemolytic-uremic syndrome is a common cause of acute renal failure in childhood. The disease process is usually associated with gastroenteritis or hemorrhagic colitis, followed by a triad of symptoms consisting of microangiopathic hemolytic anemia, thrombocytopenia, and acute nephropathy. Although the age most frequently affected by this disease is between 6 months and 5 years, hemolytic-uremic syndrome can occur in children throughout the teenage years. The long-term sequelae of this disease include residual hypertension and chronic renal failure, which may require dialysis and/or kidney transplantation *(Gregory: Pediatric Anesthesia, ed 3, p 597).*

639. **(A)** Several anti-cancer agents may have adverse side effects which may alter the anesthetic management of this patient. These include doxorubicin, bleomycin, busulfan, and cyclophosphamide. Doxorubicin can cause severe cardiac depression, which is especially likely when the cumulative dose exceeds 250 mg/m^2 (or 150 mg/m^2 with mediastinal radiation). Bleomycin can cause pulmonary fibrosis, which may be exaggerated in patients who are mechanically ventilated or administered high concentrations of oxygen. Both busulfan and cyclophosphamide inhibit plasma cholinesterases, which may affect the metabolism of succinylcholine *(Gregory: Pediatric Anesthesia, ed 3, pp 184).*

Obstetric Physiology and Anesthesia

DIRECTIONS (Questions 640 through 686): Each of the questions or incomplete statements in this section is followed by answers or by completions of the statement, respectively. Select the ONE BEST answer or completion for each item.

640. A 38-year-old primiparous patient with placenta previa and active vaginal bleeding arrives in the operating room with a blood pressure of 75 mm Hg systolic. A cesarean section is planned. The patient is lightheaded and scared. Which of the following anesthetic plans would be most appropriate for this patient?

   A. Spinal anesthetic with 8 mg of tetracaine
   B. Epidural anesthetic with 20 cc 3% 2-chloroprocaine
   C. General anesthetic induction with 3-4 mg/kg thiopental, intubation with 100 mg succinylcholine
   D. General anesthesia induction with 0.5-1 mg/kg ketamine, intubation with 100 mg succinyl-choline
   E. Replace lost blood volume first, then do any anesthetic the patient wishes

641. Which of the following lung volumes or capacities change the **LEAST** during pregnancy?

   A. Tidal volume
   B. Functional residual capacity
   C. Expiratory reserve volume
   D. Residual volume
   E. Vital capacity

642. General anesthesia is induced in a 35-year-old patient for elective cesarean section. No part of the glottic apparatus is visible after two unsuccessful attempts to intubate, but mask ventilation is adequate. The most appropriate step at this point would be

   A. Wake up the patient
   B. Use an esophageal-tracheal combitube (ETC)
   C. Attempt a blind nasal intubation
   D. Continue mask ventilation and cricoid pressure
   E. Use a laryngeal mask airway

643. Which of the following vasopressors does not decrease uterine blood flow?

   A. Phenylephrine
   B. Methoxamine
   C. Epinephrine
   D. Mephentermine
   E. Ephedrine

644. An 18-year-old patient receiving subcutaneous heparin develops a Horner's syndrome on the left side after placement of an epidural for labor analgesia. On physical exam a T5 anesthetic level is noted, but aside from the Horner's syndrome no other findings are revealed. The most appropriate course of action at this time would be

    A. Remove the epidural
    B. Consult a neurosurgeon
    C. Obtain a CT scan
    D. Secure the airway
    E. None of the above

645. What percent of all pregnancies are affected by preeclampsia?

    A. 2%
    B. 7%
    C. 12%
    D. 19%
    E. 24%

646. In a malpractice action, the final determination of culpability is determined by the defendant physician's

    A. Reputation in the community
    B. Credentials and education
    C. Rapport with the patient and family
    D. Adherence to the standards of practice
    E. History of previous lawsuits

647. Magnesium sulfate is used as an anticonvulsant in patients with preeclampsia and may produce any of the following effects **EXCEPT**

    A. Sedation
    B. Analgesia
    C. Hypotension
    D. Respiratory paralysis
    E. Tocolysis

648. Normal fetal heart rate is

    A. 60 to 100 beats/min
    B. 100 to 140 beats/min
    C. 120 to 160 beats/min
    D. 150 to 200 beats/min
    E. None of the above

649. The leading cause of maternal death in the United States is

    A. General anesthesia (failed intubation or aspiration)
    B. Hemorrhage
    C. Pulmonary embolism
    D. Pregnancy-induced hypertension
    E. Infection

650. Drugs useful in the treatment of uterine atony in an asthmatic with preeclampsia include

    A. Oxytocin, 15 methyl $PGF_{2\alpha}$ and ergonovine
    B. Oxytocin and 15 methyl $PGF_{2\alpha}$
    C. Oxytocin and ergonovine
    D. 15 methyl $PGF_{2\alpha}$ only
    E. Oxytocin only

651. What is the P_{50} of fetal hemoglobin at term?

    A. 15
    B. 19
    C. 26
    D. 31
    E. 37

652. Side effects of ritodrine include all of the following **EXCEPT**

    A. Tachycardia
    B. Hypertension
    C. Hyperglycemia
    D. Pulmonary edema
    E. Hypokalemia

653. Cardiac output returns to nonpregnant levels by how many weeks postpartum?

    A. 1
    B. 2
    C. 4
    D. 6
    E. 10

654. A 32-year-old parturient with a history of severe asthma who is wheezing is brought to the OR for emergency cesarean section under general anesthesia. Which of the following induction agents would be most appropriate for this induction?

    A. Etomidate
    B. Midazolam
    C. Ketamine
    D. Thiopental
    E. Propofol

655. Uterine blood flow at term pregnancy is

    A. 50 mL/min
    B. 250 mL/min
    C. 700 mL/min
    D. 1,000 mL/min
    E. 1,500 mL/min

656. Toxic side effects of magnesium sulfate when used to treat preeclampsia include all the following **EXCEPT**

    A. Cardiac arrest
    B. Neonatal hypotonia
    C. Potentiation of neuromuscular blockade with pancuronium
    D. Renal failure
    E. Hypoventilation

657. Somatic pain associated with the second stage of labor can be controlled by any of the following regional nerve blocks **EXCEPT**

    A. Paracervical block
    B. Saddle block
    C. Lumbar epidural
    D. Pudendal block
    E. Caudal

658. Which of the following signs and symptoms is **NOT** associated with amniotic fluid embolism?

    A. Dyspnea
    B. Hypertension
    C. Bleeding (DIC)
    D. Hypoxemia
    E. Seizures

659. When is the fetus most susceptible to the effects of teratogenic agents?

    A. 1 to 2 weeks' gestation
    B. 3 to 8 weeks' gestation
    C. 7 to 21 weeks' gestation
    D. 14 to 28 weeks' gestation
    E. Anytime during the third trimester

660. A 1,000 gm male infant is born to a 24-year-old mother who is addicted to heroin. The mother admits taking an extra "hit" of heroin prior to coming to the hospital because she was nervous. The infant's respiratory depression would be best managed by

    A. 0.1 mg naloxone IV through umbilical artery catheter
    B. 0.1 mg naloxone IM
    C. 0.1 mg naloxone subcutaneously
    D. Naloxone infusion 0.4 mg/h
    E. None of the above

661. Cardiac output is greatest

     A. During the first trimester of pregnancy
     B. During the second trimester of pregnancy
     C. During the third trimester of pregnancy
     D. During labor
     E. Immediately following delivery of the newborn

662. A 1,000 gram cyanotic infant born with a heart rate of 85, completely limp, making no respiratory effort and showing no response to stimulation would receive a one-minute Apgar score of

     A. 0
     B. 1
     C. 2
     D. 3
     E. 4

663. Which of the following respiratory parameters is not increased in the parturient?

     A. Minute ventilation
     B. Tidal volume
     C. Arterial P_aO_2
     D. Oxygen consumption
     E. Serum bicarbonate

664. A lumbar epidural catheter is placed in a healthy 23-year-old gravida 1, para 0 parturient for cesarean section. Twenty-five minutes after the full dose of local anesthetic is administered, the patient states that she has difficulty breathing through her nose. The most likely explanation for this is

     A. A total spinal from inadvertent subarachnoid injection of local anesthetic
     B. A total sympathectomy and nasal congestion from a high level of blockade
     C. Volume overload
     D. Amniotic fluid embolism
     E. Intravascular injection of local anesthetic

665. Which of the following pharmacologic agents decreases uterine contraction in a dose-dependent fashion?

     A. Barbiturates
     B. Diazepam
     C. Ketamine
     D. Nitrous oxide
     E. Local anesthetics

666. In a term fetus the normal oxygen consumption is approximately

     A. 7 mL/min
     B. 14 mL/min
     C. 21 mL/min
     D. 32 mL/min
     E. 45 mL/min

667. A 24-year-old gravida 2, para 1 parturient is anesthetized for emergency cesarean section. On emergence from general anesthesia, the endotracheal tube is removed and the patient becomes cyanotic. Oxygen is administered by positive-pressure mask-bag ventilation. High airway pressures are necessary to ventilate the patient and wheezing is noted over both lung fields. The patient's blood pressure falls from 120/80 mm Hg to 60/30 mm Hg and heart rate increases from 105 beats/min to 180 beats/min. The most likely cause of these manifestations is

   A. Venous air embolism
   B. Amniotic fluid embolism
   C. Mucous plug in trachea
   D. Pneumothorax
   E. Aspiration

668. A 29-year-old gravida 1, para 0 parturient at 25 weeks' gestation is to undergo an emergency appendectomy under general anesthesia with isoflurane, N_2O, and O_2. Which of the following is a proven untoward consequence of general anesthesia in the unborn fetus?

   A. Nephroblastoma
   B. Cleft palate
   C. Mental retardation
   D. Behavioral defects
   E. None of the above

669. A lumbar epidural is placed in a 24-year-old gravida 1, para 0 parturient with myasthenia gravis for labor. Select the true statement regarding neonatal myasthenia gravis.

   A. The newborn is usually affected
   B. The newborn is affected by maternal IgM antibodies
   C. The newborn may require anticholinesterase therapy for up to 3 weeks
   D. The newborn will need life-long treatment
   E. Only female newborns are affected

670. A 45-year-old gravida 9, para 6 parturient presents to the emergency room in labor. This patient has an increased risk for each of the following **EXCEPT**

   A. Placenta previa
   B. Uterine atony after delivery
   C. Placental abruption
   D. Preeclampsia
   E. Amniotic fluid embolism

671. A 28-year-old gravida 1, para 0 parturient with Eisenmenger's syndrome (pulmonary hypertension with an intracardiac right-to-left or bidirectional shunt) is to undergo placement of a lumbar epidural for analgesia during labor. It is best to avoid a local anesthetic with epinephrine in this patient because it

   A. Raises pulmonary vascular resistance
   B. Lowers systemic vascular resistance
   C. Increases heart rate
   D. Acts as a tocolytic agent
   E. Causes excessive increases in systolic blood pressure

672. Early decelerations are prevented by

   A. Atropine
   B. Increasing fetal oxygenation
   C. Methoxamine
   D. Morphine
   E. Epidural anesthesia

673. The most common injury in obstetric anesthetic claims is

   A. Headache
   B. Pain during anesthesia
   C. Maternal nerve damage
   D. Maternal brain damage
   E. Maternal death

674. Morphine is not used routinely for labor epidurals because it

   A. Increases uterine tone
   B. Causes excessive neonatal respiratory depression
   C. Has a slow onset
   D. Decreases uterine blood flow
   E. Adversely affects fetal heart rate variability

675. High concentrations of lidocaine which might be achieved with an accidental intravascular injection would have what effect on the uterus during labor?

   A. An increase in rate of contraction
   B. An increase in uterine blood flow
   C. Uterine artery vasodilatation
   D. An increase in intrauterine pressure
   E. None of the above

676. Under which of the following conditions would the smallest quantity of diazepam reach the placenta?

   A. At the onset of a contraction
   B. During the peak of a contraction
   C. At the end of a contraction
   D. Between contractions
   E. No relationship exists between drug concentration and uterine contractions

677. Which of the following substances is responsible for the occasional patient experiencing relentless excruciating backache associated with epidural administration of 3% 2-chloroprocaine in volumes greater than 23-25 ml?

    A. Ethylenediaminetetraacetic acid (EDTA)
    B. Sodium bisulfite
    C. Metabisulfite
    D. Paraaminobenzoic acid
    E. 4-amino-2-chlorobenzoic acid

678. A 19-year-old mother is brought to the operating room for emergency cesarean section under epidural anesthesia. 25 cc of 3% 2-chloroprocaine are used to provide surgical anesthesia. One hour after the baby is delivered, the mother complains of excruciating back pain. Neurologic exam is normal. The most appropriate treatment at this choice would be

    A. Epidural blood patch
    B. CT scan
    C. Emergency laminectomy
    D. Administer 100 µg of epidural fentanyl
    E. Observe

679. If 2-chloroprocaine is accidentally injected into maternal blood, it will be rapidly hydrolyzed by pseudocholinesterase. If a patient is homozygous, atypical cholinesterase, the half-life for this drug in the blood would be expected to be

    A. Greater than 1 hr
    B. Approximately 30 minutes
    C. Approximately 15 minutes
    D. Approximately 5 minutes
    E. Approximately 2 minutes

680. Which of the following properties of epidurally administered local anesthetics determines the extent to which epinephrine will prolong the duration of blockade?

    A. Molecular weight
    B. Lipid solubility
    C. pKa
    D. Amide versus ester structure
    E. Concentration

681. Which of the following opioids is unique in that it has both local anesthetic and narcotic properties?

    A. Morphine
    B. Nalbuphine
    C. Hydrocodone
    D. Meperidine
    E. Oxymorphone

682. A 23-year-old parturient in the first trimester is brought to the OR for emergency appendectomy. General anesthesia is planned. An increased risk of congenital malformation associated with which drug has been suggested and should almost always be avoided?

A. Thiopental
B. Nitrous oxide
C. Isoflurane
D. Diazepam
E. None of the above

683. True statements regarding inclusion of intrathecal opioids in obstetric anesthesia practice include each of the following **EXCEPT**

A. Their chief site of action is the substantia gelatinosa of the dorsal horn of the spinal column
B. There is no motor blockade
C. There is no sympathetic blockade
D. Pain relief is adequate for the second stage of labor
E. Lipophilic narcotics are associated with less respiratory depression than nonlipophilic narcotics

684. The most common side effect of intraspinal narcotics in the obstetric population is

A. Pruritus
B. Nausea and vomiting
C. Respiratory depression
D. Urinary retention
E. Headache

685. A 250 lb G1PO has a blood pressure of 180/95 during an office visit at the 18th week of gestation and a pressure 1 week later of 170/95. She has some ankle but no facial edema, and no protein detected in her urine. These findings would be classified as

A. Preeclampsia
B. Chronic hypertension
C. Chronic hypertension with superimposed preeclampsia
D. Gestational hypertension
E. A normal finding

686. An epidural is placed into a 32-year-old parturient receiving magnesium therapy for preeclampsia. Minutes after administration of the test dose, the bolus infusion is interrupted because of a contraction. After the contraction subsides, a slow epidural injection of bupivacaine is resumed. At the same time the patient complains of shortness of breath. She is panic stricken and wrestles violently with the nurses who are trying to reassure her. She repeats that she cannot breathe and becomes cyanotic and loses consciousness. During resuscitation oozing is noted from the IV sites and a pink froth is noted in the endotracheal tube. The most likely diagnosis is

A. Amniotic fluid embolism
B. High spinal
C. Intravascular bupivacaine injection
D. Magnesium overdose
E. Eclampsia

DIRECTIONS (Questions 687 through 720): For each of the items in this section, ONE or MORE of the numbered options is correct. Select the answer:

Select A if options *1, 2 and 3* are correct,
Select B if options *1 and 3* are correct,
Select C if options *2 and 4* are correct,
Select D if only option *4* is correct,
Select E if *all* options are correct.

687. Which of the following intraspinal opioid dose(s) would be acceptable to administer in combination with 12 mg bupivacaine to a parturient about to undergo a cesarean section?

    1. 15 µg fentanyl
    2. 10 µg sufentanil
    3. 0.25 mg morphine
    4. 15 µg fentanyl and 0.25 mg morphine

688. Which of the following is decreased during pregnancy?

    1. Creatinine
    2. MAC for volatile anesthetics
    3. Pseudocholinesterase
    4. Amount of local anesthetics required for lumbar epidurals and spinals

689. Anesthetics which produce uterine relaxation include

    1. Halothane
    2. Isoflurane
    3. Enflurane
    4. Nitrous oxide

690. Passive diffusion of substances across the placenta is enhanced by

    1. Decreased maternal protein binding
    2. Low molecular weight of the substance
    3. High lipid solubility of the substance
    4. High degree of ionization of the substance

691. Untoward effects associated with magnesium overdose include

    1. Complete heart block
    2. Respiratory depression
    3. Hypotension
    4. Coagulopathy

Select A if options *1, 2 and 3* are correct,
Select B if options *1 and 3* are correct,
Select C if options *2 and 4* are correct,
Select D if only option *4* is correct,
Select E if *all* options are correct.

692. Statements which correctly describe differences between fetal and maternal blood include which of the following?

    1. Fetal blood has a lower hemoglobin concentration than does maternal blood
    2. Fetal hemoglobin has a greater affinity for O_2 than does maternal hemoglobin
    3. The fetal oxyhemoglobin dissociation curve is shifted to the right of the maternal oxyhemoglobin dissociation curve
    4. Fetal blood has a lower pH than does maternal blood

693. Which of the following antihypertensive drugs used to treat pregnancy-induced hypertension by virtue of smooth muscle relaxation is (are) capable of causing increased postpartum hemorrhage?

    1. Nitroprusside
    2. Labetalol
    3. Dantrolene
    4. Trimethaphan

694. Preeclampsia is designated as "severe preeclampsia" if any one of the following conditions exists

    1. Proteinuria greater than 5 g/day
    2. Visual disturbances
    3. Urine output less than 400 ml in the 24-hour period
    4. WBC count greater than 15,000

695. Side effects of intraspinal narcotics include

    1. Pruritus
    2. Nausea and vomiting
    3. Sedation
    4. Urinary retention

696. During the second stage of labor, complete pain relief can be obtained with

    1. Paracervical block
    2. Spinal block
    3. Pudendal nerve block
    4. Lumbar epidural block

Select A if options *1, 2 and 3* are correct,
Select B if options *1 and 3* are correct,
Select C if options *2 and 4* are correct,
Select D if only option *4* is correct,
Select E if *all* options are correct.

697. Tocolytics useful in the treatment of preterm labor include

    1. Magnesium sulfate
    2. Terbutaline
    3. Nifedipine
    4. Indomethacin

698. 15 methyl-PGF$_{2\alpha}$ is administered directly into the myometrium to treat uterine atony in a 28-year-old mother. Possible complications from treatment with this drug include

    1. Nausea and vomiting
    2. Bronchospasm
    3. Fever
    4. Hypoxemia

699. True statements regarding magnesium sulfate therapy for preeclampsia include which of the following?

    1. Serum magnesium levels can be estimated by changes in deep-tendon reflexes
    2. Excessive serum magnesium levels cause motor weakness
    3. The therapeutic range for serum magnesium is 4 to 7 mEq/L
    4. The antidote for magnesium toxicity is neostigmine

700. During an emergency cesarean section under spinal anesthesia the parturient develops cough, wheezing, stridor, and becomes cyanotic. The trachea is intubated and food is noted in the pharynx. Appropriate treatment in this patient should consist of

    1. Tracheal suctioning
    2. Steroids
    3. 100% oxygen and PEEP
    4. Saline lavage

701. Antacid premedication in the parturient should be carried out with

    1. Aluminum hydroxide
    2. Magnesium trisilicate
    3. Magnesium hydroxide
    4. Sodium citrate

Select A if options *1, 2 and 3* are correct,
Select B if options *1 and 3* are correct,
Select C if options *2 and 4* are correct,
Select D if only option *4* is correct,
Select E if *all* options are correct.

702. Agents useful for raising the gastric pH just prior to induction of general anesthesia for emergency cesarean section include

1. Cimetidine
2. Metoclopramide
3. Ranitidine
4. Sodium citrate

703. Which of the following decrease(s) fetal heart rate beat-to-beat variability?

1. Morphine
2. Ephedrine
3. Fetal asphyxia
4. Glycopyrrolate

704. The rationale for inserting the epidural needle into the epidural space with the cutting edges parallel to the dural fibers during placement of a labor epidural is

1. It reduces the incidence of cannulation of a dural vein with the epidural catheter
2. It reduces the incidence of dural puncture (wet tap)
3. It reduces the incidence of accidental subdural cannulation with the epidural catheter
4. It reduces the incidence of postdural puncture headache if puncture of the dura inadvertently occurs

705. True statements regarding pregnant diabetic patients include which of the following?

1. Incidence of cesarean section is higher in diabetics
2. Insulin requirements during the second trimester are increased
3. Preeclampsia is more common in diabetics
4. Insulin readily crosses the placenta

706. Signs and symptoms of a postdural puncture headache may include

1. Exacerbation by standing
2. Fever
3. Relief by recumbency
4. Nausea and vomiting

707. Variable decelerations may occur in response to

1. Fetal head compression
2. Uteroplacental insufficiency
3. Maternal hypotension
4. Umbilical cord compression

Select A if options *1, 2 and 3* are correct,
Select B if options *1 and 3* are correct,
Select C if options *2 and 4* are correct,
Select D if only option *4* is correct,
Select E if *all* options are correct.

708. Agents which are useful in decreasing the incidence of shivering during labor in which epidural analgesia is employed include

    1. Administration of epidural sufentanil
    2. Warming of intravenous fluids
    3. Administration of epidural meperidine
    4. Warming the epidural anesthetic solutions to body temperature

709. Appropriate agents for aspiration prophylaxis in parturients who are to be anesthetized for an emergency surgical procedures include

    1. Metoclopramide
    2. Mylanta
    3. Sodium citrate
    4. Ranitidine

710. Possible causes of late decelerations during fetal heart monitoring include

    1. Maternal hypotension
    2. Umbilical cord compression
    3. Excessive uterine activity
    4. Fetal head compression

711. The following drugs and dosages used in newborn resuscitation include

    1. Epinephrine, 0.1-0.3 ml/kg of 1:10,000 solution
    2. 5% albumin, 10 ml/kg
    3. Sodium bicarbonate, 2 mEq/kg
    4. Naloxone, 0.1 mg/kg

712. Useful pharmacologic agents in the treatment of preeclampsia include

    1. Magnesium sulfate
    2. Prostaglandin inhibitors
    3. Nifedipine
    4. Ritodrine

713. Factors which lead to an increased response to inhaled anesthetics during pregnancy include

    1. Increased minute ventilation
    2. Decreased functional residual capacity
    3. Decreased minimum alveolar concentration
    4. Increased cardiac output

Select A if options *1, 2 and 3* are correct,
Select B if options *1 and 3* are correct,
Select C if options *2 and 4* are correct,
Select D if only option *4* is correct,
Select E if *all* options are correct.

714. Adverse effects associated with compression of the **aorta** by the gravid uterus include

    1. Nausea and vomiting
    2. Pallor
    3. Changes in cerebration
    4. Decreases in uterine blood flow

715. Appropriate maneuvers for prevention of aortocaval compression include

    1. Manual displacement of the uterus to the left
    2. Placing a wedge under the patient's left side
    3. Placing a wedge under the patient's right side
    4. Placement of the patient is Trendelenburg position

716. Physiologic factors in the mother that lead to an increase in oxygen delivery to the uterus include

    1. Increased minute ventilation
    2. Hemoglobin P_{50} of 30
    3. Increased cardiac output
    4. Increased hematocrit

717. A decrease in uterine blood flow can occur with

    1. Aortocaval compression
    2. Uterine contractions
    3. Drug induced hypotension
    4. Local anesthetics in high concentrations

718. Addition of epinephrine to the following local anesthetic(s) administered epidurally will reduce the peak maternal local anesthetic concentration by 30-50%

    1. Lidocaine
    2. Etidocaine
    3. Mepivacaine
    4. Bupivacaine

719. The action of which of the following agents is antagonized by the prior or concomitant administration of epidurally administered 2-chloroprocaine?

    1. Fentanyl
    2. Bupivacaine
    3. Morphine
    4. Butorphanol

Select A if options *1, 2 and 3* are correct,
Select B if options *1 and 3* are correct,
Select C if options *2 and 4* are correct,
Select D if only option *4* is correct,
Select E if *all* options are correct.

720. Advantages of spinal anesthesia over epidural anesthesia for cesarean section include

1. Decreased dose of local anesthetic
2. Predictability of segmental analgesic spread
3. Speed of onset of analgesia
4. Less marked hypotension

DIRECTIONS (Questions 721-725): Match the local anesthetics with their specific characteristics in obstetric anesthesia

A. Lidocaine
B. Bupivacaine
C. Prilocaine
D. Etidocaine
E. Chloroprocaine

721. Recalcitrant cardiac arrest

722. Excruciating back pain

723. Motor block outlasts sensory block

724. Methemoglobinemia

725. Rapid metabolism in maternal and fetal blood

OBSTRETRIC PHYSIOLOGY AND ANESTHESIA
ANSWERS, REFERENCES, AND EXPLANATIONS

640. (D)

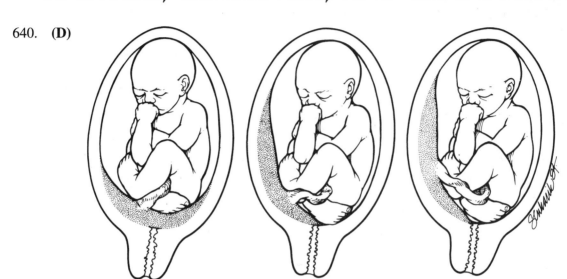

Placenta previa occurs when the placenta implants on the lower uterine segment so that all or part of the placenta covers the internal cervical os. It occurs in about 0.5% of all pregnancies and has a maternal mortality less than 1% but a fetal mortality of about 20% (primarily due to prematurity and intrauterine asphyxia). Patients typically present with painless vaginal bleeding that stops spontaneously (the first bleed). Delivery is cesarean and is often made a few weeks after the "first" bleed when the baby's lungs are more mature. A later bleed can be uncontrolled and accompanied by significant hypovolemia and hypotension. Regional anesthesia is contraindicated in severely hypovolemic patients. Replacing blood loss may not be practical since bleeding may be quicker than replacement. A rapid sequence general anesthetic (assuming an acceptable airway) is preferred. Ketamine supports the cardiovascular system better than thiopental *(Chestnut: Obstetric Anesthesia, pp 700-703; Chantigian: Antepartum Hemorrhage in Datta: Common Problems in Obstetric Anesthesia, pp 236-244).*

641. (E) At term pregnancy tidal volume (TV) increases about 45% and the inspiratory reserve volume (IRV) increases about 5%. A decrease occurs in both the expiratory reserve volume (ERV) 25% and the residual volume (RV) 15%. A capacity is defined as two or more lung volumes. Functional residual capacity (ERV + RV) is decreased about 20% and is partly responsible for the rapid fall in maternal oxygenation that occurs with apnea during the induction of general anesthesia. Total lung capacity (TV + IRV + ERV + RV) decreases slightly in 5% whereas vital capacity (TV + IRV + ERV) remains unchanged *(Chestnut: Obstetric Anesthesia, pp 18-19).*

642. (A) Evaluation of the airway should be performed before the induction of any general anesthetic. In cases where an unrecognized difficult airway exists (unable to perform endotracheal intubation early) the patient should be awakened if the procedure is purely elective. A regional anesthetic or awake intubation can then be safely performed. In cases of fetal or maternal distress other options for securing the airway may be necessary *(Chestnut: Obstetric Anesthesia, pp 589-599).*

643. **(E)**   Uterine blood flow increases dramatically during pregnancy and a generalized reduction in the sensitivity to vasoconstrictors exists. In animal studies ephedrine did not decrease uterine blood flow whereas the other drugs listed in the question did. Recent human studies have shown that drugs with alpha agonist activity (such as phenylephrine, methoxamine, and epinephrine) may give comparatively good results in treating regional anesthetic induced hypotension. However in most cases, ephedrine is still chosen as the vasopressor of choice. In cases of hypotension refractory to ephedrine, epinephrine may prove useful since raising the perfusion pressure may outweigh the risk of increasing the vascular tone *(Chestnut: Obstetric Anesthesia, pp 44-52).*

644. **(E)**   This benign condition occasionally develops after a lumbar epidural anesthetic even when the highest dermatome level blocked is below T_5. It may be related to the superficial anatomic location of the descending spinal sympathetic fibers that lie just below the spinal pia of the dorsolateral funiculus which is within diffusion range of subanesthetic concentrations of local anesthetics in the cerebrospinal fluid *(Shnider: Anesthesia for Obstetrics, ed 3, p 440).*

645. **(B)**   Preeclampsia is a disorder that rarely occurs before the 20th week of gestation (unless a hydatidiform mole is present) and is characterized by the triad of hypertension, generalized edema, and proteinuria. It occurs with an overall incidence of approximately 7% and occurs most frequently in primigravidas. The incidence of preeclampsia is significantly higher in parturients with a hydatidiform mole, multiple gestations, obesity, polyhydramnios, and diabetes. Mothers with preeclampsia during their first pregnancy have a 33% chance of having preeclampsia in subsequent pregnancies. Preeclampsia can progress to eclampsia (preeclampsia accompanied by a seizure not related to other conditions) anytime during pregnancy, labor and delivery, or within the first 24 hours following delivery. Approximately 5% of untreated parturients with preeclampsia will develop eclampsia *(Shnider: Anesthesia for Obstetrics, ed 3, pp 305-306; Stoelting: Anesthesia and Co-existing Disease, ed 2, p 783).*

646. **(D)**   The Physician's Insurers Association of America conducted a study in 1992 wherein they analyzed malpractice claims reported by physician-owned insurance companies which were closed between January 1985 and June 1991. Fewer than 5 percent of all reported claims were made against anesthesiologists, and those which resulted in payments to the plaintiff comprised fewer than 1 percent of the total paid claims against physicians of all specialties. The most common type of claim was that made against anesthesiologists who were participating in the care of patients for pregnancy and childbirth. The final determination of culpability or lack thereof is contingent on determining whether the physician did or did not follow standards of practice for his or her specialty *(Shnider: Anesthesia for Obstetrics, ed 3, pp 468-469).*

647. **(B)**   Magnesium sulfate is used either as a tocolytic agent to prevent premature labor or to prevent seizures in parturients with preeclampsia. Magnesium sulfate has many other pharmacologic properties which include sedation, hypotension, loss of deep tendon reflexes (10 mEq/L), respiratory paralysis (15 mEq/L) and cardiac arrest (25-35 mEq/L). It does not, however, have any analgesic properties *(Shnider: Anesthesia for Obstetrics, ed 3, pp 315 & 350).*

648. **(C)**   Fetal monitors consist of a two-channel recorder for simultaneous recording of fetal heart rate and uterine activity. In looking at the fetal heart rate (FHR) one assesses the baseline rate, the FHR variability and the periodic changes (accelerations or decelerations) that occur with uterine contraction. The normal fetal heart rate ranges between 120 and 160 beats/min. Some

extend the lower limit of normal to 110 beats/min. Baseline fetal heart rates < 120 beats/min (bradycardia) and >160 beats/min (tachycardia) have been associated with fetal asphyxia. Causes of fetal bradycardia include hypoxia, acidosis, congenital heart block, and some drugs; causes of fetal tachycardia include infection, fever, maternal smoking, fetal PSVT, and some drugs [ritodrine]. Normal heart rate beat-to-beat variability ranges between 5 and 20 beats/min. Lack of fetal heart rate beat-to-beat variability may be caused by drugs, such as benzodiazepines, opiates, volatile anesthetics, anticholinergics, fetal asphyxia, anemia, and prematurity *(Barash: Clinical Anesthesia, ed 2, p 1287)*.

649. **(B)** The leading cause of maternal death in the United States is hemorrhage (30%). Next is pulmonary embolism at 24%, pregnancy-induced hypertension 18%, and infection approximately 8%. Anesthesia is involved in only 3% of maternal deaths. Most of these relate to general anesthetic complications like aspiration or failure to intubate and ventilate the patient *(Atrach HK: Maternal mortality in the United States, 1979-1986. Obstet Gynecol 76:1055-1060, 1990; Shnider: Anesthesia for Obstetrics, ed 3, pp 458-460)*.

650. **(E)** Uterine atony is a common cause of postpartum hemorrhage. Treatment consists of uterine massage, drugs, and in rare cases hysterectomy. Drugs commonly used include oxytocin, ergot alkaloids (ergonovine, methylergonovine) and prostaglandins (PGE_2, $PGF_{2\alpha}$ and 15 methyl $PGF_{2\alpha}$). The ergot alkaloids not infrequently cause elevations in blood pressure and are relatively contraindicated in patients with hypertension (such as preeclampsia). Ergot alkaloids have been associated with bronchospasm and may not be appropriate in asthmatics. The prostaglandin 15-methyl $PGF_{2\alpha}$ is the only prostaglandin currently approved for treatment of uterine atony in the U.S. and may cause significant bronchospasm in susceptible patients *(Shnider: Anesthesia for Obstetrics, ed 3, p 531; Chestnut: Obstetric Anesthesia, p 973)*.

651. **(B)** The term P_{50} denotes the blood oxygen tension (P_aO_2) that produces 50% saturation of erythrocyte hemoglobin. The P_{50} value of fetal blood (75-85% of fetal blood is hemoglobin F) is around 19 mm Hg versus the adult value of 26 mm Hg. Thus fetal hemoglobin has a higher affinity for oxygen than does maternal hemoglobin *(Shnider: Anesthesia for Obstetrics, ed 3, pp 26 & 27; Chestnut: Obstetric Anesthesia, p 80)*.

652. **(B)** Ritodrine and terbutaline are beta adrenergic agonists with tocolytic properties. Side effects are similar to other beta adrenergic drugs and include tachycardia, hypotension, hyperglycemia, pulmonary edema, and hypokalemia *(Chestnut: Obstetric Anesthesia, pp 652-655)*.

653. **(B)** The numerous changes that take place in the cardiovascular system during pregnancy provide for the needs of the fetus and prepare the mother for labor and delivery. During the first trimester of pregnancy, cardiac output increases by approximately 30% to 40%. At term the cardiac output is 50% increased over nonpregnant values. This increase in cardiac output is caused by an increase in stroke volume and an increase in heart rate. During labor, cardiac output increases 15% during the latent phase, 30% during the active phase, and 45% during the expulsive stage of labor and delivery. The greatest increase in cardiac output occurs immediately following delivery of the newborn where the cardiac output can increase to greater than 80% above prelabor values. This final increase in cardiac output is attributed primarily to autotransfusion and increased venous return associated with uterine involution. Cardiac output then grad-

ually declines to nonpregnant levels by approximately 2 weeks after delivery *(Shnider: Anesthesia for Obstetrics, ed 3, pp 8 & 9; Chestnut: Obstetric Anesthesia, pp 20-23).*

654. **(C)** Asthma occurs in about 1% of all pregnancies. When inducing general anesthesia in an asthmatic patient, it is imperative to establish an adequate depth of anesthesia before placing an endotracheal tube. If the patient is "light", then severe bronchospasm may occur. In patients with mild asthma, induction may work with any of these drugs. In a patient with severe asthma, ketamine which has inherent bronchodilator properties is preferred. In patients with mild asthma that do not need the accessory muscles of respiration, regional anesthesia should be strongly considered since it would eliminate the need for endotracheal intubation *(Shnider: Anesthesia for Obstetrics, ed 3, p 533; Chestnut: Obstetric Anesthesia, pp 974-975).*

655. **(C)** Uterine blood flow increases dramatically from 50-100 ml/min before pregnancy to about 700 ml at term. Ninety percent of the uterine blood flow at term goes to the intervillous spaces. Uterine blood flow is related to the perfusion pressure (uterine arterial pressure minus uterine venous pressure) divided by uterine vascular resistance. Thus, factors that decrease uterine blood flow include systemic hypotension, aortocaval compression, uterine contraction, and vasoconstriction *(Chestnut: Obstetric Anesthesia, pp 44-47; Shnider: Anesthesia for Obstetrics, ed 3, p 23).*

656. **(D)** Magnesium sulfate overdose can lead to both maternal and neonatal complications including muscle weakness, respiratory depression, and cardiac failure. If renal failure occurs (as a result of severe preeclampsia and not as a result of magnesium sulfate), plasma magnesium concentrations should be monitored closely since magnesium is excreted by the kidneys. The therapeutic range for plasma magnesium concentration is 4 to 8 mEq/L. Plasma magnesium concentrations of 10 mEq/L can result in loss of deep-tendon reflexes and plasma magnesium concentrations of 15 mEq/L can result in sinoatrial and atrioventricular block, and respiratory paralysis. Should plasma magnesium concentrations increase to 20 to 25 mEq/L, cardiovascular collapse and cardiac arrest may ensue *(Stoelting: Basics of Anesthesia, ed 3, p 371; Shnider: Anesthesia for Obstetrics, ed 3, p 350).*

657. **(A)** Pain during the first stage of labor is visceral in nature and is related to uterine contractions and dilation of the cervix. Pain impulses enter the spinal cord at the T10 to L1 level. Second stage pain includes the visceral pain of the first stage but adds the somatic pain created with pelvic floor distention. The somatic pain is transmitted via the pudendal nerve and enters the spinal cord at the S2-4 level. The paracervical block only blocks the visceral first stage pathways. A true saddle block (sacral dermatomes only) and the pudendal block work for second stage somatic pain only whereas a lumbar epidural or a caudal epidural can be used for both first and second stage analgesia *(Chestnut: Obstetric Anesthesia, pp 181, 420-429).*

658. **(B)** Amniotic fluid embolism is a serious complication of labor and delivery that results from the entrance of amniotic fluid and constituents of amniotic fluid into the maternal systemic circulation. For this to occur, the placental membranes must be ruptured and abnormal open sinusoids at the uteroplacental site or lacerations of endocervical veins must exist. The onset of amniotic fluid embolism is associated with dyspnea, severe hypotension, and hypoxemia. DIC occurs in as many as 40% of these patients, whereas seizures occasionally occur *(Chestnut: Obstetric Anesthesia, pp 727 & 728).*

659. **(B)** Organogenesis occurs between the 15th to 56th days (3-8 weeks) of gestation in humans and is the time during which the fetus is most susceptible to teratogenic agents. There is no conclusive evidence to implicate any local, IV induction agents, or volatile anesthetic agents in the causation of congenital anomalies *(Chestnut: Obstetric Anesthesia, pp 275-283)*.

660. **(E)** Opioid abuse includes morphine, heroin, methadone, meperidine, and fentanyl. The problems associated with abuse are many and include the drug effect itself, substances mixed with the narcotics (e.g., talc, corn starch) as well as infection, and malnutrition. Newborn respiratory depression as manifested by a low respiratory rate is treated with controlled ventilation but not with naloxone. Naloxone might precipitate an acute withdrawal reaction. The dose of naloxone to treat narcotic induced respiratory depression in the non-addicted newborn is 0.1 mg/kg *(Chestnut: Obstetric Anesthesia, pp 146, 987, & 988)*.

661. **(E)** Immediately after delivery, the cardiac output can increase up to 80% above prelabor values. This is thought to result from autotransfusion secondary to increased venous return to the heart associated with involution of the uterus *(Shnider: Anesthesia for Obstetrics, ed 3, p 9)*.

662. **(B)** The Apgar score is a subjective scoring system used to evaluate the newborn and is commonly performed at 1 and 5 minutes after delivery. A value of 0, 1, or 2 is given to each of 5 signs (heart rate, respiratory effort, muscle tone, reflex irritability, and color) and totaled. A cyanotic neonate gets a 0 for color, acrocyanosis receives a 1, and a pink baby gets a 2 for color. A heart rate of 0 receives a score of 0. Fewer than 100 beats per minute receives a 1; greater than 100 beats per minute receives a 2. Completely limp muscle tone would warrant a score of 0 whereas some movement of extremities would receive a 1 and vigorous active movement would receive a 2. No respiratory effort is scored as a 0. Shallow, slow gasping efforts would receive a 1 while robust breathing or crying earns a 2. No response to stimulation, i.e., manual stimulation, suctioning, etc. would receive a 0. A grimace in response to these maneuvers would receive a 1 whereas active coughing and sneezing would receive a 2. A score of 7-10 is normal, 4-6 moderate depression, and 0-3 severe depression. Weight is not a factor in the scoring system *(Chestnut: Obstetric Anesthesia, pp 140 & 141)*.

663. **(E)** The respiratory system undergoes many changes during pregnancy with an increase in minute ventilation about 45%, tidal volume 40-45%, and arterial P_aO_2 increases slightly due to a fall in $PaCO_2$. Oxygen consumption increases about 20%. The serum bicarbonate level falls an average of 4 mEq/L to help keep the pH in the normal range due to the respiratory alkalosis ($PaCO_2$ to approximately 30) that occurs *(Chestnut: Obstetric Anesthesia, pp 18-20; Shnider: Anesthesia for Obstetrics, ed 3, p 3)*.

664. **(B)** The sympathetic nerve fibers exit the spinal cord through T1-L2. A high spinal or high epidural can block all of the sympathetic fibers causing hypotension, bradycardia, and venodilation. Venodilation of the veins in the nasal mucosa causes nasal stuffiness and swelling *(Cousins: Neural Blockade in Clinical Anesthesia and Management of Pain, ed 2, pp 279, 283)*.

665. **(A)** Barbiturates cause a dose-dependent reduction in uterine contractions. Diazepam and nitrous oxide have no effect. Ketamine produces a dose-related oxytocic effect on uterine tone during the second trimester of pregnancy but no increase in tone at term. Local anesthetics injected

intravenously cause an increase in uterine tone and at high levels can lead to tetanic contractions *(Shnider: Anesthesia for Obstetrics, ed 3, pp 54-57).*

666. **(C)** The normal term (approximately 3 kg) fetus has an oxygen consumption of about 21 ml/min. Since the fetal store of oxygen is about 42 mL it would in theory take 2 minutes to completely deplete it during an interruption in the normal blood supply of oxygen. In reality, the fetus has several compensatory mechanisms that allow it to survive for longer periods of time during periods of hypoxia *(Shnider: Anesthesia for Obstetrics, ed 3, p 25; Chestnut: Obstetric Anesthesia, p 79).*

667. **(E)** All of the choices are consistent with the scenario described in this question. From the temporal perspective gastric acid aspiration is the most likely cause. Morbidity and mortality following gastric acid aspiration is determined by both the amount and the pH of the aspirated material. Aspiration of a gastric volume greater than 0.4 mL/kg with a pH less than 2.5 causes severe pneumonitis with high morbidity and mortality. Bronchospasm and wheezing are suggestive of gastric acid aspiration and not amniotic fluid embolism. Other signs and symptoms suggestive of gastric acid aspiration include sudden coughing or laryngospasm, dyspnea, tachypnea, the presence of foreign material in the mouth or posterior pharynx, chest wall retraction, cyanosis that is not relieved by oxygen supplementation, tachycardia, hypotension, and the development of pink frothy exudate. The onset of these signs and symptoms is usually rapid *(Stoelting: Anesthesia and Co-existing Disease, ed 3, p 567; Shnider: Anesthesia for Obstetrics, ed 3, pp 410 & 411).*

668. **(E)** The primary objectives in the anesthetic management of parturients undergoing general anesthesia for nonobstetric surgery are to 1) ensure maternal safety, 2) avoid teratogenic drugs, 3) avoid intrauterine fetal asphyxia, and 4) prevent the induction of preterm labor. Premature onset of labor is the most common complication associated with surgery during the second trimester of pregnancy. Performance of an intra-abdominal procedure in which the uterus is manipulated is the most significant factor in causing preterm labor in these patients. Neurosurgical, orthopedic, thoracic, or other surgical procedures that do not involve manipulation of the uterus do not cause preterm labor. No anesthetic agent or technique has been found to be significantly associated with a higher or lower incidence of preterm labor. Furthermore, there is no evidence that the risk of developing any of the conditions listed in this question is increased for the offspring of patients who receive general anesthesia during pregnancy *(Shnider: Anesthesia for Obstetrics, ed 3, pp 268-270; Stoelting: Anesthesia and Co-existing Disease, ed 3, p 569).*

669. **(C)** Myasthenia gravis (MG) is an autoimmune neuromuscular disease in which IgG antibodies are directed against the acetylcholine receptors in skeletal muscle causing patients to present with general muscle weakness and easy fatigability. Smooth muscle and cardiac muscle are not affected. About 10-20% of newborns born to mothers with myasthenia gravis are transiently affected since the IgG antibody is transferred through the placenta. Neonatal myasthenia gravis is characterized by muscle weakness (e.g., hypotonia, respiratory difficulty) and may present within the first 4 days of life (80% present within the first 24 hours). Anticholinesterase therapy may be required for a few weeks until the maternal IgG antibodies are metabolized *(Chestnut: Obstetric Anesthesia, pp 925-927; Shnider: Anesthesia for Obstetrics, ed 3, p 575).*

670. **(D)** High parity is a risk factor for each of the conditions listed in this question except preeclampsia. Primigravid patients are at greatest risk for preeclampsia, although this disease is not limited to this group. The lack of adequate prenatal care is the most frequent condition associated with preeclampsia-eclampsia, which most likely accounts for the more frequent occurrence of this condition in parturients of lower socioeconomic status *(Shnider: Anesthesia for Obstetrics, ed 3, pp 305, 379, 385, 389, & 393; Stoelting: Anesthesia and Co-existing Disease, ed 3, pp 566 & 567)*.

671. **(B)** Eisenmenger's syndrome may develop in patients with left-to-right intracardiac shunting such as ASD, VSD, or patent ductus arteriosus. In this syndrome the pulmonary and vascular tone and right ventricular muscle undergo changes in response to the shunt producing pulmonary hypertension and a change in the direction of the shunt to a right-to-left or bidirectional type with peripheral cyanosis. The maternal mortality rate is 30-50%. Approximately 3% of all newborns with congenital heart defects will develop this condition. Because the pulmonary vascular resistance is fixed in these patients, this condition is not amenable to surgical correction; thus, survival beyond age 40 is uncommon. Any event or drug that increases pulmonary vascular resistance or decreases systemic vascular resistance will worsen the right-to-left shunt, exacerbate peripheral cyanosis, and may precipitate right ventricular heart failure in these patients. Controversy exists regarding pain management for these patients. Most prefer a narcotic based analgesic (spinal or epidural). If local anesthetics are needed, careful titration is important. Low-dose epinephrine, which is commonly used to decrease absorption of local anesthetics, can cause a decrease in systemic vascular resistance, which will exacerbate the right-to-left shunt and should not be added to the local anesthetic *(Chestnut: Obstetric Anesthesia, pp 748-750; Stoelting: Anesthesia and Co-existing Disease, ed 3, pp 559 & 560)*.

672. **(A)** Early decelerations are caused by compression of the fetal head and are not associated with fetal distress. The head compression causes an increase in intracranial pressure and results in a reflex bradycardia via the vagus nerve. This pattern can be blocked with atropine although treatment is not needed. There decelerations begin with the onset of the uterine contraction and reflect the shape of the contractions. Generally the rate does not go below 90-100 beats/min. Frequency in the first stage of labor is 20% *(Chestnut: Obstetric Anesthesia, p 128; Stoelting: Anesthesia and Co-existing Disease, ed 3, p 569)*.

673. **(E)** In obstetric claims the mean maternal age is 28 years. Sixty-seven percent of cases involves cesarean section, 33% vaginal deliveries. Of the obstetric claims, 65% were associated with regional anesthesia and 33% with general anesthesia. The most common injury was maternal death which comprised 27% of all claims. Fifteen percent of claims involved headache, 11% pain during anesthesia, 11% maternal nerve damage, 9% maternal brain damage, 8% emotional distress, and 6% back pain *(Shnider: Anesthesia for Obstetrics, ed 3, pp 476 & 477; Chestnut: Obstetric Anesthesia, p 557)*.

674. **(C)** The main reason morphine is not routinely used for labor epidurals is its long onset time (40-50 minutes after 4-5 mg epidural morphine). Morphine has little effect on uterine tone, uterine blood flow, or fetal heart rate. The doses used epidurally do not cause significant neonatal depression *(Shnider: Anesthesia for Obstetrics, ed 3, pp 44, 56, & 93)*.

675. **(D)** A large dose of lidocaine intravascularly can cause uterine artery vasoconstriction, a decrease in uterine blood flow, and an increase in intrauterine pressure. In vitro studies have shown that local anesthetics produce an increase in the tone of uterine muscle but decrease the rate and strength of contractions *(Shnider: Anesthesia for Obstetrics, ed 3, pp 35, 57; Chestnut: Obstetric Anesthesia, p 211).*

676. **(B)** During the peak of a uterine contraction, uterine arterial blood flow ceases. If the drug arrives at the uterus during the onset or decline of a contraction when only the uterine venous outflow was decreased, then the drug could be sequestered in the intervillous space and potentially could cross the placenta to a greater extent *(Shnider: Anesthesia for Obstetrics, ed 3, p 71).*

677. **(A)** In the 1980s some patients who received chloroprocaine intrathecally rather than epidurally developed arachnoiditis. The cause of the arachnoiditis was felt to be related to sodium bisulfate which was in the formulation of chloroprocaine. Recently, the bisulfate was replaced with EDTA, which may produce a severe, unrelenting backache that may last several hours when doses greater than 20 ml of chloroprocaine are used *(Shnider: Anesthesia for Obstetrics, ed 3, p 85; Chestnut: Obstetric Anesthesia, p 209).*

678. **(D)** The severe back pain that some patients develop after 25 ml of chloroprocaine can be relieved by a further dose of local anesthetic or by 100 to 200 µg of epidural fentanyl *(Shnider: Anesthesia for Obstetrics, ed 3, p 85).*

679. **(E)** Chloroprocaine breaks down rapidly in the blood by normal pseudocholinesterase. In vitro plasma half-life is 21 seconds in maternal blood and 43 seconds in fetal blood. In patients who are homozygous for the atypical cholinesterase, the half-life is prolonged to about 2 minutes *(Shnider: Anesthesia for Obstetrics, ed 3, pp 85-86).*

680. **(B)** Epinephrine is primarily added to local anesthetics to increase the intensity and duration of the block. The more lipid soluble the drug the less effect epinephrine has *(Shnider: Anesthesia for Obstetrics, ed 3, p 92; Chestnut: Obstetric Anesthesia, p 215).*

681. **(D)** Meperidine in addition to its narcotic effects also demonstrates local anesthetic actions *(Shnider: Anesthesia for Obstetrics, ed 3, p 92).*

682. **(D)** An increased risk of congenital malformations has been suggested by several studies with the use of minor tranquilizers such as diazepam, meprobamate, and chlordiazepoxide during the first trimester of pregnancy. The cause and effect relationship has not been proven but the Food and Drug Administration recommends that these drugs not be used in the first trimester of pregnancy *(Shnider: Anesthesia for Obstetrics, ed 3, pp 276 & 718; Chestnut: Obstetric Anesthesia, pp 275-283).*

683. **(D)** Intrathecal opiates are very effective in relieving the visceral pain during the first stage of labor. However, they do not provide adequate pain relief for the second stage somatic pain *(Shnider: Anesthesia for Obstetrics, ed 3, pp 157-164; Chestnut: Obstetric Anesthesia, pp 526 & 527).*

684. **(A)** The most common side effect of intraspinal narcotics is pruritus. The next most common is nausea and vomiting followed by urinary retention. Respiratory depression and postdural puncture headaches may also occur but are relatively infrequent *(Shnider: Anesthesia for Obstetrics, ed 3, pp 164 & 165).*

685. **(B)** Hypertension (systolic BP > 140 or a rise > 30 mm Hg over baseline, diastolic BP > 90 or a rise of 15 mmHg over baseline) occurs in about 5-7% of all pregnancies. It is commonly classified by the American College of Obstetricians and Gynecologists as one of four types (preeclampsia-eclampsia, chronic hypertension, chronic hypertension plus preeclampsia-eclampsia, or gestational hypertension). Preeclampsia rarely occurs before 24 weeks EGA except in patients with gestational trophoblastic neoplasms (e.g., molar pregnancy) and manifests as a triad of hypertension, generalized edema (not just dependent edema) and proteinuria. Chronic hypertension is persistent hypertension before, during, and after pregnancy (e.g., >6 weeks). Some patients develop gestational hypertension which is an increase in blood pressure without generalized edema or proteinuria which resolves by 2-6 weeks *(Shnider: Anesthesia for Obstetrics, ed 3, pp 305-307; Chestnut: Obstetric Anesthesia, p 876).*

686. **(A)** The four cardinal features of amniotic fluid embolism are dyspnea, hypoxemia, cardiovascular collapse, and coma. The patient may also develop DIC, seizures and pulmonary edema from left ventricular failure. Patients with a high spinal or epidural may complain of dyspnea, but they also have marked weakness and would certainly not be able to wrestle or struggle with their health care providers. Patients experiencing an intravascular injection of local anesthetic present with CNS signs of toxicity (lightheadedness, visual or auditory disturbances, muscular twitching, convulsion, coma) or at higher levels cardiovascular collapse. Magnesium overdosage is also associated with muscle weakness. The typical eclamptic seizure is tonic clonic, patients do not complain of dyspnea, although an associated aspiration may produce similar symptoms *(Chestnut: Obstetric Anesthesia, pp 727 & 728: Shnider: Anesthesia for Obstetrics, ed 3, pp 377-384).*

687. **(E)** Intrathecal opioids are often mixed with local anesthetics to provide better intraoperative and postoperative pain. Fentanyl is commonly used in doses of 10-25 µg, sufentanil in doses of 5-10 µg, and morphine in doses of 0.2-0.4 mg. Some anesthesiologists add both fentanyl and morphine since morphine is slow in onset and fentanyl has a comparatively shorter duration of action *(Shnider: Anesthesia for Obstetrics, ed 3, pp 92-95; Chestnut: Obstetric Anesthesia, pp 468 & 469).*

688. **(E)** The decrease in pseudocholinesterase activity of about 25% during pregnancy is not clinically significant in terms of prolonging the half-life of drugs such as succinylcholine. Plasma creatinine is decreased because cardiac output and renal blood flow are increased. Parturients are more sensitive to volatile and local anesthetics than are nonpregnant patients. The mechanism of this reduction in anesthetic requirement is not known but may be related to elevated progesterone levels *(Chestnut: Obstetric Anesthesia, pp 24, 31-34; Shnider: Anesthesia for Obstetrics, ed 3, 12-14).*

689. **(A)** All halogenated anesthetic agents cause a dose-related relaxation of uterine smooth muscle. With anesthetic concentrations of 0.5 MAC, halothane, enflurane, and isoflurane significantly decrease uterine activity. The uterine response to oxytocin at this low concentration, however,

remains intact. Nitrous oxide does not interfere with uterine activity *(Chestnut: Obstetric Anesthesia, pp 264, 265, & 349; Shnider: Anesthesia for Obstetrics, ed 3, p 54)*.

690. **(A)** Drugs with a molecular weight less than 500 daltons pass through the placenta more readily than do drugs with larger molecular weights. Decreased maternal protein binding makes more drug available to pass through the placenta. Lipid-soluble drugs penetrate the placenta more readily than water-soluble drugs, i.e. drugs with a high degree of ionization *(Miller: Anesthesia, ed 4, p 2039)*.

691. **(A)** As the blood level of magnesium increases, different adverse reactions can be seen. At 10 mEq/L deep tendon reflexes are lost. At 15 mEq/L sinoatrial, and atrioventricular block as well as respiratory paralysis occur. At 25 mEq/L cardiac arrest can develop. Magnesium sulfate does not cause coagulopathy; however, a coagulopathy may develop in patients with pregnancy-induced hypertension (who may be simultaneously receiving $MgSO_4$) *(Shnider: Anesthesia for Obstetrics, ed 3, pp 314-316)*.

692. **(C)** The fetus has several compensatory mechanisms for dealing with low O_2 pressures (umbilical vein PO_2 approximately equal to 30 mm Hg) to which it is exposed. These include a higher hemoglobin concentration (15-20 gm/dl) and the presence of fetal hemoglobin which has a greater affinity for oxygen (the oxyhemoglobin dissociation curve is shifted to the left of maternal hemoglobin) than maternal hemoglobin. Fetal blood has a lower pH than maternal blood which may be related to the higher $PaCO_2$ levels *(Shnider: Anesthesia for Obstetrics, ed 3, pp 25-27)*.

693. **(B)** Nitroprusside and dantrolene have direct effects on smooth muscle (such as the uterus) and may be associated with increased postpartum hemorrhage. Nitroprusside's effects are short lived after discontinuation. Labetalol (adrenergic blocker) and trimethaphan (ganglionic blocker) do not affect uterine contractions significantly *(Shnider: Anesthesia for Obstetrics, ed 3, pp 316-318)*.

694. **(A)** Preeclampsia occurs in about 7% of all pregnancies and is associated with hypertension, proteinuria and/or generalized edema. It usually occurs after the 20th week of gestation but may present earlier in cases of gestational trophoblastic disease (e.g., molar pregnancy). It is clarified either as mild or severe. It becomes severe if any of the following conditions coexist:

BP ≥ 160 systolic or ≥ 110 diastolic
proteinuria > 5 gm/24 hours
urine output < 400 ml/24 hours
CNS disturbances (seizures, altered consciousness, headaches, blurred vision)
pulmonary edema
coagulopathy
hepatic rupture

Most patients have increased cardiac output, normal or increased systemic vascular resistance, and normal or decreased blood volumes and filling pressures *(Shnider: Anesthesia for Obstetrics, ed 3, pp 307-309; Chestnut: Obstetric Anesthesia, p 847, Box 44-3)*.

695. (E)   The most common side effect of intraspinal narcotics is pruritus (which appears unassociated with histamine release). Respiratory depression occasionally develops and is associated with a gradual progression of increasing sedation and decreasing respiratory rate. Nausea and vomiting as well as urinary retention are other untoward effects *(Shnider: Anesthesia for Obstetrics, ed 3, p 178)*.

696. (C)   The first stage of labor starts with the onset of labor and ends with complete cervical dilation (10 cm). It is associated with uterine contractions and dilation of the cervix and is transmitted via the autonomic nervous system through the sympathetic fibers that pass through the paracervical region and enter the CNS at T10-L1 segments. The second stage of labor includes these pathways and adds the somatic fibers of the birth canal that are transmitted via the pudendal nerve entering the CNS at S2-S4. Spinal and epidural anesthesia can cover both areas and can produce complete anesthesia during the second stage of labor. If a low spinal or saddle block is performed (covering only sacral areas) the contraction pain will still be felt. Paracervical blocks only block the first stage pain. Pudendal blocks block the somatic component during the second stage but not visceral pain of contractions *(Chestnut: Obstetric Anesthesia, pp 316-317, 181)*.

697. (E)   There are several drugs that can be used for tocolytic therapy for preterm labor. Most commonly magnesium sulfate and/or beta-adrenergic agonists (ritodrine, terbutaline) are used. Indomethacin and nifedipine have recently been used in selected cases *(Chestnut: Obstetric Anesthesia, pp 647 & 648)*.

698. (E)   15-methyl $PGF_{2\alpha}$ is the preferred prostaglandin for use in the treatment of refractory uterine atony (after oxytocin). It has several important side effects such as bronchospasm, V/Q mismatch with an increase in intrapulmonary shunting and hypoxemia. Other side effects include nausea, vomiting, fever, and diarrhea *(Chestnut: Obstetric Anesthesia, p 709)*.

699. (A)   Magnesium sulfate is the anticonvulsant of choice in the preeclamptic patient in North America and is more effective than phenytoin. In addition to its anticonvulsant effect, $MgSO_4$ exerts a peripheral effect at the neuromuscular junction. The therapeutic range for serum $MgSO_4$ is 4-7 mEq/L. Loss of deep tendon reflexes occurs at 10 mEq/L, respiratory arrest at 12-16 mEq/L, and asystole at >20 mEq/L. The treatment for magnesium toxicity is calcium *(Chestnut: Obstetric Anesthesia, pp 859-860)*.

700. (B)   Three different aspiration syndromes have been described: aspiration of particulate matter, aspiration of acid fluid, and aspiration of fecal material. Aspiration of fecal material can occur with bowel obstruction and rarely is a problem in obstetrics. Symptoms of aspiration include coughing, tachypnea, tachycardia, bronchospasm, and hypoxemia. Treatment is supportive and includes suctioning the airway, administration of increased concentration of oxygen and the application of PEEP as needed. Use of saline lavage will not remove acid from the airway and can worsen hypoxemia. Steroids have not been effective in limiting the inflammation that occurs and may increase the risk of secondary bacterial infection *(Chestnut: Obstetric Anesthesia, pp 569-570)*.

701. **(D)** All of the choices listed are antacids, however, clear nonparticulate antacids (sodium citrate) are preferred over particulate antacids (aluminum hydroxide, magnesium trisilicate, magnesium hydroxide), since they cause less pulmonary damage if aspirated *(Chestnut: Obstetric Anesthesia, pp 571-572)*.

702. **(D)** Sodium citrate is the only drug listed that will raise gastric pH quickly. Cimetidine and ranitidine are H2 receptor antagonists which will increase gastric pH but take at least 30 minutes to work. Metoclopramide is not an antacid but may be useful by increasing the lower esophageal sphincter tone *(Chestnut: Obstetric Anesthesia, pp 571-573)*.

703. **(B)** Morphine and fetal asphyxia both decrease fetal heart rate beat-to-beat variability. Ephedrine increases fetal heart rate beat-to-beat variability. Glycopyrrolate, because it does not cross the placenta, has no effect on fetal heart rate beat-to-beat variability *(Barash: Clinical Anesthesia, ed 2, p 1287)*.

704. **(D)** Postdural puncture headaches are less common in patients after dural puncture when the bevel of the epidural needle is oriented parallel to the long axis of the vertebral canal as compared to perpendicular placement. One must, however, rotate the epidural needle 90° prior to catheter insertion to obtain a midline placement of the catheter. The other factors listed in this question are not related to epidural needle bevel placement relative to the dural fibers *(Shnider: Anesthesia for Obstetrics, ed 3, p 437; Chestnut: Obstetric Anesthesia, p 197)*.

705. **(A)** Diabetes mellitus is the most common endocrine problem associated with pregnancy. Type I diabetes mellitus (due to a decrease in insulin secretion) occurs in one of every 700-1,000 gestations. Gestational diabetes, i.e. that which occurs only during pregnancy, is seen in about 5% of all pregnancies. Although substantial advances in the obstetric and anesthetic management of diabetic parturients have been made, maternal and fetal mortality are still higher in these patients than in parturients without diabetes. One important goal of insulin therapy in these patients is to avoid both hyperglycemia and hypoglycemia. In general, insulin requirements are reduced during the first trimester of pregnancy and are increased during the second trimester of pregnancy. Insulin does not readily cross the placenta and therefore does not have any direct effects on glucose metabolism in the fetus. Preeclampsia and large-for-gestational-age fetus occur more frequently in parturients with diabetes *(Shnider: Anesthesia for Obstetrics, ed 3, p 539-550; Chestnut: Obstetric Anesthesia, pp 780-791)*.

706. **(B)** Postdural puncture headaches are positional headaches (worse with the head up and relieved with recumbency). They are bilateral and typically located in the fronto-occipital regions. They are sometimes associated with tinnitus, deafness, photophobia and diplopia (6th cranial nerve palsy). Nausea and vomiting, seizures, lethargy, fever, nuchal rigidity, unilateral location suggest other headache etiologies *(Chestnut: Obstetric Anesthesia, pp 606-608)*.

707. **(D)** There are several periodic fetal heart rate (FHR) patterns. Accelerations in FHR in response to fetal movement signify fetal well-being. Early decelerations are decreases in FHR usually less than 20 beats per minute (bpm) and occur concomitantly with uterine contractions. Typically they are smooth and are mirror images of the uterine contractions. They are caused by head compression which produces a vagal slowing of the FHR. They are not associated with fetal compromise. Late decelerations are decreases in FHR that occur 10-30 seconds after the onset

of a contraction and end 10-30 seconds after the end of a contraction. They are due to utero-placental insufficiency and can result whenever uterine blood flow decreases (see 717). The delayed onset is due to the time required to sense a low oxygen tension. The decrease in FHR may be a vagal reflex (mild cases) or due to direct myocardial depression from hypoxia (severe cases). Typically, in the severe cases beat-to-beat variability is decreased or absent. Variable deceleration are decreases in FHR that vary in shape, depth, and duration from contraction to contraction. They are thought to be due to umbilical cord compression. A sinusoidal pattern is a regular smooth wavelike pattern with no short-term variability. It may be caused by severe fetal anemia or as a result of the maternal administration of narcotics *(Chestnut: Obstetric Anesthesia, p 128)*.

708. **(A)** Shivering occurs in 20-75% of patients receiving epidural or spinal anesthesia for labor or cesarean deliveries. Use of epidural narcotics such as sufentanil or meperidine and warming the intravenous fluid can help decrease the incidence of shivering. Warming the epidural anesthesia solution to body temperature has no effect *(Shnider: Anesthesia for Obstetrics, ed 3, pp 439-440)*.

709. **(B)** Nonparticulate antacids (sodium citrate) and particulate antacids (e.g., Maalox, Mylanta) both raise gastric pH rapidly and can help neutralized gastric pH. However if particulate antacids are aspirated, significant pulmonary damage may result whereas nonparticulate antacids are relatively benign. H_2 receptor antagonists (such as cimetidine or ranitidine) raise gastric pH but take time (greater than 30 minutes) to exert their effect. Metoclopramide helps increase gastric emptying (in as little as 15 minutes) but also increases lower esophageal sphincter tone and may help decrease the chance of aspiration *(Chestnut: Obstetric Anesthesia, pp 570-574)*.

710. **(B)** See answers to questions 707 & 717 *(Shnider: Anesthesia for Obstetrics, ed 3, pp 658-665)*.

711. **(E)** All listed drugs and dosages are correct. Epinephrine and naloxone are given rapidly. Sodium bicarbonate given over at least 2 minutes and only after adequate ventilation is provided. Volume expanders (blood, albumin, saline, or lactated Ringers) are usually given over 5-10 minutes. Drugs used in newborn resuscitation that can be given down the endotracheal tube include *o*xygen, *n*aloxone, and *e*pinephrine (ONE) *(American Academy of Pediatrics and American Heart Association's Textbook, "Neonatal Resuscitation", 1994)*.

712. **(A)** The ultimate treatment of preeclampsia-eclampsia is delivery of the fetus. Many different drugs may be used before delivery. Magnesium sulfate is used to prevent and to treat seizures. Although it also has tocolytic properties, they may be overcome with an oxytocin infusion. These patients have increased levels of thromboxane (prostaglandin). Thromboxane produces vasoconstriction, platelet aggregation, and decreased uterine blood flow. Aspirin (a prostaglandin inhibitor) decreases the incidence and severity of preeclampsia. Nifedipine, a calcium channel blocker, has been used as an antihypertensive agent although hydralazine and labetalol are more commonly used. Caution must be utilized when magnesium sulfate and nifedipine are used since magnesium and calcium are antagonistic. Ritodrine is a tocolytic and is not useful in the treatment of preeclampsia *(Shnider: Anesthesia for Obstetrics, ed 3, pp 314-318)*.

713. **(A)** An increased minute ventilation hastens the entry of inhalation drugs into the lung and hastens the uptake of the more soluble inhalation agents. The decrease in functional residual capacity increases the uptake of the more insoluble inhalation agents. MAC during pregnancy decreases 25-40% in animal studies so that absorbed drug has an increased effect. An increase in cardiac output leads to a slower induction of inhalation agent since the concentration of anesthetic reaching the brain is lower *(Shnider: Anesthesia for Obstetrics, ed 3, pp 6-8; Chestnut: Obstetric Anesthesia, pp 29-31).*

714. **(D)** Compression of the vena cava reduces venous return and may result in shock in up to 15% of pregnant patients near term producing symptoms of hypotension, nausea and vomiting, pallor, and changes in cerebration. Compression of the aorta decreases uterine blood flow *(Shnider: Anesthesia for Obstetrics, ed 3, pp 9 & 10).*

715. **(A)** Prevention of aortocaval compression consists of left uterine displacement manually, by placing a wedge under the patient's right side or by rotating the OR table to the left. In about 10% of women right uterine displacement (wedge under left side) is more effective. Trendelenburg position without uterine displacement may actually worsen the condition since it shifts the uterus further back on the great vessels *(Shnider: Anesthesia for Obstetrics, ed 3, pp 10-11; Chestnut: Obstetric Anesthesia, p 29).*

716. **(A)** Despite a decrease in maternal hematocrit, oxygen delivery to the uterus is increased during normal pregnancies by several mechanisms. An increase in cardiac output as well as vasodilation of uterine blood vessels increases blood flow to the uterus. An increase in minute ventilation not only lowers the P_aCO_2 to 30-32 torr but raises the P_aO_2 to about 103 torr. In addition, the oxyhemoglobin dissociation curve is shifted to the right (P_{50} from 27 to 30 torr) *(Shnider: Anesthesia for Obstetrics, ed 3, p 11).*

$$(UBF)\ Uterine\ blood\ flow = \frac{Uterine\ artery\ pressure - uterine\ venous\ pressure}{Uterine\ vascular\ resistance}$$

717. **(E)** A decrease in uterine blood flow may result from a decrease in uterine artery pressure (aortocaval compression, hemorrhage, drug-induced hypotension), an increase in uterine venous pressure (uterine contractions, vena cava obstruction), an increase in uterine vascular tone (catecholamines), and by local anesthetics in high concentrations *(Shnider: Anesthesia for Obstetrics, ed 3, p 23; Chestnut: Obstetric Anesthesia, p 43-47).*

718. **(B)** Epinephrine in a dose of 5 μg/ml (1:200,000) reduces the peak blood levels of some local anesthetics such as lidocaine and mepivacaine but not others such as etidocaine and bupivacaine. The different effects may be related to the high lipid solubility of etidocaine and bupivacaine which results in a greater uptake by the adipose tissue *(Shnider: Anesthesia for Obstetrics, ed 3, pp 72-73).*

719. **(A)** 2-Chloroprocaine administered epidurally appears to decrease the quality and duration of subsequently administered fentanyl, morphine, or bupivacaine. The exact mechanism is unclear but does not seem to be related to the acid pH of chloroprocaine (since neutralization with bicarbonate has similar antagonistic properties). Butorphanol (a kappa receptor agonist) does not appear to be antagonized *(Shnider: Anesthesia for Obstetrics, ed 3, p 85; Chestnut: Obstetric Anesthesia, pp 212-213 & 363).*

720. **(B)** Advantages to using spinal instead of epidural anesthesia for cesarean section include faster onset of action, a significant decrease in total amount of anesthetics needed, and less time spent with the patient. However, because of the faster onset of action of spinal anesthesia, hypotension is more frequent and vasopressor treatment more commonly needed despite "adequate hydration". The spread of spinal anesthesia is less controlled and hence more unpredictable than with epidural anesthesia *(Shnider: Anesthesia for Obstetrics, ed 3, p 94).*

721. **(B)** Several cases of maternal cardiac arrest have occurred in pregnant women who were administered bupivacaine. Typically, the patients received unintentional intravenous bolus of 3/4% bupivacaine intended for the epidural space. They had a brief grand mal seizure followed by cardiovascular collapse. Successful treatment may be prolonged and involves basic resuscitation (intubation, ventilation with 100% oxygen, cardiac compression with left uterine tilt, defibrillation, epinephrine, bicarbonate) as well as rapid delivery of the fetus (if possible). Delivery of the fetus make successful resuscitation of the mother more likely. Incremental small injections of local anesthetics looking for toxicity should decrease the chance for cardiovascular collapse. Etidocaine, another very lipid soluble anesthetic, has also been reported to produce recalcitrant cardiac arrest *(Shnider: Anesthesia for Obstetrics, ed 3, pp 88-90, & 462-463).*

722. **(E)** Some patients who receive volumes of greater than 23-25 ml of chloroprocaine develop severe backache that may last several hours. The pain can be relieved by the epidural administration of local anesthetics or narcotics. This appears to be related to the addition of disodium ethylenediamine tetraacetic acid (EDTA) used in its formulation *(Shnider: Anesthesia for Obstetrics, ed 3, p 85).*

723. **(D)** Although all local anesthetics in high enough doses can cause significant motor block, etidocaine with its propensity to block large fibers produces motor blockade that outlasts sensory blockade *(Shnider: Anesthesia for Obstetrics, ed 3, p 91).*

724. **(C)** The metabolic product of prilocaine (α-orthotoluidine) has been shown to produce methemoglobinemia. This occurs when doses greater than 600 mg of prilocaine are used *(Shnider: Anesthesia for Obstetrics, ed 3, p 87).*

725. **(E)** Chloroprocaine (ester) has a very fast half-life in both maternal and fetal blood. The in vitro half-life is 21 records for maternal and 43 seconds for fetal blood *(Shnider: Anesthesia for Obstetrics, ed 3, pp 85-86).*

Neurologic Physiology and Anesthesia

DIRECTIONS (Questions 726 through 760): Each of the questions or incomplete statements in this section is followed by answers or by completions of the statement, respectively. Select the ONE BEST answer or completion for each item.

726. Which of the following is the most useful in improving neurologic outcome after cardiac arrest?

    A. Steroids
    B. Hypothermia
    C. Barbiturates
    D. Ibuprofen
    E. Calcium

727. Intracranial hypertension is defined as a sustained increase in intracranial pressure (ICP) above

    A. 5 mm Hg
    B. 15 mm Hg
    C. 25 mm Hg
    D. 40 mm Hg
    E. None of the above

728. An unconscious 19-year-old woman with a closed head injury is in the intensive care unit after a motor vehicle accident. The following hemodynamic parameters are noted: blood pressure 110/80 mm Hg, heart rate 96 beats/min, right atrial pressure 10 mm Hg, ICP 40 mm Hg. What is the cerebral perfusion pressure?

    A. 80 mm Hg
    B. 70 mm Hg
    C. 50 mm Hg
    D. 40 mm Hg
    E. 35 mm Hg

729. The afferent input for somatosensory evoked potentials (SSEPs) is carried through which spinal cord tract?

    A. Spinocerebellar
    B. Spinothalamic
    C. Dorsal columns
    D. Corticospinal
    E. Vestibulospinal

730. By what percent does cerebral blood flow change for each mm Hg increase in P_aCO_2?

     A. 1%
     B. 2%
     C. 7%
     D. 10%
     E. 25%

731. Which of the following intravenous anesthetics is contraindicated in patients with intracranial hypertension?

     A. Diazepam
     B. Fentanyl
     C. Thiopental
     D. Midazolam
     E. Ketamine

732. The term "luxury perfusion" refers to a situation which occurs in the brain when

     A. Blood flow has resumed after a period of ischemia
     B. When blood flow is directed from a normal region of the brain to an ischemic region
     C. When vasoparalysis exists
     D. When the Robinhood phenomenon exists
     E. When a zone of ischemic penumbra exists

733. A 62-year-old patient is scheduled to undergo resection of a bifrontal intracranial tumor under general anesthesia. Preoperatively, the patient is alert and oriented, and has no focal neurologic deficits. Within what range should P_aCO_2 be maintained?

     A. 15 and 20 mm Hg
     B. 20 and 25 mm Hg
     C. 25 and 30 mm Hg
     D. 30 and 35 mm Hg
     E. 35 and 40 mm Hg

734. A 2-year-old child is anesthetized for resection of a posterior fossa tumor. Preoperatively, the patient is lethargic and disoriented. Which of the following is most likely to adversely alter ICP?

     A. 5% dextrose in water
     B. Normal saline
     C. Lactated Ringer's solution
     D. 5% Albumin
     E. Fresh-frozen plasma

735. A 22-year-old patient is anesthetized for resection of a temporal lobe tumor. Preoperatively, he is lethargic and confused. Which of the following would be the most appropriate drug to control systemic blood pressure during direct laryngoscopy and tracheal intubation after induction of anesthesia?

    A. Trimethaphan
    B. Nitroglycerin
    C. Hydralazine
    D. Halothane
    E. Nitroprusside

736. Normal global CBF is

    A. 25 mL/100 g/min
    B. 50 mL/100 g/min
    C. 75 mL/100 g/min
    D. 100 mL/100 g/min
    E. 150 mL/100 g/min

737. The lower and upper limits of CBF autoregulation (mean arterial pressure) are, respectively,

    A. 25 and 125 mm Hg
    B. 25 and 200 mm Hg
    C. 40 and 250 mm Hg
    D. 50 and 150 mm Hg
    E. 50 and 200 mm Hg

738. How much will CBF increase in a patient whose P_aCO_2 is increased from 35 mm Hg to 45 mm Hg?

    A. There is no relationship between P_aCO_2 and CBF
    B. 10 mL/100 g/min
    C. 25 mL/100 g/min
    D. 40 mL/100 g/min
    E. 50 mL/100 g/min

739. Select the **FALSE** statement concerning autonomic hyperreflexia.

    A. Distention of a hollow viscus below the level of the spinal cord transection can elicit autonomic hyperreflexia
    B. Up to 85% of patients with a spinal cord transection above the T6 dermatome will exhibit autonomic hyperreflexia under general anesthesia
    C. Propranolol is effective in treating hypertension associated with autonomic hyperreflexia
    D. Spinal anesthesia is effective in preventing autonomic hyperreflexia
    E. Cutaneous stimulation below the level of the spinal cord transection can elicit autonomic hyperreflexia

740. What is the normal oxygen consumption in the brain per minute?

    A. 0.5 ml/100 g brain tissue
    B. 2.0 ml/100 g brain tissue
    C. 3.5 ml/100 g brain tissue
    D. 7.5 ml/100 g brain tissue
    E. 10 ml/100 g brain tissue

741. A 14-year-old girl with severe scoliosis is to undergo spinal surgery. Anesthesia is maintained with fentanyl, N_2O, 50% in O_2, vecuronium, and isoflurane. Neurologic function of the spinal cord is monitored by SSEPs. In reference to the SSEP waveform, ischemia would be manifested as

    A. Increased amplitude and increased latency
    B. Decreased amplitude and increased latency
    C. Decreased amplitude and decreased latency
    D. Increased amplitude and decreased latency
    E. Increased amplitude and no change in latency

742. For each 1°C decrease in body temperature, how much will $CMRO_2$ be diminished?

    A. 3%
    B. 5%
    C. 7%
    D. 10%
    E. 20%

743. A 24-year-old carpenter is treated for a closed head injury sustained 3 days earlier after falling from a roof. He has been hemodynamically stable, but despite aggressive efforts to pharmacologically reduce ICP, he is now unconscious and unresponsive to painful stimuli. All of the following are clinical criteria consistent with a diagnosis of brain death in this patient **EXCEPT**

    A. Persistent apnea for 10 minutes
    B. Absence of pupillary light reflex
    C. Persistent spinal reflexes
    D. Decorticate posturing
    E. Absence of oropharyngeal reflex

744. Which of the following is the most sensitive means of detecting venous air embolism (VAE)?

    A. EEG
    B. Pulmonary artery catheter
    C. Transesophageal echocardiography
    D. Mass spectrometry
    E. Right atrial catheterization

745. When intracranial hypertension exists, the main compensatory mechanism from the body is

    A. Increased absorption at the intracranial arachnoid villi
    B. Increased absorption of CSF in the spinal arachnoid villi
    C. Shifting of CSF into the spinal subarachnoid space
    D. Reduction of cerebral blood volume from compression of cerebral veins
    E. Decreased production of CSF at the choroid plexus

746. Select the correct order from greatest to least for the sensitivity of the following neurophysiologic monitoring techniques to volatile anesthetics (SSEP, somatosensory evoked potentials; VEP, visual evoked potentials; BAEP, brainstem auditory evoked potentials).

    A. SSEP > VEP > BAEP
    B. VEP > SSEP > BAEP
    C. BAEP > VEP > SSEP
    D. SSEP > BAEP > VEP
    E. SSEP = VEP > BAEP

747. Which of the following substances under normal circumstances exists in both the CSF and blood at the same concentration?

    A. Potassium
    B. Chloride
    C. Glucose
    D. Sodium
    E. Albumin

748. What is the minimum quantity of intraatrial air which can be detected by a precordial Doppler?

    A. 0.1 mL
    B. 0.5 mL
    C. 5.0 mL
    D. 10 mL
    E. 25 mL

749. With regard to regulation of blood flow, the correct order of vascular responsiveness to P_aCO_2 from most to least sensitive is

    A. Cerebrum > spinal cord > cerebellum
    B. Cerebrum > cerebellum > spinal cord
    C. Cerebellum > cerebrum > spinal cord
    D. Cerebellum > spinal cord > cerebrum
    E. Spinal cord > cerebrum > cerebellum

750.   A 67-year-old patient is scheduled to undergo posterior cervical fusion in the sitting position under general anesthesia. A central venous catheter is inserted from the right basilic vein and advanced toward the heart. Intravascular electrocardiography (with the exploring electrode attached to the V lead) is utilized to aid in placement of the catheter. After the catheter is advanced 45 cm, the tracing shown in the figure is noted on the ECG. At this time the anesthesiologist should

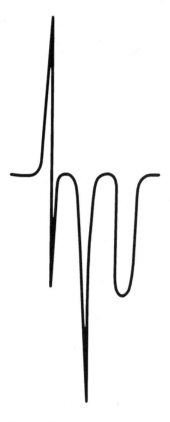

A.   Advance the catheter 5 cm
B.   Advance the catheter slightly
C.   Leave the catheter in the present position
D.   Withdraw the catheter 1 cm
E.   Remove the catheter and defibrillate the heart

751.   Select the **TRUE** statement concerning administration of glucose-containing solutions to the patient with a closed head injury versus a patient with a spinal cord injury.

A.   Glucose-containing solutions are contraindicated in both patient groups
B.   Glucose-containing solutions are contraindicated in patients with closed head injury but acceptable in patients with spinal cord injuries
C.   Glucose-containing solutions are acceptable in patients with closed head injuries but contraindicated in patients with spinal cord injuries
D.   Glucose-containing solutions may be given to either patient group if blood glucose concentrations do not exceed 200 mg/dl
E.   Glucose-containing solutions are acceptable in both patient groups

752. Critical CBF in patients anesthetized with isoflurane is

    A. 5 mL/100 g/min
    B. 10 mL/100 g/min
    C. 18 mL/100 g/min
    D. 25 mL/100 g/min
    E. 32 mL/100 g/min

753. What effect does cerebral ischemia have on CBF autoregulation?

    A. CBF autoregulation is ablated
    B. CBF autoregulation is ablated at low cerebral perfusion pressures, but remains intact at high cerebral perfusion pressures
    C. CBF autoregulation is ablated at high cerebral perfusion pressures, but remains intact at low cerebral perfusion pressures
    D. The CBF-autoregulatory curve is shifted to the right
    E. The CBF-autoregulatory curve is shifted to the left

754. The most rapid maneuver available for lowering intracranial pressure in a patient with a large intracranial mass is

    A. Mannitol, 1 g/kg IV
    B. Ketamine, 1 mg/kg IV
    C. Hyperventilation to 25 mm Hg P_aCO_2
    D. Furosemide, 1 mg/kg IV
    E. Methylprednisolone, 30 mg/kg IV

755. What effect does thiopental have on the CO_2 responsiveness of the cerebral vasculature?

    A. Thiopental attenuates the effect of hypocarbia on CBF
    B. Thiopental attenuates the effect of hypercarbia on CBF
    C. Thiopental augments the effect of hypercarbia on CBF
    D. Thiopental augments the effect of hypocarbia on CBF
    E. Thiopental does not affect CO_2 reactivity at a dose used clinically

756. Each of the following is a relative contraindication to the sitting position **EXCEPT**

    A. Ventriculoatrial shunt
    B. Platypnea-orthodeoxia
    C. Right-to-left intracardiac shunt
    D. Ventriculoperitoneal shunt
    E. Patent foramen ovale

757. A 72-year-old patient undergoing resection of an astrocytoma in the sitting position suddenly develops hypotension. Air is heard on the precordial Doppler ultrasound. Each of the following therapeutic maneuvers to treat VAE is appropriate **EXCEPT**

   A. Discontinue N_2O
   B. Apply jugular venous pressure
   C. Implement PEEP
   D. Administer epinephrine to treat hypotension
   E. Flood the surgical wound with saline

758. Calculate cerebral perfusion pressure based on the following data: intracranial pressure 25 mm Hg, central venous pressure 15 mm Hg, systolic blood pressure 120, diastolic pressure 90 mm Hg, pulmonary artery occlusion pressure 10 mm Hg

   A. 95 mm Hg
   B. 85 mm Hg
   C. 75 mm Hg
   D. 65 mm Hg
   E. 55 mm Hg

759. A 55-year-old business executive is scheduled for colonoscopy and polypectomy under general anesthesia. A bruit is auscultated over the right carotid artery on physical examination. The patient is otherwise healthy. Which of the following would be the most appropriate course of action?

   A. Cancel surgery and obtain a carotid angiogram
   B. Cancel surgery and obtain Doppler ultrasound carotid blood flow studies
   C. Cancel surgery and consult a neurologist
   D. Proceed with surgery and obtain a carotid angiogram postoperatively
   E. Proceed with surgery

760. How long after a stroke can anesthesia for surgery be carried out with about the same risk of a perioperative occlusive vascular accident as existed immediately before the previous stroke?

   A. 1 week
   B. 1 month
   C. 6 months
   D. 9 months
   E. 1 year

761. A 13-year-old boy is anesthetized with 0.5% isoflurane, 50% N_2O and fentanyl for scoliosis repair. SSEP monitoring is conducted during the procedure. Which of the following structures is not involved in conveyance of the stimulus from the posterior tibial nerve to the cerebral cortex?

   A. Corticospinal tract
   B. Medial lemniscus
   C. Brainstem
   D. Internal capsule
   E. Dorsal root ganglion

762. A 19-year-old woman is undergoing surgery for a Harrington rod placement. General anesthesia is administered with desflurane, nitrous oxide, and fentanyl. After completion of spinal instrumentation, a wake-up test is undertaken. Four thumb twitches are present when the nerve stimulator attached to the ulnar nerve is activated. The volatile anesthetic and nitrous oxide have been discontinued for ten minutes when the patient is asked to move her hands and feet. After repeated commands, the patient still does not move her hands or feet. The most appropriate intervention at this time would be

   A. 3 mg neostigmine plus 0.6 mg glycopyrrolate IV
   B. 20 μg naloxone IV
   C. 0.1 mg flumazenil IV
   D. Institute SSEP monitoring
   E. Reduce the distraction on the rods

763. A 75-year-old patient is undergoing craniotomy for resection of a large astrocytoma. During administration of isoflurane anesthesia, arterial blood gas sampling reveals a P_aCO_2 of 30 mm Hg. At this time, this patient's global cerebral blood flow would be approximately

   A. 10 ml · 100 g brain weight^{-1} · min^{-1}
   B. 20 ml · 100 g brain weight^{-1} · min^{-1}
   C. 30 ml · 100 g brain weight^{-1} · min^{-1}
   D. 40 ml · 100 g brain weight^{-1} · min^{-1}
   E. 50 ml · 100 g brain weight^{-1} · min^{-1}

764. A 24-year-old patient is brought to the intensive care unit after sustaining a closed head injury in a motor vehicle accident. Each of the following would be useful in managing intracranial hypertension in this patient **EXCEPT**

   A. Corticosteroids
   B. Barbiturates
   C. Hyperventilation
   D. Osmotic diuresis
   E. Placement of the patient in the head up position

765. Preoperative treatment of subarachnoid hemorrhage patients, without concomitant cerebral vasospasm, might include any of the following **EXCEPT**

   A. Induced hypertension (to 20 percent above baseline)
   B. Administration of nimodipine
   C. Sedation
   D. Analgesic therapy
   E. Administration of antiepileptic drugs

766. Which of the following pharmacologic agents would have the **LEAST** effect on somatosensory evoked potentials?

    A. Isoflurane
    B. Nitrous oxide
    C. Sodium thiopental
    D. Etomidate
    E. Vecuronium

767. A 75-year-old patient with signs and symptoms of a leaking cerebral aneurysm is brought to the emergency room for evaluation. T-wave inversion, a prolongation of the QT interval, and U waves are noted on the preoperative EKG. Appropriate action at this point would be

    A. Begin infusion of nitroglycerin
    B. Check serum calcium and potassium
    C. Administer esmolol
    D. Place a pulmonary artery catheter
    E. Delay surgery until myocardial infarction has been ruled out

768. Which of the following pharmacologic agents would have the **LEAST** effect on transcranial motor evoked potentials?

    A. Isoflurane
    B. Nitrous oxide
    C. Etomidate
    D. Diazepam
    E. Fentanyl

DIRECTIONS (Questions 769 through 787): For each of the items in this section, ONE or MORE of the number options is correct. Select the answer:

Select A if options *1, 2 and 3* are correct,
Select B if options *1 and 3* are correct,
Select C if options *2 and 4* are correct,
Select D if only option *4* is correct,
Select E if *all* options are correct.

769. Ketamine

    1. Decreases CBF
    2. Augments the CO_2 responsiveness of the cerebral vasculature
    3. Reduces CMR
    4. Increases cerebral blood volume

Select A if options *1, 2 and 3* are correct,
Select B if options *1 and 3* are correct,
Select C if options *2 and 4* are correct,
Select D if only option *4* is correct,
Select E if *all* options are correct.

770. CMR is increased by

    1. Seizure
    2. Hyperthermia
    3. Ketamine
    4. Isoflurane

771. Anesthetics that impair CBF autoregulation include

    1. Halothane, 1 MAC
    2. Enflurane, 1 MAC
    3. Isoflurane, 1 MAC
    4. Thiopental, 4 mg/kg

772. An 18-year-old patient is brought to the intensive care unit after sustaining a cervical spine injury, and quadriplegia, during a motor vehicle accident. In the first 24 hours after the injury, the patient is at risk for

    1. Pulmonary edema
    2. Hypothermia
    3. Hypotension
    4. Autonomic hyperreflexia

773. Signs and symptoms of intracranial hypertension include

    1. Papilledema
    2. Headache
    3. Nausea and vomiting
    4. Decreased mentation

774. An 89-year-old man with a history of transient ischemic attacks is scheduled to undergo a carotid endarterectomy under general anesthesia. Which of the following would be appropriate in the anesthetic management of this patient?

    1. Hyperventilation of the lungs to a P_aCO_2 of 30 mm Hg to reduce ICP
    2. Injection of a local anesthetic around the carotid body to prevent bradycardia
    3. Initiation of deliberate hypotension after induction of anesthesia to reduce bleeding
    4. Induction of anesthesia with sodium thiopental

Select A if options *1, 2 and 3* are correct,
Select B if options *1 and 3* are correct,
Select C if options *2 and 4* are correct,
Select D if only option *4* is correct,
Select E if *all* options are correct.

775.   Anesthetics that increase ICP include

   1. Enflurane
   2. N_2O
   3. Halothane
   4. Fentanyl-droperidol (Innovar)

776.   Five days after clipping of a cerebral aneurysm, a 68-year-old female patient develops clinical evidence of vasospasm. Therapy that is useful in the treatment of cerebral vasospasm includes

   1. Blood pressure reduction
   2. Hemodilution
   3. Diuretics
   4. Calcium channel blockers

777.   Conditions that are associated with cerebral aneurysms include

   1. Polycystic kidney disease
   2. Fibromuscular dysplasia
   3. Coarctation of the aorta
   4. Hypertension

778.   The CBF-autoregulatory curve is shifted to the right by

   1. Hypoxia
   2. Volatile anesthetics
   3. Hypercarbia
   4. Chronic hypertension

779.   Autoregulation is abolished by

   1. Hyperbaric oxygen
   2. Cardiopulmonary bypass with core temperature 27°C
   3. Chronic hypertension
   4. 3% isoflurane

780.   Etomidate

   1. Reduces $CMRO_2$
   2. Is a direct cerebral vasoconstrictor
   3. Reduces cerebral blood flow
   4. Abolishes CO_2 reactivity

Select A if options *1, 2 and 3* are correct,
Select B if options *1 and 3* are correct,
Select C if options *2 and 4* are correct,
Select D if only option *4* is correct,
Select E if *all* options are correct.

781. Following a motor vehicle accident, a 25-year-old male patient is brought to the operating room for repair of facial lacerations and fractures, and abdominal exploration. The patient is extremely micrognathic and weighs 328 pounds. Acceptable techniques for securing the airway include

    1. Awake fiberoptic intubation
    2. Blind nasal intubation
    3. Awake tracheostomy
    4. Direct laryngoscopy with rapid sequence induction

782. A 22-year-old college student involved in a motor vehicle accident sustains numerous injuries, including a closed head injury. He is unconscious and unresponsive to all external stimuli. Disadvantages of using urea compared with mannitol to reduce ICP include

    1. A higher incidence of rebound intracranial hypertension with urea
    2. A higher incidence of venous thrombosis with urea
    3. An increased ability of urea to penetrate an intact blood-brain barrier
    4. A higher incidence of myocardial depression with urea

783. Anesthetic agents that both decrease the amplitude and increase the latency of SSEPs include

    1. Isoflurane
    2. Diazepam
    3. Etomidate
    4. Nitrous oxide

784. CBF autoregulation is altered by

    1. Ischemia
    2. Chronic hypertension
    3. Halothane
    4. N_2O

785. A 45-year-old man is undergoing a posterior cervical fusion in the sitting position. Induction of anesthesia and tracheal intubation are uneventful. Anesthesia is maintained with N_2O, 50% in O_2, and enflurane. Suddenly, air is heard on the precordial Doppler ultrasound. Other observations consistent with VAE include

    1. Decreased P_aO_2
    2. Increased end-tidal nitrogen
    3. Decreased arterial blood pressure
    4. Decreased P_aCO_2

Select A if options *1, 2 and 3* are correct,
Select B if options *1 and 3* are correct,
Select C if options *2 and 4* are correct,
Select D if only option *4* is correct,
Select E if *all* options are correct.

786. In patients with increased intracranial pressure, hyperventilation is typically limited to a P_aCO_2 of 25 mm Hg because additional hyperventilation

    1. Is virtually impossible
    2. May result in clinically significant hypokalemia
    3. Could result in paradoxical cerebral vasodilation
    4. Could result in cerebral ischemia

787. A 62-year-old male patient presents for resection of a supratentorial meningioma. An intravenous induction with propofol is planned. Propofol shares which property (properties) with sodium thiopental

    1. Reduction in CMR
    2. Reduction in CBF
    3. Reduction in cerebral blood volume
    4. Reduction in ICP

NEUROLOGIC PHYSIOLOGY AND ANESTHESIA ANSWERS, REFERENCES, AND EXPLANATIONS

726. **(B)** Global brain ischemia occurs when there is an inadequate supply of oxygen and nutrients to the entire brain. Global ischemia may be stratified into incomplete (e.g., systemic shock with persistent low blood flow to the brain) or complete (e.g., cardiac arrest). In contrast, focal brain ischemia occurs when there is ischemia to only a portion of the brain (e.g., classic stroke). Although corticosteroids are thought to possess antioxidant properties, investigators evaluating their effectiveness during cardiac arrest have reported either no improvement or a worsening of neurologic outcome. Worsening of outcome is thought to be due to corticosteroid-induced hyperglycemia. During focal brain ischemia, barbiturates provide neuronal protection by decreasing cerebral metabolism (i.e., EEG activity) and redistributing regional CBF. However, since the EEG becomes isoelectric (i.e., maximal depression of electrical activity and metabolism) within 20 seconds of cardiac arrest and there is no cerebral blood flow to redistribute, studies demonstrating barbiturate-mediated brain protection during or following cardiac arrest are lacking. The use of ibuprofen for brain protection has not been demonstrated in cardiac arrest patients. During ischemia, calcium accumulates within neurons and contributes to irreversible cell death. Thus, in the setting of a disrupted blood brain barrier, i.v. calcium may worsen post-ischemic neurologic outcome. Hypothermia, at the time of either focal or global brain ischemia, has consistently been demonstrated to provide brain protection during cardiac arrest. The mechanisms of hypothermia-mediated brain protection are discussed in the references cited below (Wass: Improving Neurology Outcome Following Cardiac Arrest, Anesthesiology Clinics of North America, 1995;13:869-903; Cottrell: Anesthesia and Neurosurgery, ed 3, pp 59-92).

727. **(B)** Elevated intracranial pressure (ICP) frequently is the final stage of a pathologic cerebral insult (e.g., head injury, intracranial tumor, subarachnoid hemorrhage, metabolic encephalopathy, or hydrocephalus). The intracranial contents consist of three components: brain parenchyma (80% to 85%), blood (3% to 6%), and CSF (5% to 15%). None of these components is compressible; accordingly, an increase in the volume of any of these requires a compensatory decrease in the volume of one or both of the other components to avoid the development of intracranial hypertension. Normal ICP is < 15 mm Hg. As measured in the supine position, intracranial hypertension is defined as a sustained increase in ICP above 15 to 20 mm Hg *(Miller: Anesthesia, ed 4, pp 1910, 1911; Stoelting: Pharmacology and Physiology in Anesthetic Practice, ed 2, pp 631-632).*

728. **(C)** Cerebral perfusion pressure is defined as the difference in mean arterial pressure and right atrial pressure; however, when ICP exceeds right atrial pressure, cerebral perfusion pressure is defined as the difference in mean arterial pressure and ICP. Thus, cerebral perfusion pressure in this patient is 50 mm Hg *(Miller: Anesthesia, ed 4, p 1911; Stoelting: Basics of Anesthesia, ed 3, p 332).*

729. **(C)** Somatosensory evoked potentials (SSEPs) are voltage signals that appear in response to electrical stimulation of peripheral nerves. The impulse elicited by electrical stimulation of a peripheral nerve ascends the ipsilateral dorsal column of the spinal cord, and is ultimately recorded on the contralateral somatosensory cortex of the brain. SSEPs are composed of negative and positive voltage deflections with specific latencies and amplitudes. In general, the earlier deflections represent impulses and synapses within the spinal cord or brain stem, while the later impulses represent thalamic and/or cortical synapses. Intraoperative monitoring of SSEPs provides the ability to assess the integrity of the peripheral nerve, e.g. posterior tibial nerve, dorsal columns, brainstem, medial lemniscus, internal capsule, and contralateral somatosensory cortex *(Miller: Anesthesia, ed 4, pp 1330-1331)*.

730. **(B)** Hyperventilation of the lungs causes constriction of cerebral blood vessels, which reduces global cerebral blood flow and cerebral blood volume. This effect is mediated by changes in the pH induced in the extracellular fluid. In contrast to autoregulation, CO_2 reactivity is preserved in most patients with severe brain injury, and thus, hyperventilation can rapidly lower intracranial pressure through the reduction in cerebral blood volume. Although the effects of hyperventilation on cerebral blood volume and intracranial pressure are almost immediate, the duration of effect wanes after 6 to 10 hours of hyperventilation and may last up to 24 to 36 hours, since the pH of the extracellular fluid equilibrates to the lower P_aCO_2 level. Generally speaking, cerebral blood flow decreases by approximately 2 percent for each mmHg increase in P_aCO_2 *(Barash: Clinical Anesthesia, ed 2, p 850)*.

731. **(E)** Of the choices listed in this question, ketamine is the only intravenous anesthetic not recommended for patients with intracranial hypertension, since it increases cerebral metabolism (CMR), cerebral blood flow (CBF), cerebral blood volume (CBV), and intracranial pressure (ICP). Barbiturates, etomidate, and propofol decrease CMR, CBF, CBV, and ICP. All three of these agents indirectly decrease cerebral blood flow by their inhibitory effect on cerebral metabolic rate. However, unlike thiopental, etomidate also has a direct vasoconstrictor effect on the cerebral vasculature. One potential advantage of etomidate over thiopental is that it does not produce significant cardiovascular depression. Although not as pronounced as the barbiturates, benzodiazepines, such as midazolam also reduce cerebral metabolic rate and cerebral blood flow. Flumazenil, a benzodiazepine antagonist, has been reported to reverse the effect of midazolam on CMR, CBF, CBV, and ICP. Consequently, flumazenil should be avoided in midazolam-anesthetized patients known to have intracranial hypertension. Generally speaking, the opioid anesthetics, such as morphine and fentanyl, cause either a minor reduction or have no effect on cerebral blood flow and cerebral metabolic rate *(Barash: Clinical Anesthesia, ed 2, pp 879-880)*.

732. **(C)** During acute focal cerebral ischemia, vasoparalysis results in impaired coupling between cerebral blood flow and metabolism. Consequently, cerebral blood flow is usually greater than cerebral metabolic rate and is passively associated with systemic blood pressure. This is known as "luxury perfusion". Under these circumstances, autoregulation and the reactivity of the cerebrovasculature to carbon dioxide is also disturbed. Thus, tight control of systemic blood pressure is extremely important in the management of patients with focal ischemia, since cerebral perfusion is tightly dependent on mean arterial pressure *(Cottrell: Anesthesia and Neurosurgery, ed 3, p 151)*.

733. **(C)** Cerebral ischemia has been reported in both man and experimental animals when the P_aCO_2 is reduced below 20 mm Hg. It is likely that cerebral ischemia is caused by a leftward shift of the oxyhemoglobin dissociation curve (produced by the severe alkalosis) and possibly by intense cerebral vasoconstriction. A leftward shift of the oxyhemoglobin dissociation curve increases the affinity of hemoglobin for O_2, which reduces off-loading of O_2 from hemoglobin at the capillary bed. This effect combined with the existing reduction of CBF can result in cerebral ischemia. Combined with the fact that there is very little additional benefit in terms of reducing cerebral blood volume and ICP, it is recommended to limit acute hyperventilation of the lungs to a P_aCO_2 of 25-30 mm Hg. Within this range, reduction in ICP is maximal and risk of cerebral ischemia is minimal *(Miller: Anesthesia, ed 4, p 1915)*.

734. **(A)** Five percent dextrose in water (D_5W) is contraindicated in neurosurgical patients with intracranial hypertension for two reasons. First, D_5W easily passes through the blood-brain barrier. Once in the brain tissue, the glucose is rapidly metabolized, leaving only free water, which causes cerebral edema. Secondly, hyperglycemia is associated with increased severity of neurologic damage in patients with cerebral ischemia. This is thought to result from increased lactate production during anaerobic glycolysis during the period of ischemia *(Barash: Clinical Anesthesia, ed 2, p 891)*.

735. **(A)** The symptoms described in this patient of lethargy and confusion strongly suggest the presence of intracranial hypertension. All of the drugs listed in this question are potent cerebral vasodilators. Trimethaphan blocks neurotransmission at autonomic ganglia. Compared with the other vasodilators listed in this question, for any given degree of reduction in systemic blood pressure, trimethaphan causes the least increase in cerebral blood volume and ICP *(Stoelting: Pharmacology and Physiology in Anesthetic Practice, ed 2, p 334)*.

736. **(B)** Normal global CBF is approximately 45 to 55 mL/100 g/min. Cortical CBF (gray matter) is approximately 75 to 80 mL/100 g/min and subcortical CBF (mostly white matter) is approximately 20 mL/100 g/min. Factors that regulate CBF include P_aCO_2, P_aO_2, CMR, cerebral perfusion pressure, autoregulation, and the autonomic nervous system *(Miller: Anesthesia, ed 4, pp 689-690; Stoelting: Basics of Anesthesia, ed 3, p 33; Stoelting: Anesthesia and Co-existing Disease, ed 3, pp 182-188)*.

737. **(D)** CBF autoregulation is the intrinsic capability of the cerebral vasculature to adjust its resistance to maintain CBF constant over a wide range of mean arterial pressures. In normal subjects, the lower limit of CBF autoregulation corresponds to a mean arterial pressure of approximately 50 to 60 mm Hg and the upper limit is a mean arterial pressure of 150 mm Hg. At mean arterial pressures above or below the limits of CBF autoregulation, CBF is pressure-dependent. Although the precise mechanism of CBF autoregulation is not known, it is thought to result from an intrinsic characteristic of cerebral vascular smooth muscle that has not yet been identified *(Miller: Anesthesia, ed 4, p 694; Barash: Clinical Anesthesia, ed 2, pp 875-876)*.

738. **(B)** CBF will increase by approximately 1 mL/100 g/min for every 1-mm Hg increase in P_aCO_2, i.e. approximately 2%. This effect is caused by CO_2-mediated decrease in the pH of the extracellular fluid surrounding the cerebral vessels, which causes cerebral vasodilatation. The pH changes rapidly because CO_2 diffuses freely across the cerebral vascular endothelium into the extracellular fluid. However, the change in pH wanes after 6 to 10 hours since extracellular fluid pH is gradually normalized by reabsorption of HCO_3^- and excretion of H^+ by the kidneys. An increase in P_aCO_2 of 10 mm Hg (from 35 mm Hg to 45 mm Hg) will result in an increase in CBF of approximately 10 mL/100 g/min *(Miller: Anesthesia, ed 4, pp 692-693; Stoelting: Basics of Anesthesia, ed 3, p 331).*

739. **(C)** Autonomic hyperreflexia is a neurologic disorder that occurs in association with resolution of spinal shock and a return of spinal cord reflexes. Cutaneous or visceral stimulation (such as distention of the urinary bladder or rectum) below the level of the spinal cord transection initiates afferent impulses that are transmitted to the spinal cord at this level, which subsequently elicits reflex sympathetic activity over the splanchnic nerves. Since modulation of this reflex sympathetic activity from higher centers in the central nervous system is lost (due to the spinal cord transection), the reflex sympathetic activity below the level of the injury results in intense generalized vasoconstriction and hypertension. Bradycardia occurs secondary to activation of baroreceptor reflexes. The incidence of autonomic hyperreflexia during general anesthesia depends on the level of the spinal cord transection. Approximately 85% of patients with a spinal cord transection above the T6 dermatome will exhibit this reflex during general anesthesia. In contrast, it is difficult to elicit this reflex in patients with a spinal cord transection below the T10 dermatome. Treatment of autonomic hyperreflexia is with ganglionic blocking drugs, such as trimethaphan, α-adrenergic receptor antagonists, such as phentolamine, direct-acting vasodilators, such as nitroprusside or nitroglycerin, and deep general or regional anesthesia. Patients with autonomic hyperreflexia should not be treated initially with propranolol or other ß-adrenergic receptor antagonists for two reasons. First, bradycardia can be potentiated by $ß_1$-adrenergic receptor blockade and second, $β_2$-adrenergic receptor blockade in skeletal muscle will leave the α-adrenergic properties of circulating catecholamines unopposed, causing a paradoxical hypertensive response *(Stoelting: Anesthesia & Co-existing Disease, ed 3, pp 226-228).*

740. **(C)** The brain is an obligate aerobe, as it cannot store oxygen. Under normal circumstances, there is a substantial safety margin in that the delivery of oxygen is considerably greater than demand. Oxygen consumption is in the range of 3 to 5 mL/100 g of brain tissue/minute whereas the delivery of oxygen is approximately 50 mL blood/100 g brain tissue/minute *(Stoelting: Pharmacology and Physiology in Anesthetic Practice, ed 2, p 588).*

741. **(B)** SSEPs are composed of negative and positive voltage deflections with specific latencies and amplitudes. Baseline values for latency and amplitude must be determined for each patient at the onset of surgery because the characteristics of SSEP waveforms change with recording circumstances (e.g., the latency becomes greater and the amplitude becomes smaller as the distance between the neural generator and the recording electrode is increased). A decrease in the amplitude or an increase in the latency in the SSEP waveform from baseline values may suggest ischemia along the sensory pathway in question *(Miller: Anesthesia, ed 4, pp 1330-1331).*

742. **(C)** $CMRO_2$ is closely coupled to temperature. The relationship between temperature and $CMRO_2$ is exponential. In general $CMRO_2$ decreases approximately 7% for each 1°C decrease in body temperature *(Miller: Anesthesia, ed 4, p 692)*.

743. **(D)** Brain death is defined as irreversible cessation of brain function. There are clinical and laboratory (see explanation to question 751) criteria for defining brain death. It is extremely important to identify and reverse any factors that can mimic the clinical or laboratory criteria for brain death, such as hypothermia, drug intoxication (hypnotic sedatives and major tranquilizers), or metabolic encephalopathy. Clinical criteria for brain death can be divided into those that are related to cortical function and those that are related to brainstem function. Absence of cortical function is manifested by lack of spontaneous motor activity, consciousness, and purposeful movement in response to painful stimuli. Absence of brainstem function is manifested by the inability to elicit reflexes, such as the pupillary response to light and the corneal oculocephalic, oculovestibular, oropharyngeal, and respiratory reflexes. For example, in patients without brainstem function there is no increase in heart rate when atropine is administered intravenously, and there is no respiratory effort during apnea even when the P_aCO_2 is >60 mm Hg. Decerebrate and decorticate posturing are not consistent with the diagnosis of brain death *(Miller: Anesthesia, ed 4, pp 2566, 2574; Stoelting: Anesthesia and Co-existing Disease, ed 3, pp 231-232; Barash: Clinical Anesthesia, ed 2, pp 1479-1480)*.

744. **(C)** The most common complications associated with the surgical sitting position include venous air embolism (VAE), paradoxical VAE, cardiovascular instability, pneumocephalus, subdural hematoma, peripheral neuropathy, and quadriplegia (quadriplegia is possibly caused by compression ischemia of the cervical spinal cord in patients with aberrant spinal cord blood supply). VAE occurs when air is entrained into open veins in the presence of negative intraluminal pressures (i.e., negative with respect to atmospheric pressure). Significant VAE can result in reduced cardiac output and profound hypoxia. Current devices used to detect VAE include the transesophageal echocardiograph, Doppler ultrasound, pulmonary artery mass catheter spectrometer (to monitor changes in P_ECO_2 and P_EN_2), right atrial catheter, and esophageal stethoscope (to listen for cardiac murmurs). The most sensitive means of diagnosing VAE include transesophageal echocardiography or precordial Doppler monitoring *(Miller: Anesthesia, ed 4, pp 1068-1070)*.

745. **(C)** The primarily compensatory mechanism for intracranial hypertension is translocation of cerebral spinal fluid from the intracranial vault into the spinal subarachnoid space *(Cottrell: Anesthesia and Neurosurgery, ed 3, p 151)*.

746. **(B)** Many of the commonly used anesthetic agents can alter the characteristics of evoked-potential waveforms. In general, volatile anesthetics cause a dose-dependent increase in the latency and decrease in the amplitude of somatosensory evoked potentials. Brainstem auditory evoked potentials (BAEP) are the most resistant to the depressant effects of volatile anesthetics, while visual evoked potentials (VEP) are the most sensitive. In general, up to 1 MAC of isoflurane, enflurane, or halothane is compatible with adequate SSEP monitoring *(Miller: Anesthesia, ed 4, pp 1333-1337)*.

747. **(D)** Cerebral spinal fluid is a clear aqueous solution that is formed at a rate of 0.35-0.40 ml/min or approximately 560 ml/day in the average size human. The turnover time for the total cerebral spinal fluid volume is approximately 5-7 hours, or a turnover rate of about 4 times per day. Cerebrospinal fluid is produced primarily by the choroid plexus, by the oxidation of glucose, and by ultrafiltration by cerebral capillaries. The composition of cerebral spinal fluid is markedly different from that of plasma. Only sodium exists in both the cerebrospinal fluid and plasma at approximately the same concentration. Macromolecules, such as albumin, globulin, and fibrinogen, are almost completely excluded from the cerebrospinal fluid. Compared with plasma, cerebrospinal fluid contains higher concentrations of chloride and magnesium, and lower concentrations of glucose, potassium, bicarbonate, calcium, and phosphate *(Cottrell: Anesthesia and Neurosurgery, ed 3, pp 94-95)*.

748. **(B)** Except for the transesophageal echocardiograph, the Doppler ultrasound is the most sensitive device for detection of intracardiac air. Under ideal circumstances, as little as 0.5 mL of intracardiac air can be detected by this device *(Faust: Anesthesiology Review, ed 2, pp 403-404)*.

749. **(B)** P_aCO_2 is one of the most important extracerebral biochemical factors that regulate CBF. The cerebral vasculature is most sensitive to changes in P_aCO_2 within the physiologic range for P_aCO_2 (approximately 20 to 80 mm Hg). In general, the regional sensitivity of the cerebral vasculature to changes in P_aCO_2 (i.e., CO_2 responsiveness) is directly proportional to the resting CMR for each region of the brain. Regional CO_2 responsiveness is greatest in the cerebrum, less in the cerebellum, and least in the spinal cord *(Miller: Anesthesia, ed 4, pp 692-693; Miller: Anesthesia, ed 2, p 1257)*.

750. **(D)** The tip of multiorificed right atrial catheters must be accurately placed at the junction of the superior vena cava and right atrium, because air has a tendency to localize at this junction. There are several methods that can be used to ensure that the catheter tip is accurately positioned at the junction of the superior vena cava and right atrium. For example, chest x-rays can be performed. However, there may be difficulty in interpreting the position of the tip of the catheter, and the catheter could migrate after the x-ray is performed. Cardiovascular pressures could be monitored, but this technique requires that the tip of the catheter be first introduced into the right ventricle and then pulled back into the right atrium. Introduction of the tip of the catheter into the right ventricle could cause dysrhythmias, heart block, or bleeding or rupture of cardiac structures. A technique frequently used to accurately place multiorificed catheters at the junction of the superior vena cava and right atrium is intravascular electrocardiography. The appropriate position of the catheter is confirmed when a large negative P complex is obtained on the electrocardiogram. The P complex shown in the figure of this question is biphasic, which indicates that the tip of the catheter is in the midatrial position and should be withdrawn slightly until there is a large negative downward configuration of the P complex *(Miller: Anesthesia, ed 4, pp 1904-1905)*.

751. **(A)** Both laboratory and clinical studies have reported that hyperglycemia at the time of either focal (e.g., stroke) or global (e.g., systemic shock or cardiac arrest) results in a worsening of neurologic outcome (i.e., both histologic and functional). Unfortunately, it is not widely appreciated that the administration of glucose does not need to produce high blood glucose levels to augment post-ischemic cerebral injury. Thus, glucose-containing solutions should not be administered to patients who are at risk for either cerebral or spinal cord injury *(Cottrell: Anesthesia and Neurosurgery, ed 3, pp 63, 268, & 279)*.

752. **(B)** Critical CBF is the CBF below which EEG evidence of cerebral ischemia begins to appear. Critical CBF in patients anesthetized with isoflurane is approximately 10 mL/100 g/min. In contrast, critical CBF in patients anesthetized with halothane is 18 to 20 mL/100 g/min and critical CBF in patients anesthetized with enflurane is about 15 mL/100 g/min. Based on studies that compared the requirement for shunt placement following carotid artery crossclamping in patients under isoflurane, enflurane, and halothane anesthesia, it appears that isoflurane provides some degree of cerebral protection against incomplete regional cerebral ischemia in humans *(Michenfelder: Anesthesia and the Brain, p 86)*.

753. **(A)** It is important to note that CBF autoregulation is easily impaired and modified by numerous factors, such as cerebral vasodilators (including volatile anesthetics), chronic hypertension, and cerebral ischemia. Cerebral ischemia abolishes CBF autoregulation such that CBF becomes passively dependent on the cerebral perfusion pressure *(Barash: Clinical Anesthesia, ed 2, pp 875-876)*.

754. **(C)** Changes in plasma P_aCO_2 will affect cerebral vascular tone. Hypocarbia (associated with hyperventilation) will rapidly cause vasoconstriction, thereby reducing cerebral blood flow and cerebral blood volume. Thus hyperventilation is the technique that will be most rapidly available to decrease intracranial pressure in patients with an intracranial mass *(Cottrell: Anesthesia and Neurosurgery, ed 3, p 288)*.

755. **(E)** In general, the cerebrovascular response to changes in P_aCO_2 is preserved following the administration of intravenous anesthetics. Specifically, in humans, CO_2 reactivity is maintained with barbiturate concentrations sufficient to produce burst suppression on the electroencephalogram *(Cottrell: Anesthesia and Neurosurgery, ed 3, pp 79 & 164; Michenfelder: Anesthesia and the Brain, p 95)*.

756. **(D)** There are a number of practical reasons for using the sitting position. These include better surgical exposure, less tissue retraction and bleeding, a lower incidence of cranial nerve damage, ready access to the patient's airway, chest, and extremities, and more complete resection of the lesion. Although there are minimal objective data, there are, nonetheless, some conditions considered relative contraindications to the sitting position. These include an open ventriculoatrial shunt, presence of right-to-left intracardiac shunts (because of the potential for paradoxical VAE), presence of platypnea-orthodeoxia (i.e., patients who are well oxygenated in the supine position but become hypoxic when they assume the upright position; these patients have hemodynamic-dependent right-to-left intracardiac shunts), and the tendency to develop cerebral ischemia when the patient assumes the upright position. In contrast to the situation with ventriculoatrial shunts, air cannot be entrained via a ventriculoperitoneal shunt directly into the circulation. Ventriculoperitoneal shunt is not a relative contraindication to surgery in the sitting position *(Barash: Clinical Anesthesia, ed 2, pp 894-895)*.

757. **(C)** The general approach to treating patients following venous air embolism (VAE) is to: a) stop further air entrainment, b) aspirate entrained air, c) prevent expansion of existing air, and d) support cardiovascular function. Cessation of subsequent air entrainment is achieved by flooding the surgical field with irrigation fluid. Additionally, non-collapsible veins may be sealed using electrocautery, vessel ligation, or bone wax. Neck veins may be compressed as a means of increasing jugular venous pressure, which mitigates or prevents further air entry and helps localize the source of air. A multi-orifice right atrial catheter, placed prior to the event, is the most effective means of aspirating VAE. In order to prevent expansion of the VAE, nitrous oxide is immediately discontinued. Cardiovascular function is supported using inotropes, vasopressors, and i.v. fluids as indicated. Of the response options provided, positive end-expiratory pressure (PEEP) is the least correct answer. Approximately 20-30% of humans have a probe patent foramen ovale. Initiation of PEEP may: a) increase the risk of paradoxical embolism or b) decrease venous effluent from the calvarium resulting in increased cerebral blood volume and intracranial pressure *(Cottrell: Anesthesia and Neurosurgery, ed 3, pp 348-357; Barash: Clinical Anesthesia, ed 2, pp 894-895).*

758. **(C)** Autoregulation of cerebral vasomotor tone maintains cerebral blood flow within a narrow range over a wide range of mean arterial pressures or cerebral perfusion pressures. The relationship between cerebral blood flow, cerebral perfusion pressure, and cerebrovascular resistance is expressed as follows. Cerebral perfusion pressure can be approximated as the difference in mean arterial pressure and intracranial pressure.

$$CBF = \frac{CPP}{CVR}$$

Cerebral perfusion pressure approximates mean arterial pressure when the cranium is open. Mean arterial pressure can be approximated as 1/3 the systolic blood pressure plus 2/3 the diastolic pressure. In this patient, the cerebral perfusion pressure is 75 mm Hg *(Cottrell: Anesthesia and Neurosurgery, ed 3, pp 288 & 310).*

759. **(E)** Approximately four percent of the population over 40 years of age have asymptomatic carotid bruits. There is no evidence that the incidence of postoperative neurologic complications is increased in these patients following non-neurologic surgery. Surgery should therefore proceed as planned; however, it must be remembered that the risk of postoperative cardiac complications, such as angina and myocardial infarction, is increased *(Stoelting: Anesthesia and Co-existing Disease, ed 3, pp 196-198).*

Note: It deserves mention that the National Institute of Health currently recommends carotid endarterectomy in asymptomatic patients with a $\geq 60\%$ reduction in the carotid artery diameter. In the case scenario presented in this question, it may now be considered most appropriate to further study the status of this patient's carotid artery disease prior to proceeding with an elective colonoscopy *(National Institute of Neurological Disorders and Stroke: Carotid endarterectomy for patients with asymptomatic internal carotid artery stenosis. J Neurol Sci 1995;129:76-77).*

760. **(B)** In patients who have suffered a cerebral vascular accident as a result of occlusive vascular disease, there is a loss of normal vasomotor responses to changes in P_aCO_2 and arterial blood pressure in the areas of ischemia (i.e., vasomotor paralysis). Approximately 4 to 6 weeks is required for these changes to stabilize. Therefore, it is recommended that anesthesia for elective non-neurologic surgical procedures be postponed for about a month after an occlusive vascular accident to minimize the risk of a subsequent perioperative occlusive vascular accident *(Miller: Anesthesia, ed 4, p 716)*.

761. **(A)** Somatosensory evoked potentials (SSEPs), recorded on the contralateral cerebral cortex, are the physiologic response of the nervous system to peripheral nerve stimulation. Extraction of SSEPs from the background EEG is accomplished by computerized signal averaging for summation. SSEPs assess the integrity of the peripheral nerve (usually posterior tibial or median), dorsal column, brainstem, medial lemniscus, internal capsule, and contralateral somatosensory cortex. However, they do not evaluate the integrity of the ventral or lateral spinothalamic tracts or the corticospinal tract since the latter is a motor not sensory pathway *(Cottrell: Anesthesia and Neurosurgery, ed 3, pp 212-213)*.

762. **(B)** The differential diagnosis for a non-moving patient during a wakeup test includes presence of neuromuscular blockade, inadequate volatile or nitrous oxide washout, or the presence of opiates or sedative hypnotic-type drugs like midazolam. There are also a few other extremely rare central causes such as stroke. Since gross neuromuscular blockade has worn off in this patient and the volatile anesthetic and nitrous oxide have largely been washed out, a trial of naloxone would not be unreasonable. An initial small dose such as 20 μg may be all that is needed to reverse the effects of the morphine. If this dose is not effective, it should be repeated *(Wedel: Orthopedic Anesthesia, p 187)*.

763. **(D)** Arterial CO_2 tension (P_aCO_2) is the single most potent physiologic determinant of cerebral blood flow (CBF) and cerebral blood volume (CBV). Between P_aCO_2 values of 20 and 80 mm Hg, CBF decreases 1 to 1.5 ml • 100 g brain weight^{-1} • min^{-1} and CBV decreases approximately 0.05 ml • 100 g brain weight^{-1} for each 1 mm Hg decrease in P_aCO_2. Decreasing the P_aCO_2 to 25-30 mm Hg should provide near-maximal reductions in CBF, CBV, and ICP, lasting up to 24-36 hours, without adversely affecting acid-base/electrolyte (e.g., decreases in potassium or ionized calcium) status or decreasing cerebral oxygen delivery (i.e., as a result of intense cerebral vasoconstriction and a leftward shift of the oxyhemoglobin dissociation curve). Since this patient's P_aCO_2 is 10 mm Hg below normal, CBF also would be reduced to approximately 35-40 ml • 100 g brain weight^{-1} • min^{-1} *(Faust: Anesthesiology Review, ed 2, pp 388-389; Cottrell: Anesthesia and Neurosurgery, ed 3, pp 23 & 266)*.

764. (A) Intracranial pressure (ICP) is determined by the relationship of the intracranial vault (formed by the skull), volume of brain parenchyma, volume of cerebral spinal fluid (CSF), and cerebral blood volume (CBV). Studies evaluating the effectiveness of corticosteroids in the setting of head injury, or global or focal brain ischemia, have demonstrated either no improvement or a worsening of neurologic outcome (see explanation for question 726). All intravenous anesthetics, except ketamine, cause some degree of reduction in cerebral metabolic rate (CMR), cerebral blood flow (CBF), CBV, and ICP (provided ventilation is not depressed). Of intravenous anesthetics, barbiturates are thought to be the "gold standard" for anesthetic-mediated brain protective therapy during focal or incomplete global brain ischemia. The impact of hyperventilation on ICP is discussed in question 763. Both osmotic and loop diuretics are effective in reducing ICP. Elevation of the head above the level of the heart facilitates effluent of blood from the calvarium which results in decreases in CBV and ICP *(Faust: Anesthesiology Review, ed 2, pp 388-389).*

765. (A) Following subarachnoid hemorrhage (SAH), patients may experience rebleeding, cerebral vasospasm, intracranial hypertension, and seizures. Provided the patient is not experiencing cerebral vasospasm, hypertension should be avoided. In contrast, had this patient been in vasospasm, induced hypertension would have been an appropriate therapeutic intervention (see explanation for question 776). Hypertension is avoided, in part, by the administration of sedative and analgesic medications. Antiepileptic drugs and calcium channel blockers (e.g., nimodipine) are often administered in an attempt to prevent or mitigate seizures and the sequele of cerebral vasospasm, respectively *(Cottrell: Anesthesia and Neurosurgery, ed 3, pp 367-369).*

766. (E) Somatosensory evoked potentials (SSEPs) are used to monitor the integrity of sensory pathways in the nervous system during neurosurgical or orthopedic surgery (see explanation for question 761). Volatile anesthetics (e.g., isoflurane) and barbiturates (e.g., sodium thiopental) decrease the amplitude and increase the latency SSEP waveforms. Nitrous oxide decreases the amplitude, yet has no effect on latency. Etomidate increases both the amplitude and latency. In contrast, nondepolarizing muscle relaxants (e.g., vecuronium) have no effect on sensory pathways of the nervous system, and, thus, can be used during SSEP monitoring *(Miller: Anesthesia, ed 4, p 1334).*

767. (B) In addition to EKG changes (e.g., T-wave inversion, depression of the ST segment, the appearance of U waves, prolonged QT interval, and rarely Q waves), abnormal thallium scintigraphy, regional wall motion abnormalities, and elevated creatine kinase-MB isoenzymes have been reported in patients with subarachnoid hemorrhage (SAH). Although historically considered a functionally insignificant neurogenic phenomena, there is increasing evidence that these changes may be a sign of underlying myocardial ischemia. However, even if myocardial ischemia is present, it seems to have a minimal impact on patient outcome (i.e., morbidity and mortality). Since electrolyte abnormalities (e.g., hypokalemia or hypocalcemia) may contribute to the etiology of the EKG changes, it would probably be most appropriate to quantify these electrolytes prior to initiating other therapies or canceling emergency surgery *(Cottrell: Anesthesia and Neurosurgery, ed 3, pp 379-380; Anesth Analg 1993;76:253-258).*

768. **(E)** Limitations in somatosensory evoked potential monitoring has prompted interest in monitoring the motor system. Specifically, motor evoked potentials (MEP) are used to monitor the integrity of motor pathways in the nervous system during neurosurgical, orthopedic, or major vascular (e.g., procedures that involve cross-clamping of the thoracic aorta) surgery. Electrical or magnetic stimulation of the motor cortex produces an evoked potential that is propagated via descending motor pathways and can be recorded from the spinal epidural space, spinal cord, peripheral nerve, or the muscle itself. In general, inhalational and intravenous anesthetics decrease the amplitude and increase the latency of the MEP response. Fentanyl is an exception to this rule and has little, if any, effect on MEP monitoring. *(Cottrell: Anesthesia and Neurosurgery, ed 3, p 221).*

769. **(D)** Ketamine is thought to increase cerebral blood flow and consequently, cerebral blood volume and ICP by two mechanisms: 1) there may be a direct effect on cerebral vascular smooth muscle to cause vasodilatation and 2) there may be a "coupled" effect caused by an increase in CMR (see explanation to question 768). There is some controversy regarding the effect of ketamine on CBF/CMR coupling. Animal studies in vivo indicate that CMR and CBF are increased proportionally in structures of the limbic system. In contrast, there is evidence from one human study that while ketamine increased CBF (by 62%), CMR remained unchanged. The effect of ketamine on CBF autoregulation has not been studied. The CO_2 responsiveness of the cerebral vasculature is not altered by ketamine *(Miller: Anesthesia, ed 4, p 702; Stoelting: Pharmacology and Physiology in Anesthetic Practice, ed 2, pp 137-138).*

770. **(A)** In contrast to ketamine and increased neural activity (e.g., seizures or hyperthermia), which increase CBF and CMR, volatile anesthetics cause a simultaneous, dose-dependent increase in CBF and decrease in CMR (i.e., volatile anesthetics "uncouple" global CBF and CMR) *(Miller: Anesthesia, ed 4, pp 690-692).*

771. **(A)** Maintenance of a relatively constant cerebral blood flow despite changes in systemic mean arterial blood pressure is termed autoregulation. The upper and lower limits of autoregulation, in normotensive adult humans, are cerebral perfusion pressures of 150 and 50 mm Hg, respectively. Autoregulation appears to be impaired by volatile anesthetics in a dose-dependent manner. In contrast, nitrous oxide, barbiturates, and fentanyl do not appear to disturb autoregulation *(Cottrell: Anesthesia and Neurosurgery, ed 3, pp 150 & 164).*

772. **(A)** Acute spinal cord injury above T4-T6 produces a sympathectomy below the level of injury, which decreases systemic arteriolar and venous vasomotor tone, and abolishes vasopressor reflexes (i.e., spinal shock). This pathophysiologic process may continue for up to 6 weeks after injury. As spinal shock resolves, patients with spinal cord injuries cephalad to T4-T6 may develop autonomic hyperreflexia (i.e., acute generalized sympathetic hyperactivity due to stimulation below the level of injury). Neurogenic pulmonary edema may develop during either spinal shock or autonomic hyperreflexia. Thermoregulation is lost, resulting in *poikilothermia,* because the hypothalamic thermoregulatory center is unable to communicate with the peripheral sympathetic pathways. In the cool environment of the intensive care unit, spinal cord injury patients are unable to vasoconstrict below the level of injury, and, thus, may experience hypothermia. Loss of sympathetic-mediated vasomotor tone also results in hypotension *(Cottrell: Anesthesia and Neurosurgery, ed 3, pp 649 & 725; Faust: Anesthesiology Review, ed 2, p 405).*

773. **(E)** Signs and symptoms of intracranial hypertension include nausea and vomiting, systemic hypertension, bradycardia, altered level of consciousness, irregular breathing pattern, papilledema, seizure activity, personality changes, and coma *(Stoelting: Basics of Anesthesia, ed 3, pp 333-334)*.

774. **(D)** General anesthesia can be induced safely in patients with carotid artery disease using intravenous anesthetics, such as thiopental, midazolam, or etomidate. Isoflurane, in conjunction with N_2O or opioids, is a good choice for maintenance of anesthesia in these patients, because critical CBF is reduced during isoflurane anesthesia which may provide some cerebral protection (see explanation to question 752). Arterial blood pressure and P_aCO_2 should be maintained in the normal ranges for each patient because the vasculature within ischemic regions of the brain have lost the ability to autoregulate CBF and respond to changes in P_aCO_2. Marked reductions in arterial blood pressure may reduce CBF (especially via collateral channels) to ischemic brain tissue. Theoretically, if P_aCO_2 is increased from normal, cerebral blood vessels surrounding the region of ischemia which retain normal CO_2 responsiveness will dilate, diverting rCBF away from the ischemic brain tissue (i.e., steal phenomenon). Conversely, if the P_aCO_2 is reduced from normal, the cerebral blood vessels surrounding the ischemic brain tissue will constrict, diverting rCBF to ischemic areas of the brain (inverse-steal phenomenon or Robin Hood effect). Hyperventilating the lungs in an attempt to produce the inverse-steal phenomenon is not recommended since the actual effect on rCBF to the ischemic brain has not been measured and may actually produce paradoxical and unpredictable responses. The carotid sinus (not carotid body) baroreceptor reflex can be blunted by intravenous injection of atropine or by local infiltration of the area of the carotid sinus with a local anesthetic *(Stoelting: Anesthesia and Co-existing Disease, ed 3, pp 198-202)*.

775. **(A)** The effect of N_2O on CBF, cerebral blood volume, and ICP is controversial. In a number of animal and human studies, N_2O increased CBF by 35% to 103%. Conversely, in other animal studies, N_2O was consistently found to have only minimal effects on CBF. Differences between species may be one factor contributing to these conflicting results. Since N_2O appears to increase CBF and cerebral blood volume in humans, it seems prudent to discontinue N_2O in patients in whom intracranial hypertension is not responsive to other therapeutic maneuvers *(Barash: Clinical Anesthesia, ed 2, pp 878-879)*.

776. **(C)** Following subarachnoid hemorrhage (SAH), the incidence and severity of cerebral vasospasm has been reported to correlate with the amount and location of blood in the calvarium. Angiographic evidence of vasospasm has been noted in up to 70% of SAH patients. However, clinically significant vasospasm occurs in only 20 to 30% of SAH patients. The incidence peaks approximately 7 days after SAH. Calcium channel blockers (e.g., nimodipine) decrease the morbidity and mortality associated with vasospasm, but investigators have been unable to demonstrate any significant change in the incidence or severity of vasospasm. This suggests that the beneficial effects of nimodipine may be related to inhibition of primary and secondary ischemic cascades, rather than direct cerebral vasodilation. Treatment of vasospasm also includes "triple H therapy" (i.e., hypervolemia, induced hypertension, and hemodilution) and cerebral angioplasty. The rationale of induced hypervolemia and hypertension is that ischemic regions of brain have impaired autoregulation, and, thus, cerebral blood flow (CBF) is perfusion pressure-dependent. Hemodilution is thought to increase blood flow through the cerebral microcirculation (due to improved rheology and reactive hyperemia). One argument against hemodilution is that increases in CBF are offset by concomitant decreases in the oxygen carrying

capacity. Taken together, blood pressure reductions and diuretic use are incorrect responses to this question *(Cottrell: Anesthesia and Neurosurgery, ed 3, pp 367-368 & 381-383).*

777. **(E)** There are a variety of medical conditions associated with cerebral aneurysms and subsequent subarachnoid hemorrhage (SAH). These include hypertension, coarctation of the aorta, polycystic kidney disease, and fibromuscular dysplasia. Additionally, a recent study reported a significant association between cigarette smoking and SAH *(Cottrell: Anesthesia and Neurosurgery, ed 3, p 365).*

778. **(D)** Chronic hypertension shifts the CBF-autoregulatory curve to the right. The clinical significance of this observation is that CBF could decrease and cerebral ischemia could occur at a higher mean arterial pressure in patients with chronic hypertension compared to normal patients. Chronic antihypertensive therapy to control systemic blood pressures within the normal range will restore normal CBF autoregulation *(Barash: Clinical Anesthesia, ed 2, p 875; Miller: Anesthesia, ed 4, Figure 21-5).*

779. **(D)** Cerebral autoregulation is disturbed in a number of diseases (e.g., acute cerebral ischemia, mass lesions, trauma, inflammation, prematurity, neonatal asphyxia, and diabetes mellitus). The final common pathway of dysfunction, in its most extreme form, is termed vasomotor paralysis. Autoregulation is not, or minimally, affected by hyperoxia. During normothermic and moderate hypothermic (i.e., approximately 27°C) cardiopulmonary bypass, autoregulation is well preserved. Chronic hypertension causes a rightward shift of the autoregulation curve toward higher upper and lower cerebral perfusion pressure limits. Autoregulation is impaired by volatile anesthetics (e.g., isoflurane) in a dose-dependent manner. At > 2 MAC, autoregulation is abolished *(Cottrell: Anesthesia and Neurosurgery, ed 3, pp 23-28, 150, & 164).*

780. **(A)** The cerebral pharmacologic profile of etomidate is similar to thiopental in that it produces a dose-related decrease in the cerebral metabolic rate (CMR) and cerebral blood flow (via direct cerebral vasoconstriction and coupling to decreased CMR). As noted following barbiturate administration, intravenous etomidate does not disturb cerebral autoregulation or CO_2 reactivity *(Cottrell: Anesthesia and Neurosurgery, ed 3, pp 79 & 164).*

781. **(B)** Nasal intubation should be avoided in patients with suspected basal skull fractures or sinus injuries. Since approximately 10% of head injury patients have associated cervical spine injuries, it is prudent to assume that all head injury patients have co-existing cervical spine injury until proven otherwise. Additionally, the patient described in this question may have abnormal airway anatomy due to extreme micrognathia, facial injuries, and obesity. Taken together, direct laryngoscopy with rapid sequence induction is probably not an acceptable technique for securing this patient's airway. In contrast, awake intubation by direct or fiberoptic laryngoscopy, or tracheostomy are considered appropriate techniques for tracheal intubation of this patient *(Cottrell: Anesthesia and Neurosurgery, ed 3, pp 263-266).*

782.   **(A)**   Hyperosmotic drugs, such as mannitol and urea, and loop diuretics, such as furosemide, are effective in reducing ICP since intracellular water is a significant component of the intracranial contents. The maximum reduction in ICP typically occurs in 15 to 60 minutes following administration of these agents. Mannitol should be administered intravenously in doses of 0.25 to 1.0 g/kg over 15 to 30 minutes. Doses of mannitol > 1.0 g/kg do not further increase the magnitude of ICP reduction. Urea should be administered intravenously in doses of 1.0 to 1.5 g/kg over 15 to 30 minutes. Rebound intracranial hypertension occurs more frequently following administration of urea compared with mannitol. This observation reflects the ability of urea molecules to penetrate the blood-brain barrier, which reduces the osmotic gradient and increases brain water. Another disadvantage of urea (compared with mannitol) is a high incidence of venous thrombosis should extravasation of the urea occur. Since osmotic diuretics can initially increase intravascular fluid volume, these agents should be administered carefully in patients with limited cardiac reserve. The incidence of venous thrombosis after administration of mannitol is low. Neither mannitol or urea cause myocardial depression *(Miller: Anesthesia, ed 4, pp 1913-1914; Stoelting: Anesthesia and Co-existing Disease, ed 3, pp 185-186).*

783.   **(A)**   The effects of isoflurane, nitrous oxide, and etomidate were discussed in the explanation for question 766. Diazepam, like isoflurane and etomidate, decreases the amplitude and increases the latency of the SSEP waveform *(Miller: Anesthesia, ed 4, p 1334).*

784.   **(A)**   See explanation to questions 753, 778, and 779 *(Miller: Anesthesia, ed 4, pp 694, 702-706, 716-717).*

785.   **(A)**   Progressive entrainment of air into the pulmonary microcirculation reduces lung perfusion, and increases pulmonary vascular resistance (PVR) and alveolar dead-space ventilation. The increase in PVR is reflected by increases in pulmonary arterial and central venous pressures. A large air embolus can result in right ventricular outflow obstruction, which will dramatically reduce cardiac output and cause hypotension. The increased alveolar dead space results in a decrease in P_ECO_2. In severe VAE, CO_2 cannot be eliminated and P_aCO_2 increases. P_EN_2 increases because air diffuses into the pulmonary alveoli. The sensitivity of continuous P_ECO_2 and P_EN_2 monitoring is similar *(Miller: Anesthesia, ed 4, pp 1900-1902; Barash: Clinical Anesthesia, ed 2, pp 894-895).*

786.   **(C)**   The cerebrovascular response to hyperventilation was reviewed in the explanation for question 763 *(Faust: Anesthesiology Review, ed 2, pp 388-389; Cottrell: Anesthesia and Neurosurgery, ed 3, pp 23 & 266).*

787.   **(E)**   The effects of propofol on cerebral blood flow (CBF), cerebral blood volume (CBV), cerebral metabolism (CMR), and intracranial pressure (ICP) are quite similar to those of barbiturates. That is, propofol causes reductions in CBF, CBV, CMR, and ICP (provided ventilation is not depressed) *(Miller: Anesthesia, ed 4, p 701).*

Anatomy, Regional Anesthesia, and Pain Management

DIRECTIONS (Questions 788 through 859): Each of the questions or incomplete statements in this section is followed by answers or by completions of the statement, respectively. Select the ONE BEST answer or completion for each item.

788. Tachyphylaxis to local anesthetics is most closely related to which of the following?

    A. Speed of injection
    B. Dosing interval
    C. Temperature of local anesthetic
    D. Volume of local anesthetic
    E. pH of solution

789. A 57-year-old diabetic patient is scheduled to undergo shunt placement for hemodialysis. How will the duration of action of a lidocaine axillary block be altered in this patient?

    A. Increased because of renal failure
    B. Decreased because of high plasma glucose levels
    C. Decreased because of increased cardiac output
    D. Decreased because of anemia
    E. Not affected

790. The maximum dose of lidocaine containing 1:200,000 epinephrine that can be administered to a 70-kg patient for regional anesthesia is

    A. 50 mg
    B. 100 mg
    C. 200 mg
    D. 500 mg
    E. 1,000 mg

791. Which of the following concentrations of epinephrine corresponds to a 1:200,000 mixture?

    A. 0.5 µg/mL
    B. 5 µg/mL
    C. 50 µg/mL
    D. 0.5 mg/mL
    E. None of the above

792. An anesthesia pain service consult is sought for a 78-year-old patient with a complaint of pain in the distribution of the trigeminal nerve. The patient has no other medical problems except a history of congestive heart failure for which he takes digoxin and thiazide. In addition to his chief complaint, the patient over the last 72 hours has also complained of dysesthesia in the feet as well as difficulty with vision and emesis times three. The most appropriate step at this time would be

    A. Trigeminal nerve block with bupivacaine
    B. Obtain neurologic workup for multiple sclerosis
    C. Administration of fentanyl and ondansetron
    D. Initiate therapy with carbamazepine
    E. Obtain a digoxin level

793. Which of the following is the earliest sign of lidocaine toxicity?

    A. Shivering
    B. Nystagmus
    C. Lightheadedness and dizziness
    D. Tonic-clonic seizures
    E. Nausea and vomiting

794. An analgesic effect similar to the epidural administration of 10 mg of morphine could be achieved by which dose of intrathecal morphine?

    A. 0.1 mg
    B. 1 mg
    C. 5 mg
    D. 10 mg
    E. There is no correlation

795. Clinically significant methemoglobinemia may result from administration of large doses of

    A. Chloroprocaine
    B. Bupivacaine
    C. Etidocaine
    D. Prilocaine
    E. Lidocaine

796. Which of the following is the most important disadvantage of interscalene brachial plexus block compared with other approaches?

    A. Not suitable for operations on the shoulder
    B. Large volumes of local anesthetics required
    C. Frequent sparing of the ulnar nerve
    D. Frequent sparing of the musculocutaneous nerve
    E. High incidence of pneumothorax

797. A 68-year-old woman is to undergo foot surgery under spinal anesthesia. Which of the following statements concerning the immediate physiologic response to the surgical incision is true?

   A. The cardiovascular response to stress will be blocked, but the adrenergic response will not
   B. The adrenergic response to stress will be blocked, but the cardiovascular response will not
   C. Both the adrenergic and cardiovascular responses will be blocked
   D. Neither the adrenergic or cardiovascular response will be blocked
   E. The cardiovascular response will be blocked but the adrenergic response will be augmented

798. The "snap" felt just prior to entering the epidural space represents passage through which ligament?

   A. Anterior longitudinal ligaments
   B. Posterior longitudinal ligaments
   C. Ligamentum flavum
   D. Supraspinous ligament
   E. Interspinous ligament

799. A 26-year-old woman undergoes a left-sided stellate ganglion block for treatment of her reflex sympathetic dystrophy in the left hand. Twenty minutes after the block is placed, the skin temperature in her upper extremity rises from 33°C to 36.5°C. The veins in her hand and arm are engorged, and she has a small pupil on the left side with a drooping eyelid. Her pain, however, is not relieved. Which of the following explanations for this is most plausible?

   A. The pain-carrying fibers originated from the right stellate ganglion.
   B. The pain-carrying fibers originated from the superior cervical ganglion.
   C. The pain-carrying fibers originated from the middle cervical ganglion.
   D. The pain-carrying fibers originated from the inferior cervical ganglion.
   E. The pain-carrying fibers originated from the second thoracic ganglion.

800. A sciatic nerve block is performed in a healthy 26-year-old male patient for bunion surgery. Fifteen milliliters of 1.5% mepivacaine is slowly injected after the landmarks are identified and a paresthesia is elicited in the great toe. In what order would the following nerve fibers be blocked?

   A. Sympathetic, proprioception, pain, motor
   B. Sympathetic, pain, proprioception, motor
   C. Motor, pain, proprioception, sympathetic
   D. Pain, proprioception, sympathetic, motor
   E. Pain, proprioception, motor, sympathetic

801. A 95-year-old woman has persistent and prolonged thoracic pain after a herpes zoster infection. Which of the treatments below would be **LEAST** efficacious in the treatment of her pain?

   A. Oral amitriptyline
   B. Oral clonidine
   C. Steroid epidural block
   D. Transcutaneous electrical nerve stimulation
   E. Subcutaneous injection of bupivacaine and triamcinolone

802. The deep peroneal nerve innervates the

    A. Lateral aspect of the dorsum of the foot
    B. Entire dorsum of the foot
    C. Web space between the great toe and the second toe
    D. Web space between the third and fourth toes
    E. Medial aspect of the dorsum of the foot

803. The correct arrangement of local anesthetics in order of their ability to produce cardiotoxicity from most to least is

    A. Bupivacaine, lidocaine, ropivacaine
    B. Bupivacaine, ropivacaine, lidocaine
    C. Lidocaine, bupivacaine, ropivacaine
    D. Ropivacaine, bupivacaine, lidocaine
    E. Lidocaine, ropivacaine, bupivacaine

804. A 38-year-old construction worker has received disability payments for a back injury received on the job. The patient currently takes diazepam, codeine, and hydromorphone for chronic back pain. He presents to the pain clinic for evaluation and treatment of his pain. Which of the following treatments would be most appropriate for this patient prior to diagnostic evaluation?

    A. Stop all narcotics and continue treatment with clonidine and diazepam
    B. Hospitalize and taper patient off equipotent doses of methadone
    C. Hospitalize and taper patient off equipotent doses of an agonist-antagonist narcotic
    D. Discontinue all narcotics and continue treatment with tricyclic antidepressants
    E. Stop all oral narcotics and sedative hypnotics and continue treatment with epidural steroids and narcotics

805. The primary mechanism by which the action of tetracaine is terminated when used for spinal anesthesia is

    A. Systemic absorption
    B. Uptake into neurons
    C. Hydrolysis by pseudocholinesterase
    D. Hydrolysis by nonspecific esterases
    E. Spontaneous degradation at 37°C

806. Causalgia is differentiated from reflex sympathetic dystrophy by knowledge of its

    A. Etiology
    B. Chronicity
    C. Affected body region
    D. Type of symptoms
    E. Rapidity of onset

807. The primary determinant of local anesthetic potency is

    A. pKa
    B. Molecular weight
    C. Lipid solubility
    D. Concentration
    E. Protein binding

808. Which of the following would have the greatest effect on the level of sensory blockade after a subarachnoid injection of 5% lidocaine?

    A. Coughing during placement of the block
    B. Addition of epinephrine to the local anesthetic solution
    C. Barbotage
    D. Patient weight
    E. Patient position

809. Which of the following local anesthetics would produce the lowest concentration in the fetus relative to the maternal serum concentration during a continuous lumbar epidural?

    A. Etidocaine
    B. Bupivacaine
    C. Lidocaine
    D. Chloroprocaine
    E. Mepivacaine

810. Severe hypotension associated with high spinal anesthesia is caused primarily by

    A. Decreased cardiac output secondary to decreased preload
    B. Decreased systemic vascular resistance
    C. Decreased cardiac output secondary to bradycardia
    D. Decreased cardiac output secondary to decreased myocardial contractility
    E. Increased shunting through metarterioles

811. Select the one **true** statement concerning phantom limb pain.

    A. Most phantom limb pain becomes more severe with time
    B. Most amputees do not experience phantom limb pain
    C. Nerve blocks are commonly used to treat phantom limb pain
    D. Trauma amputees have a higher incidence of phantom limb pain than non-trauma amputees
    E. The incidence of phantom limb pain increases with more distal amputations

812. Which of the following local anesthetics used for intravenous regional anesthesia (Bier block) is most rapidly metabolized and thus least toxic?

    A. Lidocaine
    B. Bupivacaine
    C. Mepivacaine
    D. Prilocaine
    E. Etidocaine

813. Select the **FALSE** statement regarding spinal anatomy and spinal anesthesia.

    A. The addition of phenylephrine to the local anesthetic will prolong spinal anesthesia
    B. A high thoracic sensory block will result in total sympathetic blockade
    C. The largest vertebral interspace is L5-S1
    D. The dural sac extends to the S3-4 interspace
    E. Dibucaine provides longer anesthesia than does tetracaine

814. Four days after a left total hip arthroplasty, an obese 62-year-old woman complains of severe back pain in the region where the epidural was placed. Over the ensuing 48 hours, the back pain gradually worsens and a severe aching pain which radiates down the left leg to the knee develops. The most likely diagnosis is

    A. Epidural abscess
    B. Epidural hematoma
    C. Anterior spinal artery syndrome
    D. Arachnoiditis
    E. Meralgia paresthetica

815. Which of the following choices is **NOT** consistent with a limb affected by chronic reflex sympathetic dystrophy?

    A. Osteoporosis
    B. Allodynia
    C. Dermatomal distribution of pain
    D. Atrophy of the involved extremity
    E. Hyperesthesia

816. The main advantage of neurolytic nerve blockade with phenol vs. alcohol is

    A. More dense blockade
    B. Blockade is permanent
    C. The effects of the block can be evaluated immediately
    D. The block is less painful
    E. Phenol is selective for sympathetic fibers

817. How much local anesthetic should be administered per spinal segment to patients between 20 and 40 years of age receiving epidural anesthesia?

    A. 0.3 to 0.5 mL
    B. 0.5 to 1.0 mL
    C. 1 to 1.5 mL
    D. 1.5 to 2 mL
    E. 2 to 2.5 mL

818. The artery of Adamkiewicz most frequently arises from the aorta at which spinal level?

    A. T1-4
    B. T5-8
    C. T9-12
    D. L1-4
    E. L5-S3

819. The anterior and posterior spinal arteries originate from the

    A. Common carotid and vertebral arteries, respectively
    B. Internal carotid and vertebral arteries, respectively
    C. Internal carotid and posterior cerebral arteries, respectively
    D. Vertebral and anterior cerebellar arteries, respectively
    E. Vertebral and posterior inferior cerebellar arteries, respectively

820. Important landmarks for performing a sciatic nerve block (classic approach of Labat) include

    A. Iliac crest, sacral hiatus, greater trochanter
    B. Iliac crest, coccyx, and greater trochanter
    C. Posterior superior iliac spine, coccyx, and greater trochanter
    D. Posterior superior iliac spine, greater trochanter and sacral hiatus
    E. Posterior superior iliac spine and greater trochanter

821. A 36-year-old female patient is undergoing thyroidectomy under a deep cervical plexus nerve block. Which of the following complications would be least likely with this block?

    A. Horner's syndrome
    B. Subarachnoid injection
    C. Blockade of the recurrent laryngeal nerve
    D. Blockade of the spinal accessory nerve
    E. Blockade of the phrenic nerve

822. A retrobulbar block anesthetizes each of the following nerves **EXCEPT**

    A. Ciliary nerves
    B. Cranial nerve IV (trochlear nerve)
    C. Cranial nerve III (oculomotor nerve)
    D. Cranial nerve VI (abducens nerve)
    E. Maxillary branch of the trigeminal nerve

823. Which of the following muscles of the larynx is innervated by the external branch of the superior laryngeal nerve?

    A. Vocalis muscle
    B. Thyroarytenoid muscles
    C. Posterior cricoarytenoid muscle
    D. Oblique arytenoid muscles
    E. Cricothyroid muscle

824. All the following agents are acceptable for use in a Bier block **EXCEPT**

   A. 0.5% Lidocaine
   B. 0.5% Mepivacaine
   C. 0.5% Procaine
   D. 0.5% Prilocaine
   E. 0.25% Bupivacaine

825. The stellate ganglion lies in closest proximity to which of the following vascular structures?

   A. Common carotid artery
   B. The internal carotid artery
   C. The vertebral artery
   D. The axillary artery
   E. The aorta

826. Which of the following structures in the antecubital fossa is the most medial?

   A. Brachial artery
   B. Cephalic vein
   C. Tendon of the biceps
   D. Median nerve
   E. Musculocutaneous nerve

827. During placement of an epidural in a 78-year-old patient scheduled for a total knee arthroplasty, the patient complains of a sharp sustained pain radiating down his left leg as the catheter is inserted to 2 cm. The most appropriate action at this time would be

   A. Leave the catheter at 2 cm, give test dose
   B. Give small dose to relieve pain then advance 1 cm
   C. Withdraw the catheter 1 cm, give test dose
   D. Withdraw needle and catheter, re-insert in a new position
   E. Abandon epidural technique, place long-acting spinal

828. Cutaneous innervation of the plantar surface of the foot is provided by the

   A. Sural nerve
   B. Posterior tibial nerve
   C. Saphenous nerve
   D. Deep peroneal nerve
   E. Superficial peroneal nerve

829. Which of the following local anesthetics has the greatest depressant effect on myocardial contractility?

   A. Tetracaine
   B. Etidocaine
   C. Bupivacaine
   D. Prilocaine
   E. Chloroprocaine

830. A 57-year-old patient is scheduled for hemorrhoidectomy. The patient has a history of mild COPD, hypertension, and traumatic foot amputation from a tractor accident. His only hospitalizations were for two suicide attempts related to excruciating phantom limb pain which resolved 10 years ago. He takes Phenelzine (Nardil), Thiazide, and Potassium. Which of the following anesthetic techniques would be most appropriate for this patient?

    A. Spinal anesthetic with 0.5% hyperbaric bupivacaine
    B. Epidural anesthetic with 0.5% bupivacaine
    C. Local infiltration with lidocaine and epinephrine, sedation with propofol and meperidine
    D. General anesthesia with pentothal, succinylcholine, nitrous oxide, isoflurane, meperidine
    E. General anesthesia with propofol, succinylcholine, nitrous oxide, fentanyl

831. If the recurrent laryngeal nerve is transected bilaterally, the vocal cords would

    A. Be paralyzed in the open position
    B. Be paralyzed in the closed position
    C. Be paralyzed in the intermediate position
    D. Not be affected unless the superior laryngeal nerve is also injured
    E. Appear exactly the same as if an intubating dose of succinylcholine were given

832. The length of the trachea in a full-term neonate is

    A. 2 cm
    B. 4 cm
    C. 6 cm
    D. 8 cm
    E. 10 cm

833. What is the correct order of structures (from cephalad to caudad) in the intercostal space?

    A. Nerve, artery, vein
    B. Vein, nerve, artery
    C. Vein, artery, nerve
    D. Artery, nerve, vein
    E. Artery, vein, nerve

834. Which of the following types of regional anesthesia is associated with the greatest serum concentration of local anesthetics?

    A. Intercostal
    B. Caudal
    C. Epidural
    D. Brachial plexus
    E. Femoral nerve block

835. Differences in which of the following local anesthetic properties accounts for the fact that the onset of an epidural block with 3% 2-chloroprocaine is more rapid than 2% lidocaine?

    A. Protein binding
    B. pKa
    C. Lipid solubility
    D. Concentration
    E. Ester vs. amide structure

836. A 69-year-old man with a history of diabetes mellitus and chronic renal failure is to undergo placement of a dialysis fistula under regional anesthesia. During needle manipulation for a supraclavicular brachial plexus block, the patient begins to cough and to complain of chest pain and shortness of breath. The most likely diagnosis is

    A. Angina
    B. Pneumothorax
    C. Phrenic nerve irritation
    D. Intravascular injection of local anesthetic
    E. Intrathecal injection of local anesthetic

837. Which of the following nerves is located immediately lateral to the trachea?

    A. Vagus
    B. Recurrent laryngeal
    C. Phrenic
    D. Long thoracic
    E. Spinal accessory

838. If a needle is introduced 2 cm inferior and lateral to the pubic tubercle, to which nerve will it lie in close proximity?

    A. Obturator nerve
    B. Femoral nerve
    C. Lateral femoral cutaneous nerve
    D. Sciatic nerve
    E. Ilioinguinal nerve

839. The most common complication associated with a supraclavicular brachial plexus block is

    A. Blockade of the phrenic nerve
    B. Intravascular injection into the vertebral artery
    C. Spinal blockade
    D. Blockade of the recurrent laryngeal nerve
    E. Pneumothorax

840. Which portion of the upper extremity is not innervated by the brachial plexus?

    A. Posterior medial portion of the arm
    B. Elbow
    C. Lateral portion of the forearm
    D. Medial portion of the forearm
    E. Anterolateral portion of the arm

841. Which section of the brachial plexus is blocked with a supraclavicular block?

    A. Roots
    B. Trunks
    C. Divisions
    D. Cords
    E. Branches

842. A celiac-plexus block would not effectively treat pain resulting from a malignancy involving which of the following organs?

    A. Ureter
    B. Adrenal gland
    C. Stomach
    D. Pancreas
    E. Gallbladder

843. A 72-year-old female with insulin-dependent diabetes mellitus and coronary artery disease is to undergo debridement of an ulcer on her right great toe. An ankle block is planned. Which nerves must be adequately blocked in order to perform the surgery?

    A. Sural, posterior tibial, saphenous, deep peroneal
    B. Deep peroneal, superficial peroneal, sural, saphenous
    C. Posterior tibial, sural, deep peroneal, superficial peroneal
    D. Saphenous, deep peroneal, superficial peroneal, posterior tibial
    E. Saphenous, posterior tibial, deep peroneal

844. A 54-year-old man is administered morphine via patient-controlled analgesia (PCA) pump after a left total hip arthroplasty. The pump is programmed to deliver a maximum dose of 2 mg every 15 minutes (lockout time) as needed for patient comfort. The total maximum dose which can be delivered in 4 hours is 30 mg. On the first day the patient receives 15 doses every 4 hours by pressing the delivery button every 15 to 18 minutes. How should his pain control be further managed?

    A. Discontinue the PCA pump and administer intramuscular morphine
    B. Increase the lockout time from 15 to 25 minutes
    C. Change the analgesic from morphine to fentanyl
    D. Increase the dose to 3 mg every 15 minutes as needed up to a total maximum dose of 40 mg every 4 hours
    E. Make no changes

845. The mechanism of the transcutaneous electrical nerve stimulator (TENS) unit in relieving pain is

   A. Direct electrical inhibition of type Aδ and C fibers
   B. Depletion of neurotransmitter in nociceptors
   C. Hyperpolarization of spinothalamic tract neurons
   D. Activation of inhibitory neurons
   E. Distortion of nociceptors

846. Epidural use of which of the following narcotics would result in the greatest incidence of delayed respiratory depression?

   A. Sufentanyl
   B. Fentanyl
   C. Morphine sulfate
   D. Hydromorphone
   E. Meperidine

847. A 21-year-old patient reports tingling in her thumb during cesarean section under epidural anesthesia. To which dermatomal level would this correspond?

   A. C4
   B. C5
   C. C6
   D. C7
   E. C8

848. Which of the following would hasten the onset and increase the clinical duration of action of a local anesthetic, and provide the greatest depth of motor and sensory blockade when used for epidural anesthesia?

   A. Addition to 1:200,000 epinephrine
   B. Increasing the volume of local anesthetic
   C. Increasing the concentration of local anesthetic
   D. Increasing the dose
   E. Placing the patient in the head-down position

849. Select the **FALSE** statement concerning neurolytic nerve blocks

   A. There is little difference in the efficacy between alcohol and phenol
   B. Destruction of peripheral nerves can be followed by a denervation hypersensitivity which is worse than the original pain
   C. Neurolytic blocks should be reserved for patients with short life expectancies
   D. Neurolytic blockade with phenol is permanent
   E. Intrathecal neurolysis may be an effective management for certain pain conditions

850. The addition of epinephrine to epidural bupivacaine will

    A. Prolong motor blockade only
    B. Prolong sensory blockade only
    C. Prolong motor and sensory blockade
    D. Shorten duration of sensory blockade
    E. Will have no effect on either duration of motor or sensory blockade

851. The epidural administration of a mixture of chloroprocaine and bupivacaine would have

    A. A latency similar to chloroprocaine with a duration of action similar to bupivacaine
    B. A latency shorter than chloroprocaine with a duration of action longer than bupivacaine
    C. A latency shorter than chloroprocaine with a duration of action similar to bupivacaine
    D. A latency longer than chloroprocaine with a duration of action similar to chloroprocaine
    E. A latency longer than chloroprocaine with a duration of action shorter than bupivacaine

852. Each of the following is associated with an increased incidence of headache after spinal anesthesia **EXCEPT**

    A. Young age
    B. Female gender
    C. Early ambulation
    D. Pregnancy
    E. Large needle size

853. Each of the following items describes pain in the abdominal viscera **EXCEPT** which one?

    A. Pain is transmitted via the vagus nerve
    B. The nerve fibers are type C vs. Aδ
    C. Pain is not in a dermatomal distribution
    D. Pain is characterized by a dull aching or burning sensation
    E. Distention of the transverse colon causes more pain than surgical transection

854. A 24-year-old man undergoes repair of a right anterior shoulder dislocation under interscalene brachial plexus block. Anesthesia is produced with 30 mL of 0.5% bupivacaine with 5 µg/mL of epinephrine. The next day the patient complains of numbness in his right arm and hand. The most likely cause of these complaints is

    A. Excessive retraction by the surgeon
    B. Prolonged pressure on the brachial plexus from malpositioning
    C. Pressure on the right medial epicondyle from malpositioning
    D. Pressure on the right posterior humerus from malpositioning
    E. Residual anesthesia

855. Which of the following patients would be **LEAST** likely to develop a decrease in heart rate with a high (C8) placement of spinal anesthesia?

    A.   A 15-year-old female patient with history of Wolff-Parkinson-White syndrome
    B.   A 73-year-old patient with glaucoma treated with pilocarpine eyedrops
    C.   A 33-year-old with a T6 paraplegia
    D.   A 45-year-old diabetic man with a history orthostatic hypotension
    E.   A 47-year-old patient who had a myocardial infarction 1 month ago, now taking procainamide

856. A 35-year-old woman receives a sciatic nerve block for foot surgery. Which other nerve must be blocked in order to have complete anesthesia of the foot?

    A.   Deep peroneal nerve
    B.   Superficial peroneal nerve
    C.   Sural nerve
    D.   Saphenous nerve
    E.   Posterior tibial nerve

857. The most common complication of a celiac plexus block is

    A.   Hypotension
    B.   Seizure
    C.   Subarachnoid injection
    D.   Retroperitoneal hematoma
    E.   Constipation

858. The occipital portion of the skull receives sensory innervation from

    A.   Spinal accessory nerve (nerve XI)
    B.   Facial nerve (nerve VII)
    C.   Ophthalmic branch of trigeminal nerve (nerve V)
    D.   Maxillary branch of trigeminal nerve (nerve V)
    E.   None of the above

859. Each of the following is a potential complication of lumbar sympathetic block EXCEPT

    A.   Puncture of the renal pelvis
    B.   Intravascular injection
    C.   Seizure
    D.   S1 nerve block
    E.   Accidental subarachnoid injection

DIRECTIONS (Questions 860 through 895): For each of the items in this section, ONE or MORE of the number options is correct. Select the answer:

Select A if options *1, 2 and 3* are correct,
Select B if options *1 and 3* are correct,
Select C if options *2 and 4* are correct,
Select D if only option *4* is correct,
Select E if *all* options are correct.

860. After placement of an epidural catheter in a 55-year-old patient for total hip arthroplasty, an entire epidural dose is administered into the subarachnoid space. Physiologic effects consistent with subarachnoid injection of large volumes of local anesthetic include

    1. Hypotension
    2. Bradycardia
    3. Apnea
    4. Dilated pupils

861. A 49-year-old patient with a long history of dull aching pain in the right lower extremity receives a spinal anesthetic with 100 mg of procaine with 5% dextrose. The patient reports no relief in symptoms, but has complete bilateral motor blockade. What diagnosis is consistent with this differential blockade examination?

    1. Central pain
    2. Myofascial pain
    3. Malingering
    4. Reflex sympathetic dystrophy

862. An 18-year-old man has a seizure during placement of an interscalene brachial plexus block with 2% lidocaine. The anesthesiologist begins to hyperventilate the patient's lungs with 100% O_2 using an anesthesia bag and mask. The rationale for this therapy is to

    1. Decrease delivery of lidocaine to the brain
    2. Prevent hypoxia
    3. Hyperpolarize the nerve membranes
    4. Convert of lidocaine to the protonated (ionized) form

863. Para-aminobenzoic acid is a metabolite of

    1. Mepivacaine
    2. Benzocaine
    3. Bupivacaine
    4. Tetracaine

Select A if options *1, 2 and 3* are correct,
Select B if options *1 and 3* are correct,
Select C if options *2 and 4* are correct,
Select D if only option *4* is correct,
Select E if *all* options are correct.

864. True statement(s) concerning peripheral nerve structure and function include which of the following?

   1. Both nonmyelinated and myelinated nerves are surrounded by Schwann cells
   2. The speed of propagation of an action potential along a nerve axon is greatly enhanced by myelin
   3. Generation of an action potential is an "all-or-nothing" phenomenon
   4. Propagation of an action potential along myelinated nerve axons occurs by saltatory conduction via the Nodes of Ranvier

865. The seizure threshold for local anesthetics is raised by

   1. Hypokalemia
   2. Hyperoxia
   3. Hypocarbia
   4. Acidosis

866. Factor(s) which determine the proportion of local anesthetic that exists in the un-ionized (free base) and ionized (cation) forms include

   1. Local anesthetic concentration
   2. Tissue pH
   3. Local anesthetic volume
   4. pKa of the local anesthetic

867. Sensory innervation to the larynx is derived from

   1. Internal branch of the superior laryngeal nerve
   2. External branch of the superior laryngeal nerve
   3. Recurrent laryngeal nerve
   4. Glossopharyngeal nerve

868. The incidence of postdural puncture headache is increased in which of the following situations?

   1. Pregnancy
   2. Young age
   3. Use of large-bore spinal needle
   4. Use of paramedian instead of midline approach

Select A if options *1, 2 and 3* are correct,
Select B if options *1 and 3* are correct,
Select C if options *2 and 4* are correct,
Select D if only option *4* is correct,
Select E if *all* options are correct.

869. True statement(s) concerning the metabolism of local anesthetics include which of the following?

    1. Plasma clearance of ester-type local anesthetics is decreased in patients who are homozygous for atypical pseudocholinesterase
    2. Plasma clearance of ester-type local anesthetics is decreased in patients with severe cirrhotic liver disease
    3. Plasma clearance of amide-type local anesthetics is decreased in patients with severe cirrhotic liver disease
    4. Plasma clearance of amide-type local anesthetics is decreased in patients with severe renal insufficiency

870. Through which of the following would a spinal needle pass during the placement of a subarachnoid block in the L3-4 lumbar space?

    1. Supraspinous ligament
    2. Interspinous ligament
    3. Ligamentum flavum
    4. Anterior longitudinal ligament

871. Local anesthetics metabolized by ester hydrolysis include

    1. Lidocaine
    2. Cocaine
    3. Mepivacaine
    4. Tetracaine

872. Anatomic structures involved in the oculocardiac reflex include

    1. Ciliary ganglion
    2. Gasserian ganglion
    3. Vagus nerve
    4. Facial nerve

873. Factor(s) that increase the rate of onset of local anesthetic action include

    1. Rapid stimulation rate of the nerve
    2. High extracellular calcium concentration
    3. Alkaline pH
    4. Large nerve-fiber diameter

Select A if options *1, 2 and 3* are correct,
Select B if options *1 and 3* are correct,
Select C if options *2 and 4* are correct,
Select D if only option *4* is correct,
Select E if *all* options are correct.

874.   Branches of the sciatic nerve include

    1.   Posterior tibial
    2.   Common peroneal
    3.   Sural
    4.   Saphenous

875.   The cricothyroid muscle

    1.   Is an extrinsic muscle of the larynx
    2.   Receives innervation from the recurrent laryngeal nerve
    3.   Receives innervation from the internal branch of the superior laryngeal nerve
    4.   Tenses the vocal cords

876.   Potential complication(s) of a stellate ganglion block include

    1.   Recurrent laryngeal nerve paralysis
    2.   Subarachnoid block
    3.   Brachial plexus block
    4.   Pneumothorax

877.   The duration of epidural anesthesia is affected by

    1.   Height of patient
    2.   Age of patient
    3.   Weight of patient
    4.   Addition of epinephrine (1:200,000) to the local anesthetic

878.   Which of the following local anesthetic concentrations is (are) isobaric?

    1.   2% Lidocaine
    2.   0.5% Tetracaine
    3.   0.5% Bupivacaine
    4.   0.75% Bupivacaine

879.   Epinephrine is effective in increasing the clinical duration of action of

    1.   Procaine
    2.   Lidocaine
    3.   Tetracaine
    4.   Etidocaine

Select A if options *1, 2 and 3* are correct,
Select B if options *1 and 3* are correct,
Select C if options *2 and 4* are correct,
Select D if only option *4* is correct,
Select E if *all* options are correct.

880. Local anesthetics that produce profound motor blockade with skimpy sensory blockade when injected into the epidural space include

    1. Tetracaine
    2. Prilocaine
    3. Mepivacaine
    4. Etidocaine

881. Extrinsic muscles of the larynx include

    1. Digastric
    2. Sternohyoid
    3. Thyrohyoid
    4. Cricothyroid

882. Factor(s) which antagonize local anesthetics include

    1. Tissue acidosis
    2. Presence of myelin
    3. Increasing fiber diameter
    4. Rapid firing rate

883. Factor(s) that influence systemic absorption of local anesthetics include

    1. Site of injection of the local anesthetic
    2. Lipid solubility of the local anesthetic
    3. Addition of vasoconstrictor substances to the local anesthetic
    4. Concentration of the local anesthetic

884. Duration of action of local anesthetics may be increased by

    1. Adding vasoconstrictors
    2. Adding bicarbonate
    3. Increasing the dose
    4. Use of carbonated solutions

885. Which of the following conditions is associated with decreased clearance of ester-type local anesthetics?

    1. Cirrhotic liver disease
    2. Pregnancy
    3. Renal insufficiency
    4. Severe chronic obstructive pulmonary disease

Select A if options *1, 2 and 3* are correct,
Select B if options *1 and 3* are correct,
Select C if options *2 and 4* are correct,
Select D if only option *4* is correct,
Select E if *all* options are correct.

886. Nerves that originate from the sacral plexus include

    1. Femoral nerve
    2. Obturator nerve
    3. Lateral femoral cutaneous nerve
    4. Sciatic nerve

887. Drugs that will decrease the plasma clearance of ester-type local anesthetics include

    1. Echothiophate
    2. N_2O
    3. Neostigmine
    4. Phenytoin

888. In order to perform surgery on the knee, which of the following nerves should be blocked?

    1. Femoral nerve
    2. Sciatic nerve
    3. Lateral femoral cutaneous nerve
    4. Obturator nerve

889. A 74-year-old patient undergoes a lumbar sympathetic block to improve blood flow after frostbite. Findings that suggest a successful lumbar sympathetic block include

    1. Inability to dorsiflex foot
    2. Blushing in the toes
    3. Numbness from the knee to the toes
    4. Temperature increase in the legs

890. Choose all items that correctly match anatomic structures with their level of termination in adults.

    1. Spinal cord, L1-2
    2. Preganglionic sympathetic nerves, L2
    3. Spinal canal, sacral hiatus
    4. Dural sac, S4

891. Which of the following drugs will decrease the plasma clearance of amide-type local anesthetics?

    1. Propranolol
    2. Cimetidine
    3. Halothane
    4. Phenytoin

Select A if options *1, 2 and 3* are correct,
Select B if options *1 and 3* are correct,
Select C if options *2 and 4* are correct,
Select D if only option *4* is correct,
Select E if *all* options are correct.

892. Choose all items that correctly pair local anesthetics with their maximum dose for infiltration when administered without a vasoconstrictor

   1. Lidocaine, 300 mg
   2. 2-Chloroprocaine, 600 mg
   3. Mepivacaine, 300 mg
   4. Bupivacaine, 225 mg

893. Factor(s) associated with the occurrence of neurotoxicity as a result of accidental intrathecal injection of a large volume of commercially prepared Nesacaine-CF include

   1. Methylparaben
   2. Acidic pH
   3. Ortho-toluidine
   4. Sodium bisulfite

894. True statements concerning local anesthetics include which of the following?

   1. The un-ionized form of a local anesthetic binds to the nerve membrane to actually block conduction
   2. If one node of Ranvier is blocked conduction will be reliably interrupted
   3. The ability of a local anesthetic to block nerve conduction is directly proportional to the diameter of the fiber
   4. The presence of myelin enhances the ability of a local anesthetic to block nerve conduction

895. "Postspinal" headaches

   1. Usually occur immediately following dural puncture
   2. Are relieved 8 to 12 hours after an epidural blood patch is performed
   3. Occur more frequently in nonpregnant compared with pregnant patients
   4. Can be associated with neurologic deficits

DIRECTIONS (Questions 896 through 914): These groups of questions consists of several numbered statements followed by lettered headings. For each numbered statement within each group, select the ONE lettered heading that is most closely associated with it. Each lettered heading may be selected once, more than once, or not at all.

896. Phrenic nerve

897. Cardiac accelerator fibers

898. Pudendal nerve

899.   Pain fibers to the uterus

900.   Inhibitory presynaptic fibers to the gastrointestinal tract

    A.   T10-L1
    B.   T1-4
    C.   T5-T12
    D.   C3-5
    E.   S2-4

901.   Medium diameter; efferent to muscle spindles

902.   Small diameter; preganglionic autonomic function

903.   Large diameter; fast conduction; motor function

904.   Medium diameter; pain; temperature; touch

905.   Small diameter; postganglionic autonomic function and pain, temperature, touch

906.   Large diameter; proprioception

    A.   Type A-α fibers
    B.   Type A-ß fibers
    C.   Type A- γ fibers
    D.   Type A-δ fibers
    E.   Type B fibers
    F.   Type C fibers

This group of questions consists of several numbered statements followed by lettered headings. For each numbered statement, select the ONE lettered heading that is most closely associated with it. Each lettered heading may be selected once, more than once, or not at all.

907.   Sensory innervation to the posterior one third of the tongue

908.   Motor innervation to the cricothyroid muscle

909.   Sensory innervation to the carina

910.   Sensory innervation to the mucous membranes of the false cords

911.   Motor innervation to the omohyoid muscle

912.   Sensory innervation to the posterior pharynx

913.   Motor innervation to the intrinsic muscles of the larynx

914.   Motor innervation to the superior and middle constrictor muscles

    A.   Glossopharyngeal nerve
    B.   Internal branch of the superior laryngeal nerve
    C.   External branch of the superior laryngeal nerve
    D.   Recurrent laryngeal nerve
    E.   Cranial nerve XI

ANATOMY, REGIONAL ANESTHESIA, AND PAIN MANAGEMENT ANSWERS, REFERENCES, AND EXPLANATIONS

788. **(B)** Tachyphylaxis is a well-known phenomenon associated with repetitive or continuous administration of local anesthetics. Several theories have been proposed to explain this tachyphylaxis including increased uptake of drug from the epidural space, local edema, down regulation of receptors, or spinal inhibition *(Rogers: Principles and Practice of Anesthesiology, p 1452)*.

789. **(C)** The systemic disposition of amide-type local anesthetics is not altered in patients with chronic renal failure because these drugs are metabolized by the liver. However, increased tissue blood flow in these patients shortens the clinical duration of regional anesthetic blocks. Bupivacaine anesthesia is particularly useful in these patients if a lengthy surgical procedure is anticipated, because of its long duration of action *(Stoelting: Anesthesia and Co-existing Disease, ed 2, p 427)*.

790. **(D)** The maximum dose of local anesthetics containing 1:200,000 epinephrine that can be used for major nerve blocks is: lidocaine, 500 mg; mepivacaine, 500 mg; prilocaine, 600 mg; bupivacaine, 225 mg; etidocaine, 400 mg; and tetracaine, 200 mg *(Miller: Anesthesia, ed 4, p 505)*.

791. **(B)** 1:200,000 means 1 gm (1,000 mg) (1,000,000 mcg) per 200,000 ml
    1,000,000 mcg ÷ 200,000 ml = 5 mcg/ml
    Epinephrine is commonly packaged
    1:1,000   1,000 mg ÷ 1,000 ml = 1 mg/ml
    1:10,000   1,000 mg ÷ 10,000 ml = 0.1 mg/ml

    (Barash: Clinical Anesthesia, ed 2, p 356).

792. **(E)** The early signs of digitalis toxicity include loss of appetite, nausea, vomiting, and in some patients there may be pain which is similar to trigeminal neuralgia. Pain or discomfort in the feet and pain and discomfort in the extremities may also be a feature of digitalis toxicity. Transient visual disturbances have also been reported in patients with digitalis toxicity. In this patient, therefore, it would be prudent to obtain a digoxin level as an early part of the workup for these complaints. He may also have true trigeminal neuralgia and workup for this may also be undertaken after digitalis toxicity has been ruled out *(Stoelting: Pharmacology and Physiology in Anesthetic Practice, ed 2, p 290)*.

793. **(C)** Toxic reactions to local anesthetics are usually due to intravascular or intrathecal injection or to an excessive dosage. The initial symptoms of local anesthetic toxicity are lightheadedness and dizziness. Patients may also note perioral numbness and tinnitus. Progressive CNS excitatory effects include visual and auditory disturbances, shivering, twitching, and ultimately generalized tonic-clonic seizures. CNS depression can follow leading to respiratory depression or arrest *(Miller: Anesthesia, ed 4, p 510)*.

794. **(B)** The site of action of spinally administered opiates is the substantia gelatinosa of the spinal cord. Epidural administration is complicated by factors related to dural penetration, absorption in fat and systemic uptake. Therefore, the quantity of intrathecally administered opioid required to achieve effective analgesia is typically much smaller. Morphine is typically given in doses of 3-10 mg in the lumbar epidural space. Intrathecal morphine dosage is 0.2-1.0 mg. Onset time for epidural administration is 30-60 minutes with a peak effect in 90 to 120 minutes. Onset time for intrathecal administration is shorter than epidural administration. Duration of 12-24 hours of analgesic effect can be expected by either route *(Rogers: Principles and Practice of Anesthesiology, pp 1440 & 1456).*

795. **(D)** Large doses of prilocaine can result in clinically significant methemoglobinemia. Usually greater than 600 mg epidurally. Prilocaine is metabolized by the liver to o-Toluidine which is responsible for the oxidation of hemoglobin to methemoglobin. Methemoglobinemia can be treated with IV methylene blue or it will resolve spontaneously *(Miller: Anesthesia, ed 4, p 515).*

796. **(C)** The major disadvantage of the interscalene block for hand and forearm surgery is that blockade of the inferior trunk (C8-T1) is often incomplete. Supplementation of the ulnar nerve is often required. The risk of pneumothorax is quite low but blockade of the ipsilateral phrenic nerve occurs in up to 100% of blocks. This can cause respiratory compromise in patients with significant lung disease *(Miller: Anesthesia, ed 4, p 1536-1538).*

797. **(C)** Surgical trauma includes a wide variety of physiologic responses. General anesthesia has none or only a slight inhibitory effect on endocrine and metabolic responses to surgery. Regional anesthesia inhibits the nociceptive signal from reaching the central nervous system and therefore has a significant inhibitory effect on the stress response including adrenergic, cardiovascular, metabolic, immunologic, and pituitary. This effect is most pronounced with procedures on the lower part of the body and less with major abdominal and thoracic procedures. The variable effect is probably due to unblocked afferents, i.e., vagal, phrenic, or sympathetic *(Rogers: Principles and Practice of Anesthesiology, pp 1219-1220, 1584).*

798. **(C)** The structures that are traversed by a needle prior to the epidural space are as follows: skin, i.e., subcutaneous tissue, supraspinous ligament, interspinous ligament and ligamentum flavum. The ligamentum flavum is tough and dense and often perceived as a "snap." The anterior and posterior longitudinal ligaments bind the vertebral bodies together (see explanation and diagram for 870) *(Barash: Clinical Anesthesia, ed 2, pp 816-817).*

799. **(E)** Sympathetic nerves to the upper extremity exit the spinal cord T2 to T8, travel to the sympathetic chain as white communicating rami. They will synapse at the second thoracic ganglia, first thoracic or inferior cervical ganglion. In 82% of cases the inferior cervical ganglion is fused to the first thoracic ganglion forming the stellate ganglion. The stellate ganglion supplies sympathetic innervation to the upper extremities through gray communicating rami of C7, C8, T1 and occasionally C5 and C6. Gray rami from T2 and T3 occasionally contribute fiber; these fibers do not pass through the stellate ganglion but join the brachial plexus. These fibers known as "Kuntz's nerves" have been implicated when inadequate relief of sympathetic pain occurs despite evidence of a satisfactory stellate block. These fibers can only be reliably blocked by a posterior approach *(Raj: Practical Management of Pain, ed 2, p 785).*

800. **(B)** Differential nerve blockade is a complex process where anatomical and chemical factors determine the susceptibility of fibers to blockade by local anesthetics. Diameter, myelinization, and location within the nerve trunk affect the onset and regression time. In general, the small unmyelinated sympathetic fibers are blocked first followed by unmyelinated C fibers (pain and temp) then small myelinated fibers (proprioception, touch, pressure) and finally the large myelinated fibers (motor) *(Cousins: Neural Blockade in Clinical Anesthesia and Management of Pain, ed 2, p 36).*

801. **(B)** Post-herpetic neuralgia is defined as pain persisting beyond the healing of the herpes zoster lesions. The incidence of post herpetic neuralgia increases with age and occurs in 20-50% of patients over 50 and greater than 50% in patients over 80 years. Treatment is very difficult but some success has been had with the following: tricyclic antidepressants, phenothiazines, epidural, and subcutaneous injections of local anesthetic and steroids; sympathetic and somatic nerve blocks, and anticonvulsants. Oral clonidine which is used to treat hypertension and opioid withdrawal has not been used to treat post herpetic neuralgia *(Raj: Practical Management of Pain, ed 2, pp 538-540).*

802. **(C)** The deep peroneal nerve innervates the short extensors of the toes and the skin of the web space between the great and second toe. The deep peroneal nerve is blocked at the ankle by infiltration between the tendons of the anterior tibial and extensor hallucis longus muscle *(Miller: Anesthesia, ed 4, pp 1552-1553).*

803. **(B)** All local anesthetics have a dose dependent depression effect on cardiac contractility and conduction velocity. The cardiodepressant effect generally parallels the anesthetic potency. Bupivacaine has been shown to be 16 times more toxic than lidocaine, well out of proportion to the potency ratio and 2 times more toxic than ropivacaine despite similar nerve blocking potency *(Cousins: Neural Blockade in Clinical Anesthesia and Management of Pain, ed 2, p 435; Stoelting: Pharmacology and Physiology in Anesthetic Practice, ed 2, p 79).*

804. **(B)** Diagnosis and treatment of chronic pain syndromes is quite complex, often complicated by psychological issues, disability/litigation, and drug dependence. Tapering and withdrawal from sedatives and narcotics is often best accomplished in a controlled in-patient setting. Substituting long-acting agents (i.e., methadone) then slowly tapering over time. Agonist-antagonist narcotics could cause an acute withdrawal syndrome. Tricyclic antidepressants and epidural steroids can be considered once the drug dependence issue has been dealt with *(Miller: Anesthesia, ed 4, p 2351).*

805. **(A)** Ester local anesthetics are hydrolyzed by cholinesterase enzymes which are present mainly in plasma and a smaller amount in liver. Since there is no cholinesterase enzymes present in cerebral spinal fluid, the anesthetic effect of tetracaine will persist until it is absorbed into systemic circulation. The rate of hydrolysis varies with chloroprocaine being fastest, procaine intermediate and tetracaine the slowest. Toxicity is inversely related to the rate of hydrolysis and therefore tetracaine is most toxic *(Stoelting: Pharmacology and Physiology in Anesthetic Practice, ed 2, p 155).*

806. **(A)** Reflex sympathetic dystrophy is a clinical syndrome of continuous burning pain usually occurring after an injury or surgery. Patients present with variable sensory, motor, autonomic, and trophic changes. Causalgia exhibits the same features of reflex sympathetic dystrophy but the etiology is damage to a major nerve *(Raj: Practical Management of Pain, ed 2, p 317; Stoelting: Basics of Anesthesia, ed 3, p 474)*.

807. **(C)** Potency of local anesthetics is directly related to its lipid solubility. Speed of onset is related to the pKa. The degree of protein binding is important for toxicity and metabolism *(Raj: Practical Management of Pain, ed 2, p 685)*.

808. **(E)** Many factors have an effect on the sensory level after a subarachnoid injection. The baricity of the solution and the patient position are the most important determinant of sensory level. The other listed options have little to no effect on sensory level. Patient height also has little effect on sensory level *(Miller: Anesthesia, ed 4, p 1519-1520)*.

809. **(D)** Due to the rapid hydrolysis of ester local anesthetics, very little drug is available to cross the placenta. Plasma cholinesterase activity can be reduced up to 40% in pregnant patients yet the elimination half-life of chloroprocaine is little affected (ranging from 1.5-6 minutes) *(Stoelting: Pharmacology and Physiology in Anesthetic Practice, ed 2, p 155)*.

810. **(A)** With a high spinal anesthesia, modest degrees of hypotension in normovolemic patients are due to decreased vascular resistance. Severe hypotension is due to decreased cardiac output caused by decreased preload from peripheral pooling of blood and/or hypovolemia *(Cousins: Neural Blockade in Clinical Anesthesia and Management of Pain, ed 2, p 231; Stoelting: Basics of Anesthesia, ed 3, p 171)*.

811. **(C)** The incidence of phantom limb pain is estimated to be 60-85%. The incidence of phantom limb pain does not differ between traumatic and nontraumatic amputees. The incidence of phantom pain increases with more proximal amputation. Although very difficult to treat, nerve blocks are commonly used in an attempt to treat phantom pain. These include trigger point injections, peripheral and central nerve blocks, and sympathetic blocks *(Raj: Practical Management of Pain, ed 2, p 510)*.

812. **(D)** Prilocaine is the most rapidly metabolized of the amide local anesthetics and therefore least toxic. 2-Chloroprocaine is hydrolyzed rapidly in the blood and therefore would appear to be ideal, but it has been associated with a high incidence of thrombophlebitis and is therefore not recommended. To avoid toxicity, maximum doses are as follows: Prilocaine, 3-4 mg/kg; Lidocaine, 1.5-3 mg/kg; Bupivacaine, 0.75-1.5 mg/kg *(Cousins: Neural Blockade in Clinical Anesthesia and Management of Pain, ed 2, pp 448-449; Rogers: Principles and Practice of Anesthesiology, p 1245)*.

813. **(D)** Both phenylephrine and epinephrine will prolong a spinal anesthetic. The Taylor approach for spinal anesthesia uses a paramedian approach to the L5-S1 interspace—the largest interspace of the vertebral column. The sympathetic nervous system originates in the thoracic and lumbar spinal cord T1-L3. Therefore, a high thoracic sensory level can cause a complete sympathetic block. The dural sac extends to S2-3, not S3-4. The spinal cord extends to L3 in the infant and L1-2 in adults *(Miller: Anesthesia, ed 4, pp 1518, 1519, 528, & 1507)*.

814. **(A)**   Development of an epidural abscess is fortunately an exceedingly rare complication of spinal or epidural anesthesia. When it does occur, however, prompt recognition and treatment are essential if permanent sequelae are to be avoided. Symptoms from an epidural abscess may not become apparent until several days after placement of the block. The usual symptoms include severe back pain, sensory disturbances and motor weakness. Unlike an epidural hematoma in which severe back pain is the key feature, patients with epidural abscesses will complain of radicular pain approximately three days after development of the back pain. Anterior spinal artery syndrome is characterized predominantly by motor weakness or paralysis of the lower extremities. Meralgia paresthetica is related to entrapment of the lateral femoral cutaneous nerve as it courses below the inguinal ligament and is associated with burning pain over the lateral aspect of the thigh. It is not a complication of epidural anesthesia *(Raj: Practical Management of Pain, ed 2, p 775).*

815. **(C)**   Reflex sympathetic dystrophies are associated with trauma. The main feature is burning and continuous pain which is exacerbated by normal movement, cutaneous stimulation, or stress usually weeks after the injury. The pain is not anatomically distributed. Other associated features include cool, red, clammy skin and hair loss in the involved extremity. Chronic cases may be associated with atrophy and osteoporosis *(Miller: Anesthesia, ed 4, p 2355).*

816. **(D)**   Neurolytic blockade with phenol (6% to 10% in glycerine) is painless because phenol has a dual action as both a local anesthetic and a neurolytic agent. The initial block wears off over a 24-hour period, during which time neurolysis occurs. For this reason one must wait a day to determine how effective the neurolytic block is. Alcohol (100% ethanol) is painful on injection and should be preceded by local-anesthetic injection. Unfortunately there is no neurolytic agent that affects only sympathetic fibers *(Miller: Anesthesia, ed 4, pp 2360-2361).*

817. **(C)**   Each milliliter of local anesthetic will anesthetize about one spinal segment. For example, if in a parturient undergoing caesarean section, 15 mL 3% chloroprocaine were injected through an epidural placed at L2-3, about 15 segments would be anesthetized. Two thirds of these would be above the epidural entry site and one third would be below *(Stoelting: Basics of Anesthesia, ed 3, p 175).*

818. **(C)**   The artery of Adamkiewicz is also called the arteria radicularis magna and is one of the "feeder" arteries for the anterior spinal artery. Damage to this artery can lead to ischemia in the thoracolumbar region of the spinal cord. The origin of this artery is variable as follows: T9 to T12 in 60% of cases; T5 to T8 in 12% to 15% of cases; L1 in 14% of cases; L2 in 10% of cases, and L3 in 1.4% of cases. In the remaining 0.2% of cases, the artery originates between L4 and L5. *(Barash: Clinical Anesthesia, ed 2, p 1061).*

819. **(E)**   The posterior spinal arteries are paired; they arise from the posterior inferior cerebellar arteries and have 25 to 40 radicular arteries. The anterior spinal artery is a single midline artery which arises from the union of a branch of each vertebral artery. It descends in front of the anterior longitudinal sulcus of the spinal cord. This single artery is also fed by numerous radicular arteries *(Barash: Clinical Anesthesia, ed 2, pp 993-994 & 1061).*

820. **(D)**   To perform a sciatic nerve block, first draw a line from the posterior superior iliac spine to the greater trochanter. Then draw a 5-cm line perpendicular from the midpoint of this line caudally and a second line from the sacral hiatus to the greater trochanter. The intersection of the second line with the perpendicular line marks the point of entry *(Miller: Anesthesia, ed 4, p 1550).*

821. **(D)**　Complications of deep cervical plexus block include injection of the local anesthetic into the vertebral artery, subarachnoid space, or epidural space. Other nerves which may be anesthetized as a complication of this block include the phrenic, recurrent laryngeal nerve, and the cervical sympathetic chain with resultant Horner's syndrome *(Barash: Clinical Anesthesia, ed 2, p 848)*.

822. **(E)**　A retrobulbar block anesthetizes the three cranial nerves responsible for movement of the eye. The ciliary nerves are also blocked, providing anesthesia to the conjunctiva, cornea, and uvea. The ophthalmic branch of the trigeminal nerve provides sensory innervation to the skin of the forehead, the cornea, and eyelid. This branch of the trigeminal nerve may be blocked, but the maxillary branch would be spared *(Barash: Clinical Anesthesia, ed 2, pp 1104-1105)*.

823. **(E)**　All the other muscles of the larynx are innervated by the recurrent laryngeal nerve *(Miller: Anesthesia, ed 4, p 2184)*.

824. **(E)**　Because of the potential for cardiotoxicity and since bupivacaine has no advantages over other local anesthetics in this setting, it is no longer recommended for use in intravenous regional anesthesia *(Rogers: Principles and Practice of Anesthesiology, p 2199)*.

825. **(C)**

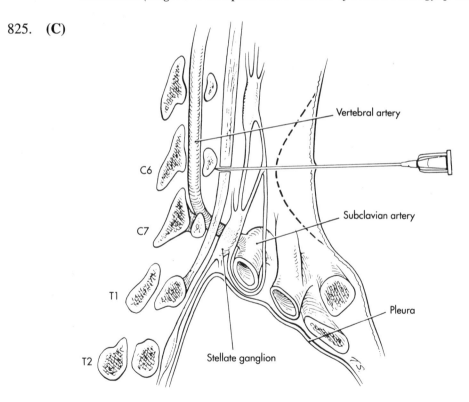

The stellate ganglion usually lies in front of the neck of the first rib. The vertebral artery lies anterior to the ganglion as it has just originated from the subclavian artery. After passing over the ganglion, it enters the vertebral foramen and lies posterior to the anterior tubercle of C6 *(Raj: Practical Management of Pain, ed 2, p 785)*.

826. **(D)** The median nerve is the most medial structure in the antecubital fossa. To block this nerve, first the brachial artery is palpated at the level of the intercondylar line between the medial and lateral epicondyles, and then a needle is inserted just medial to the artery and directed perpendicular to the skin *(Raj: Practical Management of Pain, ed 2, p 731).*

827. **(D)** Epidural placement is a blind technique. The exact location of the needle tip relative to the anatomic structures of the back can only be surmised. If malposition of either the needle or the catheter is suspected, it is prudent to withdraw the entire apparatus and reinsert a second time. In the case above, it is possible that the catheter tip has found its way into a nerve root. Under these circumstances, injection of a local anesthetic or narcotic could produce pressure which would lead to ischemia and possible neurologic damage. During placement or injection of an epidural catheter, a paresthesia is always a warning sign which should be heeded *(Raj: Practical Management of Pain, ed 2, p 775).*

828. **(B)** There are five nerves that supply the ankle and foot. These include the posterior tibial, sural, superficial and deep peroneal, and saphenous nerves. These nerves are superficial at the level of the ankle and are easy to block. The posterior branch of the tibial nerve gives rise to the medial and lateral plantar nerves, which supply the plantar surface of the foot *(Barash: Clinical Anesthesia, ed 2, p 869).*

829. **(A)** In general, in both in vivo and in vitro studies there is an overall direct correlation between anesthetic's potency and its direct depressant effect on myocardial contractility. This effect is greatest for tetracaine, slightly less for bupivacaine and etidocaine, and least with procaine *(Rogers: Principles and Practice of Anesthesiology, p 1248).*

830. **(E)** Reactivation of phantom limb pain has been reported in patients who have received both spinal and epidural anesthetics. With a history of a painful phantom limb so severe as to drive a patient to attempt suicide, it is probably wise to avoid spinal and epidural anesthetics. Any anesthetic or combination of techniques which involves meperidine is contraindicated in patients receiving monoamine oxidase inhibitors. The combination of meperidine and MAO inhibitors has been associated with hypothermia, hypotension, hypertension, ventilatory depression, skeletal muscle rigidity, seizures, and coma. Because of this unfavorable drug interaction, meperidine should be avoided in patients receiving monoamine oxidase inhibitors. Accordingly, the only acceptable anesthetic in this question would be general anesthesia with propofol, succinylcholine, nitrous oxide, and fentanyl *(Raj: Practical Management of Pain, ed 2, p 507; Stoelting: Pharmacology and Physiology in Anesthetic Practice, ed 2, p 381).*

831. **(B)** The recurrent laryngeal nerve innervates all the muscles of the larynx except the cricothyroid muscle, which tenses the vocal cords and is innervated by the external branch of the superior laryngeal nerve. One would expect that bilateral transections of the recurrent laryngeal nerve would produce tense (because the superior laryngeal nerve remains intact) closed (because the muscle which opens the cords have been denervated) vocal cords. What is actually seen are flaccid, closed cords. The cricothyroid muscle is evidently unable to tense the vocal cords without resistance from the other muscle in the larynx *(Barash: Clinical Anesthesia, ed 2, p 1114).*

832. **(C)** The length of the trachea in the neonate is 6 cm. The distance an endotracheal tube should be inserted from the lips to the midtrachea is about 11 cm in the neonate *(Stoelting: Basics of Anesthesia, ed 3, pp 151, 159).*

833. **(C)** An intercostal nerve block is performed with the patient in the prone position. The needle is inserted about 8 cm lateral to the midline posteriorly. If the needle is inserted more laterally, the lateral cutaneous branches of the intercostal nerves may be missed as they arise at the midaxillary line. The needle is then advanced until the rib is contacted and is then "walked off" the inferior border of the rib. Five milliliters of local anesthetic is injected after the needle has been advanced 2 to 3 mm. The most common complications of this block are intravascular injection and pneumothorax *(Miller: Anesthesia, ed 4, pp 1559-1560).*

834. **(A)** The site of injection of the local anesthetic is one of the most important factors influencing systemic local anesthetic absorption and toxicity. The degree of absorption from the site of injection depends on the blood supply to that site. Areas that have the greatest blood supply have the greatest systemic absorption. For this reason, the greatest plasma concentration of local anesthetic occurs after an intercostal block, followed by caudal, epidural, brachial plexus, and femoral nerve block *(Barash: Clinical Anesthesia, ed 2, p 522).*

835. **(D)** Local anesthetics are weak bases. The neutral (nonionized) form of the molecule is able to pass through the lipid nerve cell membrane, whereas the ionized (protonated) form actually produces anesthesia. Chloroprocaine has the highest pKa of local anesthetics meaning that a greater percentage of it will exist in the ionized form at any given pH than any of the other local anesthetics. In spite of this fact, 3% chloroprocaine has a more rapid onset than 2% lidocaine, presumably because of the greater number of molecules (concentration). If one compares onset time for 1.5% lidocaine against 1.5% chloroprocaine, the former will have a more rapid onset *(Miller: Anesthesia, ed 4, p 501).*

836. **(B)** The risk of pneumothorax is a significant limitation for supraclavicular brachial plexus blocks. Furthermore, the technique is difficult to teach and describe. For these reasons, this block should not be performed in patients in whom a pneumothorax or phrenic nerve block would result in significant dyspnea or respiratory distress. A pneumothorax should be considered if the patient begins to complain of chest pain or shortness of breath or begins to cough during placement of supraclavicular brachial plexus block *(Barash: Clinical Anesthesia, ed 2, pp 853-854).*

837. **(B)** The structures in the neck from medial to lateral are: recurrent laryngeal nerve, carotid artery, vagus nerve, internal jugular vein, and the phrenic nerve *(Clemente: Anatomy: Regional Atlas of the Human Body, ed 3, Fig 586).*

838. **(A)** An obturator nerve block is achieved by placement of the needle 1 to 2 cm lateral to and below the pubic tubercle. After contact with the pubic bone, the needle is withdrawn and walked cephalad to identify the obturator canal. Between 10 and 15 mL of local anesthetic should be placed in the canal *(Stoelting: Basics of Anesthesia, ed 3, p 186).*

839. **(E)**   The most common complication associated with a supraclavicular brachial plexus block is pneumothorax. Other potential complications include phrenic nerve paralysis, Horner's syndrome, nerve damage or neuritis, or intravascular injection *(Stoelting: Basics of Anesthesia, ed 3, p 182)*.

840. **(A)**   The arm receives sensory innervation from the brachial plexus except for the shoulder, which is innervated by the cervical plexus, and the posterior medial aspect of the arm, which is supplied by the intercostobrachial nerve *(Stoelting: Basics of Anesthesia, ed 3, p 181)*.

841. **(B)**   The advantages of the supraclavicular block are fourfold. The plexus is blocked where it is most compact, namely at the level of the trunks. A small volume of anesthetic is required and no part of the plexus is spared as with axillary or interscalene block. Lastly, the block can be performed with the arm in any position *(Cousins: Neural Blockade in Clinical Anesthesia and Management of Pain, ed 2, p 393)*.

842. **(A)**   The celiac plexus innervates most of the abdominal viscera, including the pancreas, liver, spleen, kidneys, adrenal glands, biliary tract, omentum, and small and large bowel. The pelvic organs are supplied by the hypogastric plexus *(Raj: Practical Management of Pain, ed 2, pp 794-795)*.

843. **(D)**   The great toe is innervated by the deep peroneal, the superficial peroneal, the posterior tibial, and occasionally the saphenous nerve. All four of these nerves should be blocked for surgery on the great toe *(Rogers: Principles and Practice of Anesthesiology, p 1339)*.

844. **(D)**   Frequent dosing by a patient receiving postoperative analgesia through a PCA pump suggests the need to increase the magnitude of the dose. It is important to keep in mind that a patient should be given a sufficient loading dose of narcotic prior to initiative therapy with a PCA pump. Otherwise, the patient will be playing the frustrating game of "catch up" *(Barash: Clinical Anesthesia, ed 2, p 1559)*.

845. **(D)**   Transcutaneous nerve stimulation is low-intensity, high-frequency (30 to 100 Hz) electrical stimulation which produces segmental analgesia by eliciting paresthesias. This technique is effective in treating nociceptive and deafferentation syndromes by a mechanism that is not reversed by naloxone. The mechanism is thought to be activation of inhibitory neurons and/or release of endogenous opiates *(Barash: Clinical Anesthesia, ed 2, pp 1567-1568)*.

846. **(C)**   Water-soluble drugs such as morphine have a very high potential for inducing delayed respiratory depression through cephalad migration in the central nervous system *(Barash: Clinical Anesthesia, ed 2, p 1564; Rogers: Principles and Practice of Anesthesiology, p 1454)*.

847. **(C)**   The thumb corresponds to dermatome C6, the middle finger corresponds to dermatome C7, and the little finger corresponds to dermatome C8 *(Stoelting: Basics of Anesthesia, ed 3, p 165)*.

848. **(D)**   Increasing the total dose (mass) of local anesthetic is more efficacious in hastening the onset and increasing the duration of an epidural anesthetic than increasing the volume or increasing the concentration (while holding the total dose constant) *(Barash: Clinical Anesthesia, ed 2, p 830)*.

849. **(D)** Alcohol and phenol are similar in their ability to cause nonselective damage to neural tissues. Neural tissue will regenerate; therefore, neurolytic blocks are never "permanent" and neurolysis can lead to a denervation hypersensitivity which can be extremely painful *(Stoelting: Basics of Anesthesia, ed 3, pp 472-473)*.

850. **(B)** Epinephrine's effect on the duration of anesthesia depends on the local anesthetic and the site. Infiltration and peripheral block duration with most agents will be prolonged with epinephrine. The addition of epinephrine to epidural 0.5% or 0.75% bupivacaine has not been shown to increase the duration of the motor blockade but does extend the duration of the sensory block *(Miller: Anesthesia, ed 4, p 502)*.

851. **(E)** Mixtures of local anesthetics have been used to take advantage of the short latency of certain agents (chloroprocaine) and the long duration of other agents (bupivacaine). Rapid onset-prolonged duration. Duration of epidural anesthesia by mixtures of chloroprocaine and bupivacaine have been shown to be shorter than bupivacaine alone and onset time longer than chloroprocaine alone *(Miller: Anesthesia, ed 4, p 503)*.

852. **(C)** Other factors that affect the incidence of spinal headache include the number of dural punctures and the position of the needle bevel. The incidence of spinal headache goes up as the number of dural punctures increases. The incidence of headache has been shown to be less when the dural fibers are split longitudinally rather than cutting them when the needle is placed in a transverse direction. The timing of ambulation relative to dural puncture has not been shown to affect the incidence of post spinal headache *(Miller: Anesthesia, ed 4, p 1521)*.

853. **(A)** Virtually all pain arising in the thoracic or abdominal viscera is transmitted via the sympathetic nervous system in unmyelinated type C fibers. Visceral pain is dull, aching, burning, and nonspecific. Visceral pain is caused by any stimulus which excites nociceptive nerve endings in diffuse areas. In this regard, distention of a hollow viscus causes a greater sensation of pain than does the highly localized damage produced by transecting the gut *(Raj: Practical Management of Pain, ed 2, pp 70-71)*.

854. **(E)** The brachial plexus is not normally retracted during repair of an anterior shoulder dislocation. Prolonged pressure on the brachial plexus will result in hand or arm numbness. This may occur if this structure becomes pinched between the clavicle and the head of the humerus, as seen in patients placed in steep Trendelenburg with the shoulders resting against shoulder braces. Prolonged pressure on the medial epicondyle may produce an ulnar neuropathy, whereas prolonged pressure against the posterior surface of the humerus may produce a radial neuropathy. Bupivacaine is a long-acting local anesthetic and may cause numbness for 24 hours or longer *(Brown: Atlas of Regional Anesthesia, p 43)*.

855. **(D)**   The cardiac accelerator fibers originate in the T1-4 segments. A high spinal, above T1, will cause bradycardia by anesthetizing these fibers. Diabetic patients who display orthostatic hypotension have an autonomic neuropathy. The cardiac accelerator fibers are essentially ablated in these patients and they will therefore not develop further heart-rate slowing with high spinals. Pilocarpine, a parasympathomimetic agent, will not prevent bradycardia with spinal anesthesia. Patients with Wolff-Parkinson-White syndrome will become bradycardic when the autonomic accelerator fibers are interrupted, as will patients with a spinal cord transection below T4. Recent myocardial infarction does not eliminate susceptibility to bradycardia with sympatholysis unless the patient has a complete heart block *(Stoelting: Anesthesia and Co-existing Disease, ed 3, p 342).*

856. **(D)**   All of the nerves of the foot with the exception of the saphenous are derived from the sciatic nerve. The saphenous nerve is a branch of the femoral nerve and provides sensory innervation to a thin medial strip of the foot *(Rogers: Principles and Practice of Anesthesiology, p 1339).*

857. **(A)**   The sympathectomy produced by a celiac plexus block causes hypotension by decreasing pre-load to the heart. This complication can be avoided by volume loading the patient with lactated Ringer's solution. Subarachnoid injection is the most serious complication of celiac plexus block. Seizure is possible with an intravascular injection. Retroperitoneal hematoma is also possible, but extremely rare. This block frequently relieves constipation by interrupting the sympathetic fibers and leaving the parasympathetic fibers unopposed *(Barash: Clinical Anesthesia, ed 2, p 863).*

858. **(E)**   The occiput receives sensory innervation from the occipital nerves, which are terminal branches of the cervical plexus. Blockade of these nerves is usually carried out as a diagnostic step in the evaluation of headache *(Barash: Clinical Anesthesia, ed 2, p 849).*

859. **(D)**   Potential complications from lumbar sympathetic block include subarachnoid injection, puncture of a major vessel or renal pelvis, neuralgia, somatic nerve damage, perforation of a disk, infection, ejaculatory failure, and chronic back pain. Blockade of nerve arising from the lumbar plexus is possible, but given the anatomic location of the sacral plexus, blockade of an S1 nerve would be extremely unlikely if not impossible *(Raj: Practical Management of Pain, ed 2, pp 807-808).*

860. **(E)**   Blockade of the sympathetic fibers (T1-L2) produces hypotension, particularly if the patient is hypovolemic. Bradycardia is produced by blocking the cardiac accelerator fibers (T1-4). The phrenic nerve (C3-5) is also blocked by a total spinal anesthetic. The pupils become dilated after intrathecal injection of large quantities of local anesthetics; they will return to normal size after the block recedes *(Miller: Anesthesia, ed 4, p 1528).*

861. **(B)**   Somatic pain in the extremities is relieved with spinal anesthesia. If a patient fails to obtain pain relief in spite of complete sympathetic, sensory, and motor blockade, a "central" mechanism for the pain is likely or the lesion causing the pain is higher in the CNS than the level of blockade achieved by the spinal. Central pain states may include encephalization, psychogenic pain, or malingering. Persistence of pain in the lower extremities after successful spinal blockade suggests a central source or psychological source of pain *(Miller: Anesthesia, ed 4, p 2354).*

862. **(A)**   During a seizure, administration of 100% O_2 helps to prevent hypoxia in a patient who might otherwise not be breathing. Hyperventilation induces hypokalemia and respiratory alkalosis both of which result in hyperpolarization of nerve membranes and elevation of the seizure threshold. Hyperventilation also causes cerebral vasoconstriction and decreased delivery of local anesthetic to the brain. Hyperventilation also raises the patient's pH (respiratory alkalosis) and converts lidocaine into the nonionized (non-protonated) form, which crosses the membrane easily. This has no beneficial effect *(Stoelting: Basics of Anesthesia, ed 3, pp 78-79).*

863. **(C)**   Para-aminobenzoic acid is a metabolite of the ester-type local anesthetics. Local anesthetics may be placed into two distinct categories based on their chemical structure, ester, or amide. All of the amides contain the letter "i" twice, once in "caine" and once elsewhere in the name: e.g. lidocaine, etidocaine, prilocaine, mepivacaine, and bupivacaine. These are metabolized in the liver. The ester local anesthetics are: cocaine, procaine, chloroprocaine, tetracaine, and benzocaine. These drugs are metabolized by the enzyme pseudocholinesterase found in the blood. Their half-lives in blood are very short, about 60 seconds. Para-aminobenzoic acid is a metabolic breakdown product of ester anesthetic and is responsible for allergic reactions in some individuals *(Rogers: Principles and Practice of Anesthesiology, p 1235).*

864. **(E)**   Peripheral nerve axons are always enveloped by a Schwann cell. The myelinated nerves may be enveloped many times by the same Schwann cell. Transmission of nerve impulses (i.e., action potentials) along nonmyelinated nerves occurs in a continuous fashion whereas transmission along myelinated nerves occurs by saltatory conduction from one node of Ranvier to the next. Myelination speeds transmission of neurological impulses; it also renders nerves more susceptible to local anesthetic blockade. An action potential is associated with an inward flux of sodium which occurs after a certain membrane threshold has been exceeded *(Miller: Anesthesia, ed 4, pp 492-496).*

865. **(B)**   Hyperventilation of the lungs and hypocarbia decrease cerebral blood flow, thus reducing delivery of local anesthetic to the brain. The alkalosis and hypokalemia that occur as a result of hyperventilation result in hyperpolarization of the resting transmembrane potential of neurons, thus increasing the seizure threshold for local anesthetics. Conversely, acidosis and hypercarbia decrease the seizure threshold for local anesthetics. Hyperoxia does nothing to prevent seizures (see answer to question 862) *(Miller: Anesthesia, ed 4, pp 510-511; Stoelting: Basics of Anesthesia, ed 3, p 79).*

866. **(C)**   Local anesthetics are weak bases with pKas which range from 7.6 to 8.9. A low pH will result in the formation of the ionized species because more protons (hydrogen ions) are available to bind to the nitrogen atoms in the local anesthetics. Local anesthetic concentration and volume have nothing to do with the fraction of anesthetics in the ionized form *(Rogers: Principles and Practice of Anesthesiology, pp 1237-1238).*

867. **(A)**   The internal branch of the superior laryngeal nerve provides sensory innervation to the larynx above the vocal cords; the external branch provides sensory innervation to the anterior subglottic mucosa. The recurrent laryngeal nerve provides sensory innervation to the larynx below the vocal cords *(Miller: Anesthesia, ed 4, p 1404).*

868. **(A)** Patients who are at increased risk of headache after dural puncture include parturients, young patients, and females. Use of large-bore needles and glucose-containing local anesthetics can also raise the risk of spinal headache. Spinal headaches result from leakage of CSF through the dural sheath. The headache is typically frontal or occipital in location and is made worse by sitting or standing up. There is some evidence that the incidence of spinal headache is less after a dural puncture made through the paramedian approach *(Barash: Clinical Anesthesia, ed 2, pp 832-833).*

869. **(A)** Ester-type local anesthetics are hydrolyzed in plasma by pseudocholinesterase, which is produced by the liver. Thus, patients with atypical pseudocholinesterase or severe liver disease will metabolize these drugs more slowly than will normal patients. Renal excretion plays only a minor role in the elimination of amide-type local anesthetics, accounting for < 1% to 6% of the dose administered to the patient. Plasma clearance of ester-type local anesthetics may be decreased in patients with impaired hepatic function because the synthesis of pseudocholinesterase by the liver is reduced *(Miller: Anesthesia, ed 4, pp 509-510; Stoelting: Pharmacology and Physiology in Anesthetic Practice, ed 2, pp 154-155).*

870. **(A)**

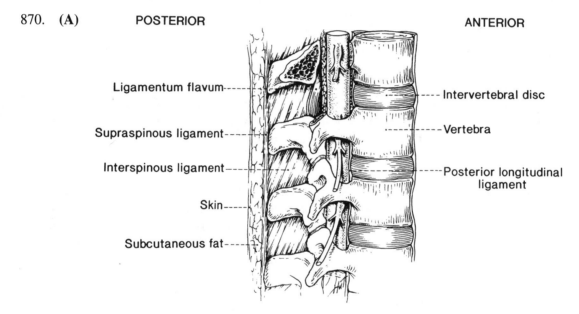

This figure shows the anatomic structures that must be traversed by the spinal needle during performance of a subarachnoid block. The structures include the skin, subcutaneous tissue, supraspinous ligament, interspinous ligament, and finally the ligamentum flavum. If one were to continue to advance the spinal needle one would encounter the dura (anteriorly) while exiting the subarachnoid space, the posterior longitudinal ligament, the periosteum of the vertebral body, and finally bone *(Cousins: Neural Blockade in Clinical Anesthesia and Management of Pain, ed 2, pp 255-263).*

871. **(C)** Cocaine and tetracaine are ester-type local anesthetics and are metabolized in part by ester hydrolysis in plasma by pseudocholinesterase (also see answer to question 863) *(Miller: Anesthesia, ed 4, p 509).*

872. **(A)** The oculocardiac reflex involves the trigeminal and vagus nerves. Afferent impulses are carried by the ophthalmic division of the trigeminal nerve through the Gasserian (trigeminal) ganglion to the main sensory nucleus in the floor of the fourth ventricle. Efferent impulses are conveyed via the vagus nerve to the sinoatrial and atrioventricular nodes of the heart. The facial nerve does not play a role in this scheme *(Miller: Anesthesia, ed 4, p 2182).*

873. **(B)** A rapid nerve-stimulation rate and alkaline pH increase the rate of onset of local anesthetic action because it is the non-ionized form of the local anesthetic molecule which passes through the neurolemma. Other factors which hasten the rate of onset include small fiber diameter, the presence of myelin, and low extracellular calcium concentration *(Stoelting: Basics of Anesthesia, ed 3, pp 73-76).*

874. **(A)** There are four main nerves in the lower extremity: the sciatic, femoral, obturator nerves, and lateral femoral cutaneous. The sciatic nerve is the largest of these and divides into the posterior tibial nerve and common peroneal nerve at the popliteal fossa. The common peroneal nerve further divides into the deep and superficial peroneal nerves. The tibial nerve divides into the posterior tibial and sural nerves. Thus, four of the five nerves which provide sensory innervation to the ankle arise from the sciatic nerve: the deep peroneal nerve, the superficial peroneal nerve, the posterior tibial nerve, and the sural nerve. The saphenous nerve is a branch of the femoral nerve and stands alone in this regard *(Miller: Anesthesia, ed 4, pp 1546 and 1552).*

875. **(D)** The cricothyroid muscle is the only intrinsic muscle of the larynx that tenses the vocal cords. It is innervated by the external branch of the superior laryngeal nerve of the vagus. All other intrinsic muscles of the larynx receive motor innervation from the recurrent laryngeal nerve *(Miller: Anesthesia, ed 4, p 2184).*

876. **(E)** All of the choices are potential complications of stellate ganglion blockade. Others include accidental injection of the local anesthetic into a vertebral artery resulting in seizure and inadvertent cervical epidural *(Barash: Clinical Anesthesia, ed 2, p 862).*

877. **(D)** Height, age, and weight of the patient do not determine the duration of epidural anesthesia. The concentration, dose, and volume of local anesthetic, and whether a vasoconstrictor is added to the local anesthetic are important factors in the determination of the duration of action of epidural blockade *(Stoelting: Basics of Anesthesia, ed 3, p 175).*

878. **(E)** All of these local anesthetic concentrations are isobaric. Tetracaine, 0.5%, is prepared by mixing equal volumes of 1% tetracaine and preservative-free saline. Hyperbaric solutions may be prepared by mixing equal volumes of 1% tetracaine and 10% dextrose, resulting in 0.5% tetracaine in 5% dextrose, or by mixing equal volumes of 0.75% bupivacaine with 10% dextrose, yielding a 0.375% solution of bupivacaine in 5% dextrose. Alternatively, factory-mixed preparations of 0.75% bupivacaine in 8.25% dextrose and 5% lidocaine in 7.5% dextrose are available. To prepare hypobaric tetracaine, 10 mg (1 mL of 1% tetracaine) are mixed with 9 mL of sterile H_2O to yield 10 mL of 0.1% tetracaine. This has a baricity of 1.0 *(Firestone: Clinical Anesthesia Procedures of the Massachusetts General Hospital, ed 3, p 194; Barash: Clinical Anesthesia, ed 2, p 827).*

879. **(A)** Epinephrine or phenylephrine is frequently added to local anesthetic solutions to produce vaso-constriction. This decreases systemic absorption of the local anesthetic and prolongs the duration of action of the local anesthetic. The extent to which epinephrine prolongs the block depends on both the site of injection and the specific local anesthetic. These beneficial effects, however, are limited when vasoconstrictors are used with epidural etidocaine and bupivacaine *(Miller: Anesthesia, ed 4, p 502)*.

880. **(B)** Etidocaine and tetracaine are poor choices for epidural analgesia in obstetrics because the concentration required to achieve sensory analgesia results in significant motor blockade. Bupivacaine has the most profound separation between sensory anesthesia and motor blockade. At low concentrations it can provide excellent sensory analgesia with little motor block. Etidocaine concentrations required for sensory analgesia also cause profound motor blockade, and the motor block may outlast the sensory block *(Shnider: Anesthesia for Obstetrics, ed 3, pp 87-91; Rogers: Principles and Practice of Anesthesiology, p 1239)*.

881. **(A)** The six pairs of extrinsic muscles of the larynx can be classified as elevators or depressors of the larynx. The stylohyoid, thyrohyoid, and digastric muscles elevate the larynx, and the omohyoid, sternothyroid, and sternohyoid muscles depress the larynx. The cricothyroid is an intrinsic muscle of the larynx *(Clemente: Anatomy: A Regional Atlas of the Human Body, ed 3, Figure 735)*.

882. **(B)** The presence of myelin and a rapid neuronal firing rate actually enhance the ability of local anesthetics to block the neuron. Local anesthetics gain access to receptors when the sodium channels are open as occurs during an action potential. Larger-diameter fibers are more difficult to block than small-diameter fibers. Tissue acidosis results in formation of the ionized form of the local anesthetics. This form does not readily transverse the lipophilic cell membrane *(Stoelting: Basics of Anesthesia, ed 3, p 76)*.

883. **(E)** All of the choices are correct. The amount of systemic absorption of a local anesthetic depends on the total dose injected, the vascularity of the injection site, the speed of injection, whether or not a vasoconstrictor is added to the local anesthetic solution, and the physicochemical properties of the local anesthetic such as protein and tissue binding, lipid solubility, and the degree of ionization at physiologic pH. For all local anesthetics, systemic absorption is greatest after injection for intercostal nerve and caudal blocks, intermediate for epidural blocks, and least for brachial plexus and sciatic nerve blocks *(Rogers: Principles and Practice of Anesthesiology, pp 1244-1245)*.

884. **(B)** Addition of CO_2 or HCO_3^- to local anesthetic solutions hastens the onset of the anesthetic block but does not increase its duration. Vasoconstrictors decrease absorption (and metabolism) of local anesthetics. A larger dose results in longer anesthetic duration as well as more dense blockade *(Miller: Anesthesia, ed 4, pp 502-503)*.

885. **(A)** Pregnancy is associated with decreased pseudocholinesterase activity; however, this reduction in activity is minimal such that the rate of hydrolysis of ester-type local anesthetics is sufficient to limit significant placental transfer to the fetus. Severe liver disease is associated with a decreased concentration of pseudocholinesterase. Likewise, uremic patients have decreased serum levels of pseudocholinesterase, which may interfere with the metabolism of ester local anesthetics. Pulmonary disease does not affect the clearance of local anesthetics, provided blood flow to the liver is not lowered by hypoxia *(Stoelting: Pharmacology and Physiology in Anesthetic Practice, ed 2, p 155).*

886. **(D)** The femoral, obturator, and lateral femoral cutaneous nerves arise from the lumbar plexus, while the sacral plexus gives rise to the sciatic nerve and its branches, common peroneal, deep and superficial peroneal, posterior tibial, and sural *(Snell: Clinical Anatomy for Anesthesiologists, pp 210-211).*

887. **(B)** Ester-type local anesthetics are broken down partly in the blood by pseudocholinesterase and red-cell esterase and partly in the liver. Anticholinesterase drugs, e.g., echothiophate, neostigmine, pyridostigmine, and edrophonium inhibit pseudocholinesterase and thus slow the plasma clearance of ester-type local anesthetics. Phenytoin is an enzyme inducer which may hasten the metabolism of amide-type local anesthetics like lidocaine, but would have little if any effect on ester-type local anesthetics and would certainly not impede their plasma clearance *(Stoelting: Pharmacology and Physiology in Anesthetic Practice, ed 2, pp 155, 227).*

888. **(E)** The knee is innervated anteriorly by the femoral nerve, medially by the obturator nerve, posteriorly by the sciatic, and laterally by the common peroneal and the lateral femoral cutaneous nerves. All of these must be blocked for operative procedures *(Rogers: Principles and Practice of Anesthesiology, p 1461).*

889. **(C)** The completeness of a lumbar sympathetic block can be ascertained by skin temperature measurements and increases in blood flow. The latter can be determined by a number of techniques which include: laser Doppler flowmeter, occlusion skin plethysmography, transcutaneous oxygen electrodes, and mass spectrometry. Numbness in the leg and inability to move it suggest an accidental subarachnoid or epidural injection, a rare but possible complication of this block *(Rogers: Principles and Practice of Anesthesiology, pp 1381-1385).*

890. **(A)** In adults the spinal cord ends at L1-2. The sympathetic nerve fiber originates in the intermediolateral grey column of the T1-L2 spinal segments. The spinal canal originates at the foramen magnum and terminates at the sacral hiatus. The dural sac terminates at S2 in adults *(Stoelting: Basics of Anesthesia, ed 3, pp 163-164 & 176; Barash: Clinical Anesthesia, ed 2, pp 813-814).*

891. **(A)** Volatile anesthetics, sympathomimetics, ß-adrenergic receptor antagonists, and the H_2-receptor antagonist cimetidine reduce hepatic blood flow, thereby reducing plasma clearance of amide-type local anesthetics. There is also evidence that propranolol directly inhibits mixed-function oxidase activity of hepatocytes. Phenytoin increases clearance of lidocaine by enzyme induction *(Stoelting: Pharmacology and Physiology in Anesthetic Practice, ed 2, pp 153-154, & 301).*

892. **(A)**   The maximum single dose of bupivacaine which can be administered to an adult (70 kg) is 175 mg. When administered with epinephrine, the dose can be somewhat higher, i.e., about 225 mg *(Stoelting: Pharmacology and Physiology in Anesthetic Practice, ed 2, p 150).*

893. **(C)**   Accidental intrathecal injections of large volumes of the commercial preparation of 2-chloro-procaine are rarely associated with neurologic injury. However, Nesacaine-CE contains higher concentrations of sodium bisulfite (an antioxidant added to local anesthetic solutions to increase their shelf life) and has a lower pH than 2-chloroprocaine. Both of these properties have been implicated as the cause of neurotoxicity when Nesacaine-CE is injected in large volume into the subarachnoid space. Ortho-toluidine is a product of prilocaine metabolism and is responsible for converting hemoglobin to methemoglobin. It has nothing to do with Nesacaine-CE. Methyl-paraben is an antimicrobial agent added to multidose vials. It is responsible for allergic reactions. Local anesthetic solutions should not contain antimicrobial agents except those used for minor infiltration *(Rogers: Principles and Practice of Anesthesiology, pp 1250-1251).*

894. **(D)**   The un-ionized form of the local anesthetic traverses the nerve membrane whereas the ionized form actually blocks conduction. About 3 nodes of Ranvier must be blocked to achieve anesthesia. The ability of a local anesthetic to block conduction is inversely proportional to the diameter of the fiber. The presence of myelin does enhance the ability of a local anesthetic to block conduction, as does rapid firing *(Stoelting: Basics of Anesthesia, ed 3, pp 75-76).*

895. **(D)**   Postspinal headaches are characterized by frontal or occipital pain, which worsens with sitting and improves with reclining. Postspinal headaches may be associated with neurologic symptoms such as diplopia, tinnitus, and reduced hearing acuity. The etiology of postspinal headaches is unclear; however, they are believed to be caused by a reduction in CSF pressure and resulting tension on meningeal vessels and nerves (which results from leakage of CSF through the needle hole in the dura mater). Factors associated with an increased incidence of postspinal headaches include female gender (especially parturients), the size and type of needle used to perform the block, age of the patient, and the number of dural punctures. Conservative therapy for a postspinal headache include bedrest, analgesics, and oral and intravenous hydration. If conservative therapy is not successful after 24 to 48 hours, it is recommended that an epidural "blood patch" with 10 to 20 mL of the patient's blood be performed. An epidural "blood patch" provides prompt relief of the postspinal headache *(Stoelting: Basics of Anesthesia, ed 3, pp 172-173).*

896. **(D)**   897. **(B)**   898. **(E)**   899. **(A)**   900. **(C)**   *(Rogers: Principles and Practice of Anesthesiology, p 258; pp 1276 & 1293; p 1361; p 1301; p 1294).*

901. (C)   902. (E)   903. (A)   904. (D)   905. (F)   906. (B) Peripheral nerves are classified according to the fiber size and physiologic properties such as the presence or absence of myelin, conduction velocity, location and function. Type A fibers range in diameter from 1-22 μm, are myelinated, and have moderate-to-fast conduction velocities. These fibers are subclassified into four groups based on their location and function. Type A-α and -ß fibers provide motor and proprioception function to muscles and joints; type A-γ fibers innervate muscle spindles and provide for muscle tone; type A-δ fibers provide pain, temperature and touch sensation. Type B fibers are preganglionic sympathetic nerves that are less than 3 μm in diameter, myelinated, and have medium conduction velocities. Type C fibers are postganglionic sympathetic nerves which are very small in diameter, not myelinated, and have slow conduction velocities. Type C fibers are also afferent sensory nerves involved in pain, temperature, and touch *(Miller: Anesthesia, ed 4, p 493).*

907. (A)   908. (C)   909. (D)   910. (B)   911. (A)   912. (A)   913. (D)   914. (E) The lingual branch of the glossopharyngeal nerve provides sensory innervation of the posterior one third of the tongue. Most of the sensory supply to the oropharynx and laryngopharynx is from the glossopharyngeal nerve. The muscles of the pharynx are supplied through the pharyngeal plexus from motor fibers from the 11th cranial nerve. With the exception of the cricothyroid muscle, the recurrent laryngeal nerve of the vagus provides motor innervation of all the intrinsic muscles of the larynx. The cricothyroid muscle is supplied by the external branch of the superior laryngeal nerve of the vagus. The sensory innervation of the mucosa of the larynx down to the vocal folds comes from the internal branch of the superior laryngeal nerve of the vagus and the sensory innervation of the mucosa of the larynx below the vocal folds comes from the recurrent laryngeal nerve of the vagus *(Rogers: Principles and Practice of Anesthesiology, pp 1021-1023; Miller: Anesthesia, ed 4, p 1404).*

Cardiovascular Physiology and Anesthesia

DIRECTIONS (Questions 915 through 963): Each of the questions or incomplete statements in this section is followed by answers or by completions of the statement, respectively. Select the ONE BEST answer or completion for each item.

915. A 46-year-old patient with Crohn's disease is scheduled for a colectomy under general anesthesia. The patient has a history of rheumatic fever with moderate mitral regurgitation. Which of the following antibiotics would be the most appropriate choice for prophylaxis against subacute bacterial endocarditis in this patient?

    A. Ampicillin and erythromycin
    B. Erythromycin and gentamycin
    C. Ampicillin and gentamycin
    D. Clindamycin
    E. Penicillin

916. A 68-year-old patient is undergoing elective coronary revascularization. Just prior to cardiopulmonary bypass, the hemoglobin concentration is 12.3 g/dL and platelet count is 253,000/mm³. After cardiopulmonary bypass is initiated, the patient is cooled to 20°C and 2 units of packed red blood cells are transfused. While on cardiopulmonary bypass, the anesthesiologist notices that the platelet count is 10,000/mm³ and the hemoglobin concentration is 9 g/dL. The most likely cause of thrombocytopenia is

    A. Sequestration
    B. A hemolytic transfusion reaction
    C. Dilutional thrombocytopenia
    D. Disseminated intravascular coagulation
    E. Heparin-induced thrombocytopenia

917. Which of the following is the most sensitive indicator of left ventricular myocardial ischemia?

    A. Wall-motion abnormalities on the echocardiogram
    B. ST-segment changes in lead V_5 of the electrocardiogram
    C. Appearance of V waves on the pulmonary capillary wedge pressure tracing
    D. Elevation of the pulmonary capillary wedge pressure
    E. A decrease in cardiac output as measured by the thermodilution technique

918. Which of the following characteristics of volatile anesthetics is necessary for calculation of the time constant?

    A. Blood:gas partition coefficient
    B. Brain:blood partition coefficient
    C. Oil:gas partition coefficient
    D. Minimum alveolar concentration
    E. Saturated vapor pressure

919. Accidental injection of air into a peripheral vein would be least likely to result in arterial air embolism in a patient with which of the following anatomic cardiac defects?

   A. Patent ductus arteriosus
   B. Eisenmenger's syndrome
   C. Teratology of Fallot
   D. Pulmonary atresia with ventricular septal defect
   E. Tricuspid atresia

920. Each of the following could be placed on the x-axis of the curve shown in the figure **EXCEPT**

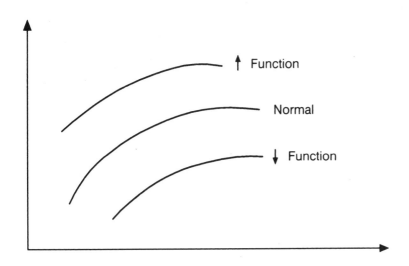

   A. Stroke volume
   B. Left ventricular end-diastolic pressure
   C. Left ventricular end-diastolic volume
   D. Left atrial pressure
   E. Pulmonary artery-occlusion pressure

921. Acetylcholine is a neurotransmitter for each of the following **EXCEPT**

   A. Neuromuscular junction
   B. Preganglionic sympathetic neurons
   C. Preganglionic parasympathetic neurons
   D. Postganglionic parasympathetic receptors on the heart
   E. Postganglionic sympathetic receptors on the heart

922. A 65-year-old patient with history of schizophrenia is anesthetized for left radical mastectomy. The patient takes chlorpromazine and atenolol. Anesthesia is induced with sodium thiopental after which time the patient's rhythm is noted to change from a sinus rhythm to a polymorphic ventricular tachycardia. Which of the treatments below would be the **LEAST** effective in the treatment of this dysrhythmia?

   A. Magnesium sulphate
   B. Defibrillation
   C. Overdrive pacing
   D. Procainamide
   E. Bretylium

923. A 78-year-old patient is anesthetized for right hemicolectomy with isoflurane and nitrous oxide. Vecuronium is administered to facilitate muscle relaxation. At the end of the operation, the neuromuscular blockade is reversed with neostigmine 4 mg and glycopyrrolate 0.8 mg. The rhythm below is noted shortly after administration of these drugs. The patient's blood pressure is 90/60. The most appropriate course of action at this point is

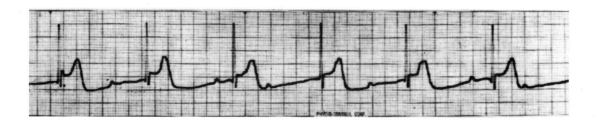

   A. DC cardioversion
   B. Isoproterenol drip
   C. Atropine
   D. Transcutaneous pacemaker
   E. Begin chest compressions

924. While on cardiopulmonary bypass during elective coronary artery revascularization, the patient is noted to have bulging sclerae. Mean arterial pressure is 50 mm Hg, temperature is 28°C, and there is no EKG activity. The most appropriate action to take at this time is to

   A. Administer mannitol, 50 gm IV
   B. Administer furosemide, 20 mg IV
   C. Decrease the cardiac index
   D. Check the position of the aortic cannula
   E. Check the position of the venous return cannula

925. Which of the following correctly describes the effect of transposition of the great arteries on the rate of induction of anesthesia?

    A. Inhalation induction is faster than normal; intravenous induction is slower than normal
    B. Inhalation induction is slower than normal; intravenous induction is faster than normal
    C. Both inhalation and intravenous induction are faster than normal
    D. Both inhalation and intravenous induction are slower than normal
    E. Inhalation induction is normal; intravenous induction is faster than normal

926. Anastomosis of the right atrium to the pulmonary artery (Fontan procedure) is a useful surgical treatment for each of the following congenital cardiac defects **EXCEPT**

    A. Tricuspid atresia
    B. Hypoplastic left heart syndrome
    C. Pulmonary valve stenosis
    D. Truncus arteriosus
    E. Pulmonary artery atresia

927. By what percent is total body O_2 consumption decreased during cardiopulmonary bypass at 30°C?

    A. 40
    B. 50
    C. 70
    D. 85
    E. 95

928. A 68-year-old smoker with a 10-year history of adult onset diabetes mellitus and recently diagnosed colon cancer is scheduled for a right hemicolectomy. Preoperative EKG reveals a right bundle branch block plus left anterior hemiblock. The most appropriate management of this patient's cardiac conduction disease would be

    A. Placement of a permanent ventricular pacemaker prior to surgery
    B. Placement of a permanent sequential pacemaker prior to surgery
    C. Placement of a temporary transvenous pacemaker after induction of general anesthesia
    D. Placement of pulmonary artery catheter with left ventricular pace port
    E. None of the above

929. Afterload reduction is beneficial during anesthesia for noncardiac surgery in patients with each of the following conditions **EXCEPT**

    A. Aortic insufficiency
    B. Mitral regurgitation
    C. Tetralogy of Fallot
    D. Congestive heart failure
    E. Patent ductus arteriosus

930. Administration of protamine to a patient who has not received heparin can result in

A. Anticoagulation
B. Hypercoagulation
C. Profound bradycardia
D. Seizure
E. Hypertension

931. The primary determinants of myocardial O_2 consumption, from most to least important, are

A. Preload > afterload > heart rate
B. Heart rate > preload > afterload
C. Afterload > preload > heart rate
D. Heart rate > afterload > preload
E. Afterload > heart rate > preload

932. The pharmacologic treatment of choice for digitalis induced ventricular dysrhythmias is

A. Verapamil
B. Procainamide
C. Esmolol
D. Lidocaine
E. Bretylium

933. Which of the following drugs should **NOT** be administered via an endotracheal tube

A. Lidocaine
B. HCO_3^-
C. Atropine
D. Propranolol
E. Isoproterenol

934. The mean arterial pressure in a patient with a blood pressure of 180/60 mm Hg is

A. 90 mm Hg
B. 100 mm Hg
C. 110 mm Hg
D. 120 mm Hg
E. 130 mm Hg

935. Hypothyroidism and hyperthyroidism could occur in patients receiving which of the following anti-dysrhythmic drugs?

A. Amiodarone
B. Bretylium
C. Phenytoin
D. Encainide
E. Procainamide

936. Calculate the systemic vascular resistance (in dynes/sec/cm^{-5}) from the following data: cardiac output 5.0 L/min, central venous pressure 8 mm Hg, mean arterial blood pressure 86 mm Hg, mean pulmonary arterial blood pressure 20 mm Hg, pulmonary capillary wedge pressure 9 mm Hg, heart rate 85 beats/min, patient weight 100 kg.

    A. 750
    B. 1,000
    C. 1,250
    D. 1,500
    E. Cannot be calculated

937. Which of the following is **NOT** included in Tetralogy of Fallot?

    A. Patent ductus arteriosus
    B. Right ventricular hypertrophy
    C. Ventricular septal defect
    D. Overriding aorta
    E. Pulmonic stenosis

938. A 65-year-old female patient with sepsis is undergoing an emergency exploratory laparotomy. After induction of anesthesia and tracheal intubation, the patient's blood pressure is noted to be 65 systolic with a heart rate of 120 beats/minute. Cardiac output determined by a thermodilution pulmonary artery catheter is 13 L/minute. Of the following vasopressors the **LEAST** appropriate choice would be

    A. Dobutamine
    B. Dopamine
    C. Norepinephrine
    D. Epinephrine
    E. Phenylephrine

939. Characteristics of beta-2 stimulation include each of the following **EXCEPT**

    A. Inhibition of insulin secretion
    B. Glycogenolysis
    C. Gluconeogenesis
    D. Renin secretion
    E. Uterine relaxation

940. A 61-year-old male patient with idiopathic hypertrophic subaortic stenosis is scheduled for left ventricular myectomy under general anesthesia. Which of the following anesthetics would provide the most stable hemodynamics in this patient?

    A. N$_2$O-narcotic
    B. Ketamine
    C. Halothane
    D. Enflurane
    E. Isoflurane

941. A healthy 59-year-old (60 kg) woman develops ventricular tachycardia during cosmetic facial surgery while under general anesthesia. Lidocaine, 180 mg IV, is administered in multiple doses, but the dysrhythmia continues. Systemic blood pressure is 120/75 mm Hg. The next step in the management of this dysrhythmia should be

A. Electrical cardioversion
B. Administration of lidocaine, 60 mg IV
C. Administration of procainamide, 20 mg/min IV
D. Administration of bretylium, 300 mg IV
E. Overdrive pacing

942. While ß-adrenergic receptor blockade is the best treatment for reentrant tachydysrhythmias associated with Romano-Ward syndrome, these dysrhythmias can also be effectively treated with

A. Lidocaine
B. Procainamide
C. Quinidine
D. Left stellate ganglion blockade
E. Right stellate ganglion blockade

943. Which of the following antidysrhythmic agents should not be used to treat wide complex tachycardia of indeterminate origin?

A. Adenosine
B. Lidocaine
C. Procainamide
D. Bretylium
E. Verapamil

944. In a normal person what percent of the cardiac output is dependent on the "atrial kick"?

A. 10
B. 20
C. 30
D. 40
E. 50

945. A 56-year-old patient has undergone a radical retropubic prostatectomy under general anesthesia. In the recovery room the hemoglobin is 8 g/dl and a transfusion with packed red blood cells is begun. Twenty minutes later the patient's temperature is noted to rise from 36.5°C to 37.8°C. Blood pressure at this time is 130/65 and heart rate is 100/minute. The patient denies chest pain, flank pain, and shortness of breath. The most appropriate course of action at this time is

A. Administer diphenhydramine
B. Administer acetaminophen
C. Administer washed RBCs
D. Administer HCO_3^-
E. Stop the transfusion

946. A 4-year-old child with Tetralogy of Fallot is to undergo elective repair of a left inguinal hernia under general anesthesia. Which of the following anesthetics would provide the most stable hemodynamics in this patient?

    A. Halothane and N_2O
    B. Enflurane and N_2O
    C. Halothane
    D. Fentanyl and N_2O
    E. Ketamine

947. The left ventricular pressure-volume loop shown in the figure depicts

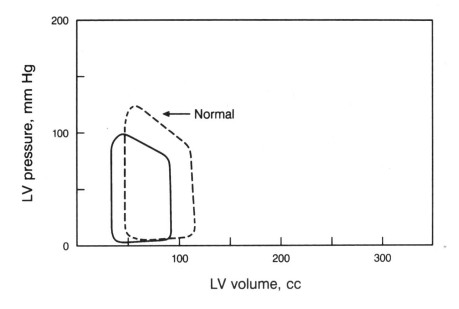

    A. Mitral stenosis
    B. Mitral regurgitation
    C. Aortic stenosis
    D. Acute aortic insufficiency
    E. Chronic aortic insufficiency

948. A 44-year-old patient is undergoing replacement of a stenotic aortic valve and two-vessel coronary artery bypass graft under general anesthesia. After induction, the pulmonary capillary wedge pressure is 15 mm Hg and pulmonary artery pressures are 26/13 mm Hg. Suddenly, new 30-mm Hg V waves appear on the oscilloscope. The systemic blood pressure is 120/70 mm Hg, heart rate is 75 beats/min, and pulmonary artery pressure is 50/35 mm Hg. Which of the following drugs should be administered to the patient?

    A. Nitroglycerin
    B. Nitroprusside
    C. Esmolol
    D. Phenylephrine
    E. Dobutamine

949. A 62-year-old patient scheduled for elective repair of an abdominal aortic aneurysm develops a wide complex tachycardia during induction of anesthesia. Blood pressure is 110/78. One hundred mg of lidocaine is administered intravenously times two with no change. According to the ACLS guidelines, which of the following steps should be taken next?

    A. Administration of procainamide, 20 mg/min
    B. Administration of bretylium, 50 mg/10 min
    C. Administration of adenosine, 6 mg rapidly over 3 seconds
    D. Verapamil, 5-10 mg IV
    E. Esmolol, 35 mg IV

950. Under maximum stress, how much cortisol is produced per day?

    A. 25 to 50 mg
    B. 50 to 100 mg
    C. 100 to 200 mg
    D. 200 to 500 mg
    E. Up to 1,000 mg

951. A VVI pacemaker programmed to pace at a rate of 70 beats/min is noted on the preoperative ECG to pace at 61 beat/min. The most likely reason for this decrease in the pacing heart rate is

    A. Decreased atrial rate
    B. Third-degree heart block
    C. Trifascicular heart block
    D. Battery failure
    E. Normal variation

952. Calculate the cardiac output from the following data: patient weight 70 kg, hemoglobin concentration 10 mg/dL. Arterial blood gases on 100% O_2: P_aO_2 450 mm Hg, P_aCO_2 32 mm Hg, pH 7.46, S_aO_2 99%; mixed venous blood gases: P_vO_2 30 mm Hg, P_aCO_2 45 mm Hg, pH 7.32, S_vO_2 60%.

    A. 2.5 L/min
    B. 3.0 L/min
    C. 3.5 L/min
    D. 4.0 L/min
    E. 4.5 L/min

953. Normal resting myocardial O_2 consumption is

    A. 2.0 mL/100 g/min
    B. 3.5 mL/100 g/min
    C. 10 mL/100 g/min
    D. 15 mL/100 g/min
    E. 25 mL/100 g/min

954. A 22-year-old man with idiopathic hypertrophic subaortic stenosis is undergoing an elective chole-cystectomy under general anesthesia. Immediately following induction with thiopental, 5 mg/kg IV, the arterial blood pressure decreases from 140/82 mm Hg to 70/40 mm Hg. What would be the most appropriate drug for treatment of hypotension in this patient?

    A. Ephedrine
    B. Mephentermine
    C. Isoproterenol
    D. Phenylephrine
    E. Epinephrine

955. A 65-year-old patient with moderate aortic stenosis develops a sudden increase in heart rate during an appendectomy under general anesthesia. The ventricular rate is 190 beats/min and is irregularly irregular, arterial blood pressure is 70/45 mm Hg, and there is 2-mm ST-segment depression in lead V_5 of the electrocardiogram. Which of the following would be the most appropriate treatment for myocardial ischemia in this patient?

    A. Electrical cardioversion
    B. Esmolol
    C. Nitroglycerin
    D. Verapamil
    E. Phenylephrine

956. After emergency repair of a ruptured abdominal aortic aneurysm, a 68-year-old patient is mechanically ventilated in the intensive care unit with 20 cm H_2O of PEEP for 3 days. Sodium nitroprusside has been infused at a rate of 1.5 µg/kg/min for 48 hours to control hypertension. Suddenly, the systemic blood pressure falls from 130/70 mm Hg to 50 mm Hg systolic and the S_aO_2 drops to 75%. The most likely cause of this scenario is

    A. Cyanide toxicity
    B. Acute myocardial infarction
    C. Tension pneumothorax
    D. Hyperventilation
    E. Methemoglobinemia

957. Normal resting coronary artery blood flow is

    A. 10 mL/100 g/min
    B. 40 mL/100 g/min
    C. 80 mL/100 g/min
    D. 120 mL/100 g/min
    E. 160 mL/100 g/min

958. Each of the following is associated with an increased incidence of pulmonary artery rupture in patients with pulmonary artery catheters **EXCEPT**

    A. Hypothermia
    B. Presence of pulmonary artery atheromas
    C. Old age
    D. Anticoagulation
    E. Pulmonary artery catheter migration

959. Risk factors for protamine allergic reactions include each of the following **EXCEPT**

   A. Diabetes treated with NPH insulin
   B. History of previous allergic reaction to protamine
   C. History of cold agglutinins
   D. Previous vasectomy
   E. Allergy to fish

960. A 66-year-old patient is undergoing a three-vessel coronary artery bypass operation. Anticoagulation is achieved with 20,000 units of heparin. How much protamine should be administered to this patient to completely reverse the heparin after cardiopulmonary bypass?

   A. 150 mg
   B. 250 mg
   C. 350 mg
   D. 450 mg
   E. 550 mg

961. The graph below represents

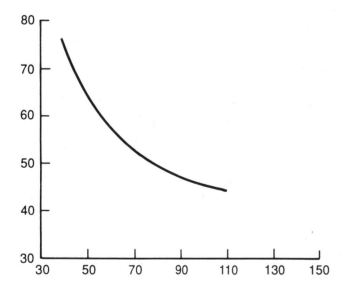

   A. Ventricular end-diastolic pressure as a function of ventricular end-diastolic volume
   B. Stroke volume as a function of end-diastolic pressure
   C. Cardiac index as a function of end-diastolic pressure
   D. Cardiac output as a function of ventricular end-diastolic volume
   E. Diastolic time (as percent of cardiac cycle) as a function of heart rate

962. A 72-year-old woman is undergoing cardiopulmonary bypass for aortic and mitral valve replacement. The surgery is uneventful; however, in the intensive care unit blood is noted to ooze from the pulmonary artery catheter and venous access sites, and the mediastinal chest tube output is 500 mL/hour. A thromboelastogram is obtained and shown in the figure. What is the most likely cause of profuse bleeding in this patient?

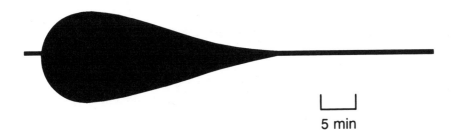

5 min

    A. Fibrinolysis
    B. Excess heparin
    C. Thrombocytopenia
    D. Factor VIII deficiency
    E. Poor surgical hemostasis

963. A 170 micron filter must be used for administration of each of the following **EXCEPT**

    A. Fresh frozen plasma
    B. Cryoprecipitate
    C. Platelets
    D. Packed red cells
    E. Albumin

964. The dose of adenosine necessary to convert paroxysmal supraventricular tachycardia to normal sinus rhythm should be initially reduced

    A. In patients receiving theophylline for chronic asthma
    B. In patients with a history of arterial thrombotic disease taking dipyridamole
    C. In patients with a history of chronic renal failure
    D. In patients with hepatic dysfunction
    E. In chronic alcoholics

965. A 56-year-old male patient is anesthetized for elective coronary revascularization. A urinary catheter is placed after induction and coupled to a temperature transducer. A pulmonary artery catheter is inserted and the temperature probe on the distal portion of the catheter is also connected to a transducer. The reason for measuring the temperature of both the bladder and the blood in the pulmonary vasculature is

A. Both are necessary for determining cardiac output by the thermodilution technique
B. The bladder temperature is more accurate prebypass; the PA catheter temperature is more accurate postbypass
C. The PA catheter temperature is more accurate prebypass; the bladder temperature is more accurate postbypass
D. It is helpful in determining the likelihood of recooling after discontinuation of cardiopulmonary bypass
E. It is the average of these two temperatures which is important in determining patient body warmth

DIRECTIONS (Questions 966 through 991): For each of the items in this section, ONE or MORE of the numbered options is correct. Select the answer:

Select A if options *1, 2 and 3* are correct,
Select B if options *1 and 3* are correct,
Select C if options *2 and 4* are correct,
Select D if only option *4* is correct,
Select E if *all* options are correct.

966. Complication(s) related to aneurysms of the ascending thoracic aorta include

1. Stroke
2. Cardiac tamponade
3. Obstruction of the coronary arteries
4. Acute mitral regurgitation

967. A 75-year-old patient in the coronary care unit 2 days following an acute anterior myocardial infarction has the following hemodynamic values: systolic arterial blood pressure 72 mm Hg, central venous pressure 24 mm Hg, pulmonary capillary wedge pressure 28 mm Hg. Conditions consistent with these hemodynamic values include

1. Left ventricular failure
2. Hypovolemia
3. Cardiac tamponade
4. Ruptured left ventricle

968. True statements concerning mitral stenosis include which of the following?

1. Symptoms do not usually occur until 20 years after acute rheumatic fever
2. Patients may be more susceptible to ventilatory depression from sedatives
3. Increased pulmonary vascular resistance and pulmonary hypertension are likely to occur when the left atrial pressure is chronically elevated above 25 mm Hg
4. Hypoxia may occur when the patient is placed in the head-down position

Select A if options *1, 2 and 3* are correct,
Select B if options *1 and 3* are correct,
Select C if options *2 and 4* are correct,
Select D if only option *4* is correct,
Select E if *all* options are correct.

969. Untoward effects associated with administration of sodium bicarbonate during cardiopulmonary resuscitation include

    1. Hyperosmolality
    2. Paradoxical CSF acidosis
    3. Hypercarbia
    4. Hyponatremia

970. Appropriate therapy for hypercyanotic "Tet spells" in patients with Tetralogy of Fallot includes

    1. Propranolol
    2. Ephedrine
    3. Phenylephrine
    4. Mephentermine

971. Administration of large doses of hetastarch (Hespan) has been associated with bleeding abnormalities. The mechanism(s) for coagulation disturbances in patients receiving hetastarch is/are:

    1. Dilution of platelets
    2. Decreased platelet function
    3. Dilution of procoagulants
    4. Interaction with antithrombin III

972. True statements regarding aortic stenosis include which of the following?

    1. Hemodynamically significant disease is associated with a gradient across the valve > 25 mm Hg
    2. Afterload reduction is beneficial during anesthesia
    3. Heart rate is not important in determining left-ventricular filling and cardiac output
    4. Angina pectoris can occur in the absence of coronary artery disease

973. A 29-year-old patient with pulmonary atresia is scheduled for an elective cholecystectomy. The patient has a Blalock-Taussig shunt (subclavian artery to pulmonary artery anastomosis) in place and functioning as well as a large ventricular septal defect. Which of the following statements regarding management of this patient is (are) true?

    1. Hyperventilation of the lungs will improve the S_aO_2
    2. Increased right to left shunting through the VSD will decrease the S_aO_2
    3. A pulmonary artery catheter should be placed to monitor cardiac output
    4. Systemic hypotension will be manifested by a decreased S_aO_2

Select A if options *1, 2 and 3* are correct,
Select B if options *1 and 3* are correct,
Select C if options *2 and 4* are correct,
Select D if only option *4* is correct,
Select E if *all* options are correct.

974. Which of the following could increase right-to-left shunting in a patient with Tetralogy of Fallot?

    1. Decreased systemic vascular resistance
    2. Curare
    3. Positive pressure ventilation
    4. Ketamine

975. A 55-year-old construction worker with a history of hypertrophic cardiomyopathy is scheduled a right hemicolectomy under general anesthesia. Appropriate steps in the management of this patient's anesthetic would include

    1. Induction with ketamine and maintenance with fentanyl and nitrous oxide
    2. Treatment of hypotension with phenylephrine
    3. Treatment of hypertension with intravenous nitroglycerine.
    4. Administration of esmolol prior to laryngoscopy

976. Which of the following factors is associated with an increased risk of morbidity and mortality after coronary artery bypass surgery?

    1. Failed angioplasty
    2. Preoperative congestive heart failure
    3. Unstable angina
    4. Male sex

977. Organs with the capability of autoregulation, i.e., maintenance of blood flow in spite of changes in perfusion pressure, include

    1. Heart
    2. Kidney
    3. Brain
    4. Liver

978. Reason(s) for cannulation of the left internal jugular vein rather than the right include

    1. A straight line to the left atrium
    2. The lower dome of the left lung than of the right lung
    3. Avoiding endangering the thoracic duct
    4. The inability to cannulate on the right

Select A if options *1, 2 and 3* are correct,
Select B if options *1 and 3* are correct,
Select C if options *2 and 4* are correct,
Select D if only option *4* is correct,
Select E if *all* options are correct.

979. Advantages of continuing of calcium channel blocker therapy in patients who are to undergo coronary artery bypass grafting surgery include

    1. Control of tachydysrhythmias
    2. Prevention of coronary artery vasospasm
    3. Reduction of hypertension
    4. Reduction in MAC

980. Electrolyte abnormalities associated with an increased QT interval and possible development of Torsades de Pointes include

    1. Hypocalcemia
    2. Hypomagnesemia
    3. Hypokalemia
    4. Hypernatremia

981. A 22-year-old woman with a history of Wolff-Parkinson-White syndrome is to undergo elective cholecystectomy under general anesthesia. Which of the following drugs may potentiate a tachydysrhythmia in this patient?

    1. Ketamine
    2. Atropine
    3. Pancuronium
    4. Droperidol

982. Ketamine and pancuronium are relatively contraindicated in patients with

    1. Aortic stenosis
    2. Mitral prolapse
    3. Mitral stenosis
    4. Aortic regurgitation

983. Effective treatments for congenital prolonged QT interval syndromes include

    1. Left stellate ganglion blockade
    2. Verapamil
    3. Propranolol
    4. Right stellate ganglion blockade

Select A if options *1, 2 and 3* are correct,
Select B if options *1 and 3* are correct,
Select C if options *2 and 4* are correct,
Select D if only option *4* is correct,
Select E if *all* options are correct.

984. For placement of a pulmonary artery catheter in a 70-kg patient, correct distances from the percutaneous insertion sites to the right atrium include which of the following?

   1. Right subclavian vein, 10 cm
   2. Right internal jugular vein, 20 cm
   3. Right antecubital vein, 50 cm
   4. Right femoral vein, 60 cm

985. A pulmonary artery catheter capable of continuously monitoring $S\overline{v}O_2$ is placed in a patient for coronary artery bypass surgery. Just prior to instituting cardiopulmonary bypass, the $S\overline{v}O_2$ falls from 85% to 71%. Which of the following could account for this change in $S\overline{v}O_2$?

   1. Cooling the patient to 27°C
   2. Acute blood loss
   3. Epinephrine, 25 µg IV
   4. Myocardial ischemia

986. The indicator dye dilution curve shown in the figure is consistent with which of the following?

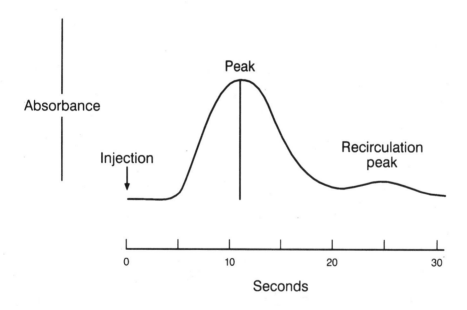

   1. Eisenmenger's complex
   2. Ventricular septal defect
   3. Tetralogy of Fallot
   4. Normal heart

Select A if options *1, 2 and 3* are correct,
Select B if options *1 and 3* are correct,
Select C if options *2 and 4* are correct,
Select D if only option *4* is correct,
Select E if *all* options are correct.

987. A 31-year-old female with primary pulmonary hypertension is in the intensive care unit awaiting heart transplantation. Pharmacologic agents that might be useful in reducing pulmonary vascular resistance include

1. Tolazoline
2. Isoproterenol
3. Nitroprusside
4. Prostaglandin E_1

988. Indication(s) for a permanent pacemaker include

1. Third degree heart block
2. Right bundle-branch block with left posterior hemiblock
3. Type II second-degree heart block
4. Type I second-degree heart block

989. Advantage(s) of membrane oxygenators over bubble oxygenators include

1. Lower cost
2. Lower priming volume
3. Simplicity
4. Less damage to erythrocytes

990. Factors which will raise the threshold for a pacemaker include

1. Stress
2. Hypoxia
3. Hypocarbia
4. Toxic levels of procainamide

991. A 54-year-old patient has 3-mm ST-segment depression on the ECG in leads II, III, and aVF during an episode of chest pain in the recovery room. Which of the following is most consistent with these findings?

1. First-degree heart block
2. Right ventricular wall-motion abnormalities
3. Third-degree heart block
4. Occlusion of the left anterior descending coronary artery

Select A if options *1, 2 and 3* are correct,
Select B if options *1 and 3* are correct,
Select C if options *2 and 4* are correct,
Select D if only option *4* is correct,
Select E if *all* options are correct.

992. Valvular heart lesions in which an increased afterload may be beneficial include

    1. Mitral insufficiency
    2. Aortic regurgitation
    3. Tricuspid insufficiency
    4. Aortic stenosis

993. Which of the following conditions would lead to erroneously high measurements of cardiac output from a pulmonary artery catheter using the thermodilution technique

    1. Too little injectate
    2. Presence of tricuspid regurgitation
    3. Ventricular septal defect with right-to-left shunting
    4. Ventricular septal defect with left-to-right shunting

994. Positive inotropic agents which increase cardiac output by direct or indirect stimulation of β_1 receptors include

    1. Digoxin (Lanoxin)
    2. Amrinone (Inocor)
    3. Calcium chloride
    4. Dopamine (Inotropin)

DIRECTIONS (Questions 995 through 997): Each group of questions consists of several numbered statements followed by lettered headings. For each numbered statement, select the ONE lettered heading that is most closely associated with it. Each lettered heading may be selected once, more than once, or not at all.

995. Widening of the QRS complex, ST segment elevation, peaked T wave

996. Increased PR interval, increased QT interval, depressed ST segments, flat T wave, U wave present

997. Increased PR interval, broadened QRS complex; short QT interval

    A. Hypokalemia
    B. Hyperkalemia
    C. Hyponatremia
    D. Hypernatremia
    E. Hypercalcemia

CARDIOVASCULAR PHYSIOLOGY AND ANESTHESIA
ANSWERS, REFERENCES, AND EXPLANATIONS

915. **(C)** Antimicrobial prophylaxis is useful in preventing bacterial endocarditis in patients with valvular heart disease, prosthetic heart valves, and other cardiac abnormalities, such as mitral prolapse, when these patients undergo procedures associated with transient bacteremia. Antimicrobial agents used for prophylaxis should be directed toward streptococci, enterococci, and staphylococci. Tracheal intubation is not an indication for prophylaxis per se. Currently, the recommended antibiotic regimen for patients needing prophylaxis for bacterial endocarditis includes ampicillin, 1-2 g IV 30 minutes prior to surgery, and gentamicin, 1.5 mg/kg IV 30 minutes prior to surgery. These doses should be repeated 8 hours after the initial dose. For patients with penicillin allergy, prophylaxis should be achieved with vancomycin, 1 g IV slowly, starting one hour prior to surgery *(Gravenstein: Manual of Complications During Anesthesia, p 250).*

916. **(A)** The effects of hypothermia on cardiovascular physiology are related in part to changes in blood viscosity and rheology, fluid and electrolyte balance, and coagulation. The overall effect of hypothermia on the coagulation system is to reduce hemostasis. For example, platelets are readily sequestered reversibly in the portal circulation and at 20°C, there is almost complete sequestration of platelets. However, upon rewarming to 35°C, the platelet count returns to normal within approximately 1 hour. These platelets function normally (as measured by bleeding time) and have a normal life span *(Miller: Anesthesia, ed 4, pp 364, 1371, & 1801).*

917. **(A)** All of the choices listed in this question occur during myocardial ischemia. However, of these choices listed, presence of left ventricular wall motion abnormalities is the most sensitive indicator.

918. **(B)** The time constant is defined as capacity divided by flow. The time constant for a volatile anesthetic is determined by the capacity of a tissue to hold the anesthetic relative to the tissue blood flow. The capacity of a tissue to hold a volatile anesthetic depends both on the size of the tissue and on the affinity of the tissue for the anesthetic. The brain time constant of a volatile anesthetic can be estimated by doubling the brain:blood partition coefficient for the volatile anesthetic. For example, the time constant of halothane (brain:blood partition coefficient of 2.6) for the brain (mass of approximately 1,500 g blood flow of 750 mL/min) is approximately 5.2 minutes *(Eger: Anesthetic Update and Action, pp 85-87).*

919. **(A)** The anesthetic management of patients with congenital heart disease requires thorough knowledge of the pathophysiology of the defect. In general, congenital heart defects can be categorized into those which result in left-to-right intracardiac shunting and into those which result in right-to-left shunting. The main feature in congenital heart defects which result in right-to-left intracardiac shunting is a reduction in pulmonary blood flow and arterial hypoxemia. The more common congenital heart defects which result in right-to-left intracardiac shunting include Tetralogy of Fallot, Eisenmenger's syndrome, Ebstein's malformation of the tricuspid valve, pulmonary atresia with a ventricular septal defect, tricuspid atresia, and patent foramen ovale. Meticulous care must be taken to avoid infusion of air via intravenous solutions, since this can lead to arterial air embolism. Patients with congenital cardiac defects which result in left-to-right intracardiac shunting, such as patent ductus arteriosus, are at minimal risk for arterial air embolism, since blood flow through the shunt is primarily from the systemic vascular system to the pulmonary vascular system *(Stoelting: Anesthesia and Co-existing Disease, ed 3, pp 42-51)*.

920. **(A)** The Frank-Starling curve relates left ventricular filling pressure to left ventricular work. Left ventricular end-diastolic volume, left ventricular end-diastolic pressure, left atrial pressure, pulmonary artery occlusion pressure (and in some instances central venous pressure) can reflect left ventricular filling pressure. Left ventricular work can be represented on the y-axis by left ventricular stroke work index, stroke volume, cardiac output, cardiac index, and arterial blood pressure *(Miller: Anesthesia, ed 4, p 1670)*.

921. **(E)** Acetylcholine functions as a neurotransmitter at the skeletal muscle neuromuscular junction, intramural sympathetic and parasympathetic ganglia, the adrenal medulla, and parasympathetic end organs, such as smooth and cardiac muscle. With the exception of the sweat glands and the adrenal medulla, all postganglionic sympathetic receptors are adrenergic *(Miller: Anesthesia, ed 4, p 524)*.

922. **(D)** Torsades de Pointes is a specific type of polymorphic ventricular tachycardia in which the QT interval is prolonged in the patient's resting EKG. Prolongation of the QT interval has numerous causes which include electrolyte abnormalities, e.g., hypomagnesemia or hypokalemia or may be the result of myocardial ischemia or infarction. Most commonly, however, the QT interval is prolonged by drugs, e.g., phenothiazines, tricyclic antidepressants, amiodarone, or class Ia antidysrhythmic agents. The latter category includes procainamide, disopyramide, and quinidine. Treatment for Torsades de Pointes is aimed at reducing ventricular repolarization time. This may be carried out in a number of ways including administration of magnesium sulphate, and overdrive pacing. Defibrillation is needed if hemodynamic deterioration occurs before successful pharmacologic intervention. Patients should not be treated with any antidysrhythmic agent which further prolongs the QT interval *(Miller: Anesthesia, ed 4, pp 2547)*.

923. **(C)** Anticholinesterase drugs may have significant cholinergic side effects including sino-atrial and atrial-ventricular node slowing, bronchoconstriction, and peristalsis. There is a high incidence of transient cardiac dysrhythmias following administration of these drugs. The cardiac effects vary from clinically unimportant atrial and junctional bradydysrhythmias, ectopic ventricular foci, to clinically important dysrhythmias such as high-grade heart block including complete heart block and cardiac arrest. The rhythm strip in this question is that of a low-grade heart block with a junctional rhythm. The most appropriate treatment of this rhythm is administration of atropine *(Stoelting: Basics of Anesthesia, ed 3, p 479; Barash: Clinical Anesthesia, ed 2, p 359)*.

924. **(E)** Incorrect positioning of the aortic perfusion and venous return cannulae is the most frequent complication associated with cardiopulmonary bypass. Facial edema (e.g., bulging sclerae) may reflect obstruction to venous drainage or inadvertent angling of the bevel of the aortic perfusion cannula toward the aortic arch vessels (e.g., innominate and left carotid arteries). Incorrect positioning of the venous return cannula can occur when the cannula is inserted too far into the superior vena cava, which causes obstruction of the right innominate vein. If the venous cannula is inserted too far into the inferior vena cava, venous return from the lower regions of the body can be impaired and abdominal distention can occur. If this happens, the vena caval cannula should be withdrawn to a more proximal position and the adequacy of the venous return from the patient to the cardiopulmonary bypass machine should be confirmed. A properly positioned venous return cannula will bleed back with nonpulsatile flow when the proximal end is lowered below the patient *(Stoelting: Basics of Anesthesia, ed 3, p 270).*

925. **(B)** Transposition of the great arteries is a congenital cardiac defect which results from failure of the truncus arteriosus to rotate during organogenesis such that the aorta arises from the right ventricle and the pulmonary artery arises from the left ventricle. As a result, the left and right ventricles are not connected in series, and the pulmonary and systemic circulations function independently. This results in profound arterial hypoxemia; survival is not possible unless there is a concomitant defect which allows intermixing of blood between the two circulations. Induction of anesthesia with volatile anesthetics will be delayed because minimal portions of inhaled drugs will reach the systemic circulation. In contrast, anesthetic drugs which are administered intravenously will be distributed with minimal dilution to the brain; therefore, doses and rates of injection should be reduced in these patients *(Stoelting: Anesthesia and Co-existing Disease, ed 3, p 48).*

926. **(D)** The Fontan procedure (usually modified Fontan) is an anastomosis of the right atrial appendage to the pulmonary artery. This procedure is most frequently performed to treat congenital cardiac defects which decrease pulmonary artery blood flow (e.g., pulmonary atresia and stenosis, and tricuspid atresia). The Fontan procedure is also used to increase pulmonary blood flow when it is necessary to surgically convert the right ventricle to a systemic ventricle (e.g., hypoplastic left heart syndrome). Truncus arteriosus occurs when a single arterial trunk which overrides both ventricles (which are connected via a ventricular septal defect) gives rise to both the aorta and pulmonary artery. Surgical treatment of this defect includes banding of the right and left pulmonary arteries and enclosure of the associated ventricular septal defect *(Stoelting: Anesthesia and Co-existing Disease, ed 3, pp 46-51).*

927. **(B)** When body temperature is lowered to 30°C, total body O_2 consumption is reduced 50% *(Kaplan: Cardiac Anesthesia, ed 2, pp 12 & 916).*

928. (E) The patient described in this question has a bifascicular heart block. Right bundle branch block plus left anterior hemiblock is the most frequent type of bifascicular block, present on about 1 percent of all electrocardiograms recorded from adults. Approximately 1 to 2 percent of these patients progressed to complete atrial-ventricular heart block annually. However, although the combination of right bundle branch block plus left posterior hemiblock is infrequent, it often progresses to third-degree atrial ventricular heart block. There is no evidence that either general or regional anesthesia exacerbate progression of bifascicular heart block to third degree atrioventricular heart block. Consequently, prophylactic placement of an artificial cardiac pacemaker is not recommended prior to anesthesia for elective surgery *(Stoelting: Anesthesia and Co-existing Disease, ed 3, pp 67-68)*.

929. (C) Afterload reduction during anesthesia is beneficial in all of the conditions listed in this question except Tetralogy of Fallot. In Tetralogy of Fallot, blood is shunted through a ventricular septal defect from the pulmonary circulation to the systemic circulation because of right ventricular outflow obstruction. A decrease in systemic vascular resistance would augment this right-to-left shunt through the ventricular septal defect, which will reduce pulmonary vascular blood flow and exacerbate systemic hypoxemia *(Stoelting: Basics of Anesthesia, ed 3, pp 259-261)*.

930. (A) Protamine is a basic compound isolated from the sperm of certain fish species and is a specific antagonist of heparin. The dose of protamine is 1.3 mg for each 100 units of heparin. If protamine is administered to a patient who has not received heparin, it can bind to platelets and soluble coagulation factors, producing an anticoagulant effect. There is no evidence that protamine has negative inotropic or chronotropic properties. Some persons (e.g., diabetics taking NPH insulin) may be allergic to protamine. Hypotension may occur when protamine is administered rapidly because it induces histamine release from mast cells *(Stoelting: Pharmacology and Physiology in Anesthetic Practice, ed 2, p 470)*.

931. (D) The primary goal in the anesthetic management of patients with coronary artery disease is to maintain the balance between myocardial O_2 supply and demand. Myocardial O_2 consumption (i.e., myocardial O_2 demand) is determined by three factors: myocardial wall tension, heart rate, and myocardial contractile state. Myocardial wall tension is directly related to the end-diastolic ventricular pressure or volume (preload) and systemic vascular resistance (afterload). In general, myocardial work in the form of increased heart rate results in the greatest increase in myocardial O_2 consumption. Also, for a given increase in myocardial work, the increase in myocardial O_2 consumption is much less with volume work (preload) than with pressure work (afterload) *(Stoelting: Pharmacology and Physiology in Anesthetic Practice, ed 2, p 698)*.

932. (D) The resting membrane potential of cells depends on the maintenance of an ion gradient between the inside and outside of the cell. This potential is largely negative and can be calculated by the Nernst equation which is mathematically expressed as follows:

$$EMF = -61 \log \frac{[Na^+]_i \, [K^+]_i}{[Na^+]_o [K^+]_o},$$

where EMF is the electromotive force (mV), $[Na^+]$ and $[K^+]$ are the concentrations of sodium and potassium (mEq/L), respectively, and the subscripts i and o represent inside and outside of the cell, respectively. The toxic effects of cardiac glycosides result from inhibition of the sodium:potassium ATPase ion transport system, which leads to an increase in $[Na^+]_i$ and a reduction in $[K^+]_i$. This results in depolarization of the cell resting membrane potential and enhancement of ventricular cell automaticity (slope of phase-4 depolarization). Electrolyte abnormalities such as hypokalemia and hypomagnesemia can predispose patients to digitalis-induced dysrhythmias. Lidocaine is the drug of choice in the treatment of digitalis-induced ventricular dysrhythmias; it reduces automaticity of subsidiary cardiac pacemakers and raises the threshold for ventricular fibrillation *(Guyton: Textbook of Medical Physiology, ed 7, pp 51 & 52; Stoelting: Anesthesia and Co-existing Disease, ed 3, pp 62 & 72).*

933. **(B)** *(Barash: Clinical Anesthesia, ed 2, p 1649).*

934. **(B)** Mean arterial pressure can be calculated using the following formula

$$Map = BP_D + 1/3 \ (BP_S - BP_D),$$

where MAP (mm Hg) is the mean arterial pressure, BP_D (mm Hg) is the diastolic blood pressure, and BP_S (mm Hg) is the systolic blood pressure *(Barash: Clinical Anesthesia, ed 2, p 1005).*

935. **(A)** Amiodarone is a benzofurane derivative with a chemical structure similar to that of thyroxine, which accounts for its ability to cause either hypothyroidism or hyperthyroidism. Altered thyroid function occurs in 2% to 4% of patients when amiodarone is administered over a long period. Amiodarone prolongs the duration of the action potential of both atrial and ventricular muscle without altering the resting membrane potential. This accounts for its ability to depress sinoatrial and atrioventricular node function. Thus, amiodarone is effective pharmacologic therapy for both recurrent supraventricular and ventricular tachydysrhythmias. In patients with Wolff-Parkinson-White syndrome, amiodarone increases the refractory period of the accessory pathway. Atropine-resistant bradycardia and hypotension may occur during general anesthesia because of the significant anti-adrenergic effect of amiodarone. Should this occur, isoproterenol should be administered or a temporary artificial cardiac pacemaker should be inserted *(Stoelting: Anesthesia and Co-existing Disease, ed 3, p 62; Stoelting: Pharmacology and Physiology in Anesthetic Practice, ed 2, pp 349-351).*

936. **(C)** Systemic vascular resistance can be calculated using the following formula:

$$SVR = \frac{\overline{MAP} - CVP}{CO} \cdot 80,$$

where SVR is the systemic vascular resistance, $\overline{MAP}$ (mm Hg) is the mean arterial pressure, CVP (mm Hg) is the central venous pressure, CO (L/min) is the cardiac output, and 80 is a factor to convert Wood units to dynes-sec-cm^{-5}. The calculation of SVR from the data in this question is as follows:

$$SVR = \frac{80 - 8}{5} \cdot 80$$

$$SVR = 1,248 \ dynes\text{-}sec\text{-}cm^{-5}$$

(Miller: Anesthesia, ed 4, p 1193).

937. **(A)** Tetralogy of Fallot is the most common congenital heart defect associated with a right-to-left intracardiac shunt. This congenital defect is characterized by a tetrad of congenital cardiac anomalies, including a ventricular septal defect, an aorta which overrides the pulmonary outflow tract, obstruction of the pulmonary artery outflow tract, and right ventricular hypertrophy. The ventricular septal defect is typically large and single, an infundibular pulmonary artery stenosis is usually prominent, and the distal pulmonary artery may be hypoplastic or even absent. Although many patients with Tetralogy of Fallot have a patent ductus arteriosus, this is not included in the definition *(Stoelting: Anesthesia and Co-existing Disease, ed 3, p 42).*

938. **(A)** The etiology of hypotension can be placed into two broad categories: decreased cardiac output and/or decreased systemic vascular resistance. In this case, cardiac output is greater than normal as one often sees in early sepsis. Treatment of this hypotension should be carried out with pharmacologic agents with strong α agonist properties. Of the choices in this question, phenylephrine is the only drug which is a pure α agonist. Dopamine in high doses has strong α activity but significant ß$_1$ activity and some ß$_2$ activity as well. Norepinephrine likewise possesses strong α activity with some ß$_1$ activity. Epinephrine also possesses α activity but has significant ß$_1$ and ß$_2$ properties. Any of the aforementioned pharmacologic agents could be used to support pressure in patients with sepsis in conjunction with definitive treatment for the septic source. Because dobutamine is a pure ß$_1$ agonist, it would be an extremely poor choice for a patient with a high cardiac output in the face of a low systemic vascular resistance *(Stoelting: Pharmacology and Physiology in Anesthetic Practice, ed 2, pp 264-267).*

939. **(A)** ß-adrenergic receptors are responsible for mediating activation of the cardiovascular system, vascular and respiratory smooth muscle relaxation, renin secretion by the kidneys, and several metabolic functions, such as lipolysis, glycogenolysis and insulin secretion. ß$_1$-adrenergic receptors primarily mediate the cardiac effects (i.e., heart rate, contractility, and conduction velocity) and the release of fatty acids from adipose tissue, whereas ß$_2$-receptors primarily mediate vascular airway, and uterine smooth muscle tone and glycogenolysis. α-Adrenergic receptors mediate intestinal and urinary bladder-sphincter tone *(Stoelting: Basics of Anesthesia, ed 3, pp 33-35).*

940. **(C)** The primary goal in the anesthetic management of patients with idiopathic hypertrophic subaortic stenosis as to reduce the gradient across the left ventricular outflow obstruction. In general, drugs which increase myocardial contractility or reduce preload or afterload increase the magnitude of this obstruction. Halothane is an ideal volatile anesthetic agent for maintaining anesthesia in these patients because it is a direct myocardial depressant, but does not decrease systemic vascular resistance. Both of these characteristics are beneficial for these patients because they do not increase the magnitude of left ventricular outflow obstruction. Should hypotension develop, phenylephrine, a pure α-adrenergic receptor agonist, should be administered to increase arterial blood pressure because it increases systemic vascular resistance, thereby reducing left ventricular outflow obstruction *(Stoelting: Basics of Anesthesia, ed 3, pp 266 & 267).*

941. **(C)**   The initial treatment for hemodynamically stable ventricular tachycardia is lidocaine, 1 mg/kg, followed by lidocaine, 0.5 mg/kg, every 8 minutes until the dysrhythmia is suppressed, up to a total dose of 3 mg/kg. If lidocaine is ineffective, procainamide, 20 mg/min IV, up to a total cumulative dose of 1 g can be administered until the tachycardia is controlled. If procainamide is ineffective, electrical cardioversion should be carried out after the patient is adequately sedated *(Miller: Anesthesia, ed 4, pp 2546 & 2547; Stoelting: Basics of Anesthesia, ed 3, p 489).*

942. **(D)**   Romano-Ward syndrome is a rare congenital abnormality characterized by prolonged QT intervals on the electrocardiogram. Jervell-Lange-Nielsen (JLN) syndrome is a congenital syndrome characterized by prolonged QT intervals on the electrocardiogram in association with congenital deafness. From 0.25% to 1% of patients with congenital deafness will have JLN. An imbalance between the right and left sides of the sympathetic nervous system may play a role in the etiology of these syndromes. This imbalance can be temporarily abolished with a left stellate ganglion block, which shortens the QT intervals. If this is successful, surgical ganglionectomy may be performed as permanent treatment *(Stoelting: Anesthesia and Co-existing Disease, ed 3, p 76).*

943. **(E)**   A wide complex tachycardia of indeterminate origin may be paroxysmal supraventricular tachycardia with aberrant conduction through an accessory pathway, such as in patients with Wolff-Parkinson-White syndrome. In these situations, verapamil would decrease atrioventricular conduction through the AV node, thus allowing conduction of electrical impulses from the atria to the ventricle exclusively via the accessory pathway. This may result in exacerbation of the ventricular rate, which may lead to hemodynamic instability *(McIntyre: Textbook of Advanced Cardiac Life Support, ed 2, pp 1-38).*

944. **(B)**   In a normal heart, approximately 20% of the cardiac output is produced by the "atrial kick." In pathologic conditions, such as aortic stenosis, the "atrial kick" may contribute more substantially to cardiac output *(Miller: Anesthesia, ed 4, p 501).*

945. **(E)**   The symptoms described in this patient are consistent with a nonhemolytic transfusion reaction. These reactions usually are not serious and are either febrile or allergic in origin. Typically, these reactions result in a mild fever, and in awake patients, they result in chills, fever, headache, malaise, nausea, and non-productive cough. Less frequently, these patients may develop hypotension, chest pain, vomiting, and dyspnea. When a nonhemolytic allergic transfusion reaction is mild and not associated with fever, or any other symptoms suggestive of a serious hemolytic reaction, it is not necessary to discontinue the transfusion. Antihistamines may be administered to the patient to relieve the symptoms of the reaction. However, when fever or other signs or symptoms suggestive of a serious hemolytic transfusion reaction are present, the transfusion should be discontinued *(Miller: Anesthesia, ed 4, p 1635).*

946. **(E)**   In patients with Tetralogy of Fallot, it is important to maintain systemic vascular resistance to reduce the magnitude of the right-to-left intracardiac shunt. Therefore, induction of anesthesia in these patients is best accomplished with ketamine 3 to 4 mg/kg IM or 1 to 2 mg/kg IV. Ketamine will usually improve arterial oxygenation, which reflects increased pulmonary blood flow due to ketamine-induced increases in systemic vascular resistance *(Stoelting: Basics of Anesthesia, ed 3, pp 260 & 261).*

947. **(A)**   Mitral stenosis in adults occurs almost exclusively in those who had rheumatic fever during childhood. Mitral stenosis causes pathophysiologic changes both proximal and distal to the abnormal valve. In general, the left ventricle is "protected" or unloaded (i.e., is not exposed to excessive volume or pressure loads), which may result in intrinsic abnormalities in myocardial contractility. In contrast, proximal to the valve, a diastolic pressure gradient develops between the left atrium and left ventricle in order to force blood across the stenotic valve orifice, which results in elevated left atrial pressures and decreased left atrial compliance and function. The elevated left atrial pressures are reflected back into the pulmonary vascular system, causing an increase in pulmonary vascular resistance and eventually poor right ventricular function. The left ventricular pressure-volume loop in patients with mitral stenosis demonstrates low to normal left ventricular end-diastolic volumes and pressures, and a corresponding reduction in stroke volume *(Stoelting: Anesthesia and Co-existing Disease, ed 3, p 24).*

948. **(A)**   Ischemia of the posterior wall of the left ventricle and posterior leaflet of the mitral valve can cause prolapse of the posterior leaflet and retrograde blood flow into the left atrium during systole. This can be manifested as V (ventricular) waves on the pulmonary capillary wedge pressure tracing even before ST segment depression can be seen on the EKG *(Stoelting: Basics of Anesthesia, ed 3, p 212).*

949. **(C)**   The patient described in this question has a wide complex tachycardia of undetermined origin. Differentiation of a ventricular from a supraventricular etiology is one of the therapeutic aims. This is accomplished by administering adenosine, 6 mg intravenously over 1 to 3 seconds. A decrease in the ventricular rate with adenosine would suggest that the origin of the tachycardia is supraventricular. If adenosine has no effect on the ventricular rate, a ventricular etiology is assumed and treated with procainamide or bretylium. Differentiation between a ventricular origin and a supraventricular origin is important because it will help guide therapy *(McIntyre: Textbook of Advanced Cardiac Life Support, ed 2, pp 1-33).*

950. **(D)**   The daily production of cortisol under normal circumstances is approximately 20 mg. Under maximum stress, daily cortisol production can increase to 200 to 500 mg *(Miller: Anesthesia, ed 4, p 921; Stoelting: Anesthesia and Co-existing Disease, ed 3, p 358).*

951. **(D)**   The anesthetic management of patients with artificial cardiac pacemakers should include electrocardiographic monitoring to confirm continued function of the pulse generators as well as emergency equipment (e.g., electrical defibrillator, external converter magnet) and drugs (atropine, isoproterenol) to maintain an acceptable intrinsic heart rate if the artificial pacemaker malfunctions. Inadvertent displacement of the endocardial electrodes by catheters has not been reported when the electrodes have been in place for four weeks or more. In general, anesthetic drugs will not alter the function of artificial cardiac pacemakers. However, the stimulation thresholds for ventricular capture are not static values and can be altered by a number of physiologic events. For example, acute hypokalemia and respiratory alkalosis will increase the threshold for ventricular capture, which could result in a loss of pacing. In contrast, acute hyperkalemia and acidosis will decrease the threshold for ventricular capture, which may make the patient vulnerable to ventricular fibrillation. A decrease in the programmed rate of the pacemaker greater than 10% is a sign of battery failure. Should this occur, elective surgery should be cancelled and a thorough evaluation of the pacemaker should be undertaken *(Stoelting: Basics of Anesthesia, ed 3, p 263).*

952. **(E)**   The Fick equation can be used to calculate cardiac output (Q) if the patient's O_2 consumption ($\dot{V}O_2$), arterial O_2 content (CaO_2), and mixed venous O_2 content ($C\bar{v}O_2$) are determined. The downfalls of this type of Q measurement are threefold: 1) sampling and analysis errors in $\dot{V}O_2$, 2) changes in Q while samples are being taken, and 3) accurate determination of $\dot{V}O_2$ may be difficult because of cumbersome equipment. The Fick equation is as follows:

$$\dot{Q} = \frac{\dot{V}O_2}{(CaO_2 - C\bar{v}O_2) \cdot 10}$$

$\dot{V}O_2 = 250$ mL/min (≈ 4 mL/kg)

$CaO_2 = 1.34 \cdot$ hemoglobin concentration $\cdot SaO_2 + (0.003 \cdot P_aO_2)$
$1.34 \cdot 10$ mg/dL $\cdot 0.99$
13.3 mL O_2/dL of blood

$C\bar{v}O_2 = 1.34 \cdot$ hemoglobin concentration $\cdot S\bar{v}O_2 + (0.003 \cdot P_vO_2)$
$1.34 \cdot 10$ mg/dL $\cdot 0.60$
8.04 mL O_2/dL of blood

$$\dot{Q} = \frac{250\ mL/\text{min}}{13.3\ mL/dL - 8.04\ mL/dL) \cdot 10^*} = 250/52.6 = 4.75\ L/\text{min}$$

*The factor 10 converts O_2 content to mL O_2/L of blood (instead of mL O_2/dL of blood) *(Miller: Anesthesia, ed 4, p 1186).*

953. **(C)**   Myocardial preservation is achieved during cardiopulmonary bypass primarily by infusing cold (4°C) cardioplegia solutions containing potassium chloride 20 mEq/L. This rapidly produces hypothermia of the cardiac muscle and a flaccid myocardium. In the normal contracting muscle at 37°C, myocardial O_2 consumption is approximately 8 to 10 mL/100 g/min. This is reduced in the fibrillating heart at 22°C to approximately 2 mL/100 g/min. Myocardial O_2 consumption of the electromechanically quiescent heart at 22°C is less than 0.3 mL/100 g/min *(Stoelting: Basics of Anesthesia, ed 3, p 271).*

954. **(D)**   All of the drugs listed in this question except phenylephrine will increase the inotropic state of the myocardium, which can increase left ventricular outflow obstruction and decrease cardiac output. Phenylephrine, because it is a pure α-adrenergic receptor agonist, has minimal direct effects on myocardial contractility *(Miller: Anesthesia, ed 4, p 1776).*

955. **(A)** The classical signs and symptoms of aortic stenosis (angina, syncope, and congestive heart failure) are related primarily to an increase in left ventricular systolic pressure, which is necessary to maintain forward stroke volume. These elevated pressures cause concentric left ventricular hypertrophy. With severe disease, the left ventricular chamber becomes dilated and myocardial contractility diminishes. The primary goals in the anesthetic management of such patients undergoing noncardiac surgery are to maintain normal sinus rhythm and avoid prolonged alterations in heart rate (especially tachycardia), systemic vascular resistance, and intravascular fluid volume. Supraventricular tachycardia should be terminated promptly by electrical cardioversion in this patient because of concomitant hypotension and myocardial ischemia *(Stoelting: Anesthesia and Co-existing Disease, ed 3, pp 31 & 32).*

956. **(C)** PEEP is produced by the application of positive pressure to the exhalation valve of the mechanical ventilator at the conclusion of the expiratory phase. PEEP is often used to increase arterial oxygenation when the F_IO_2 exceeds 0.50 to reduce the hazard of O_2 toxicity. PEEP increases lung compliance and functional residual capacity by expanding previously collapsed but perfused alveoli, thus improving ventilation/perfusion matching and reducing the magnitude of the right-to-left transpulmonary shunt. There are, however, a number of potential hazards associated with the use of PEEP. These include decreased cardiac output, pulmonary barotrauma (i.e., tension pneumothorax), increased extravascular lung water, and redistribution of pulmonary blood flow. Barotrauma, such as pneumothorax, pneumomediastinum, and subcutaneous emphysema, occurs as a result of overdistention of alveoli by PEEP. Pulmonary barotrauma should be suspected when there is abrupt deterioration of arterial oxygenation and cardiovascular function during mechanical ventilation with PEEP. If barotrauma is suspected, a chest x-ray should be performed and if a tension pneumothorax is present, a chest tube should be placed in the involved chest cavity *(Stoelting: Basics of Anesthesia, ed 3, pp 461 & 462).*

957. **(C)** Resting coronary artery blood flow is approximately 80 mL/100 g/min, or approximately 3% to 5% of the cardiac output. Resting myocardial O_2 consumption is 8 to 10 mL/100 g/min, or approximately 10% of the total body consumption of O_2 *(Stoelting: Pharmacology and Physiology in Anesthetic Practice, ed 2, p 696).*

958. **(B)** Pulmonary artery rupture is a disastrous but fortunately rare complication associated with the use of pulmonary artery catheters. The hallmark of pulmonary artery rupture is hemoptysis, which may be minimal or copious. Efforts should be made to separate the lungs. This can be achieved by endobronchial intubation with a double-lumen endotracheal tube. The presence of atheromas in the pulmonary artery is not associated with an increased risk of pulmonary artery rupture. Atheromatous changes are usually minimal or absent in the middle and distal portions of the pulmonary artery (i.e., in the segments where the tip of the pulmonary artery catheter typically reside) *(Miller: Anesthesia, ed 4, p 1185; Kaplan: Cardiac Anesthesia, ed 3, pp 841 & 842).*

959. **(C)** Allergic reactions have been described in patients who have been chronically exposed to low doses of protamine or to any molecule similar to protamine. Protamine should be avoided in patients with a history of a previous anaphylactic reaction to protamine. This presents a special problem for patients who require cardiopulmonary bypass. Heparin reversal in these patients can be carried out with the drug hexadimethrine or reversal can be omitted entirely. If heparin reversal is omitted, however, several hours may be required until adequate hemostasis can be achieved, which may lead to a substantial blood loss and multiple transfusions *(Kaplan: Cardiac Anesthesia, ed 3, pp 973-978).*

960. **(B)** Twenty thousand units of heparin is equal to 200 mg. Heparin can be neutralized by administration of 1.0 mg to 1.5 mg of protamine for each mg of heparin. Protamine is a basic protein which combines to the acidic heparin molecule to produce an inactive complex which has no anticoagulant properties. The half-life of heparin is 1.5 hours at 37°C. At 25°C metabolism of heparin is minimal *(Davison: Clinical Anesthesia Procedures of the Massachusetts General Hospital, ed 4, p 352).*

961. **(E)** Unlike most organs of the body where perfusion is continuous, coronary perfusion is somewhat intermittent. It is determined by the difference in aortic pressure, and right and left ventricular pressures. During systole, left ventricular pressure increases to or above systemic arterial pressure, resulting in almost complete occlusion of the intramyocardial portions of the coronary arteries. Thus, perfusion of the left ventricular myocardium occurs almost entirely during diastole resulting in a decrease in left ventricular coronary perfusion as heart rate increases. In contrast, the right ventricle is perfused during both systole and diastole, since right ventricular pressures remain less than that of the aorta. An increase in heart rate results in a relatively shorter diastolic period *(Morgan: Clinical Anesthesiology, ed 1, p 301).*

962. **(A)** The thromboelastograph (TEG) is a viscoelastometer that measures the viscoelastic properties of blood during clot formation. The coagulation variables measured from a thromboelastogram are the 1) R value (normal value 10 to 15 minutes), which reflects the intrinsic clotting pathway, 2) MA (maximum amplitude, normal value 50 to 60 mm), which represents maximum clot strength, and 3) MA30 (i.e., the amplitude 30 minutes after the MA; normal value MA-5 mm), which represents the rate of clot destruction (i.e., fibrinolysis). The MA is determined by fibrinogen concentration, platelet count, and platelet function. The thromboelastogram depicted in the figure of this question is consistent with fibrinolysis *(Miller: Anesthesia, ed 4, pp 1218 & 1219).*

963. **(E)** At the time of collection, an anticoagulant is added to donor blood. Nonetheless, small clots will occasionally form in the units requiring filtration at the time of transfusion. A 170 micron filter is present in standard blood administration sets for this purpose. Those filters permit rapid transfusion and should be used for infusions of platelets, fresh frozen plasma, cryoprecipitate, red blood cells, and granulocyte concentrates. Albumin does not need to be administered through a 170 micron filter as it does not contain blood clots *(Questions and Answers about Transfusion Practices, ed 2, American Society of Anesthesiologists, p 24).*

964. **(B)** Adenosine in doses of 6 to 12 mg IV can be very effective in the treatment of supraventricular tachycardias including those associated with Wolff-Parkinson-White syndrome. The drug is rapidly metabolized such that it is not influenced by liver or renal dysfunction. Its effects, however, can be markedly enhanced by drugs which interfere with nucleotide metabolism such as dipyridamole. Administration of the usual dose of adenosine to a patient receiving dipyridamole may result in asystole. Methylxanthines, e.g., caffeine, theophylline, and amrinone, are competitive antagonists of this drug and doses may need to be adjusted accordingly *(Stoelting: Pharmacology & Physiology in Anesthetic Practice, ed 2, p 337).*

965. **(A)** Temperature of the thermal compartment can be measured accurately in the pulmonary artery, distal esophagus, tympanic membrane, or nasopharynx. These temperature monitoring sites are reliable, even during rapid thermal perturbations such as cardiopulmonary bypass. Other temperature sites such as oral, axillary, rectal, and urinary bladder will estimate core temperature reasonably accurately except during extreme thermal perturbations. During cardiac surgery, the temperature of the urinary bladder is usually equal to the pulmonary artery when urine flow is high. However, it may be difficult to interpret urinary bladder temperature, since it is strongly influenced by urine flow. The adequacy of rewarming following coronary artery bypass is thus best evaluated by considering both the core and urinary bladder temperatures *(Miller: Anesthesia, ed 4, pp 1365-1366).*

966. **(A)** The clinical signs and symptoms associated with aneurysms of the ascending thoracic aorta reflect extension of the aneurysm to involve the trachea, esophagus, laryngeal nerves, vessels of the aortic arch (e.g., carotid arteries), coronary arteries, and pericardium. It is therefore extremely important to evaluate the neurologic, pulmonary, and cardiovascular systems of these patients prior to surgery. The most important complication associated with these aneurysms is retrograde dissection producing acute aortic regurgitation, not mitral regurgitation *(Stoelting: Anesthesia and Co-existing Disease, ed 3, pp 113 & 114)*

967. **(B)** Flow-directed, balloon-tipped pulmonary artery catheters provide a means to directly measure right-sided heart pressures, and with application of the thermodilution technique, cardiac output. Indications for their use include the need for assessment of intravascular fluid volume and the cardiovascular response to fluid administration, evaluation of left ventricular function, calculation of systemic and pulmonary vascular resistance (which is essential information for evaluating the response of the cardiovascular system to inotropes or vasodilators), and on rare occasions, a monitoring device for subendocardial myocardial ischemia (e.g., myocardial ischemia may be manifested by V waves on the pulmonary capillary wedge pressure tracing). The combination of systemic hypotension, low cardiac output, and increased pulmonary capillary wedge pressure is suggestive of left ventricular failure or cardiac tamponade. The combination of systemic hypotension, low cardiac output, and normal pulmonary capillary wedge pressure is suggestive of right heart failure or pulmonary embolism. The combination of systemic hypotension, low cardiac output, and decreased pulmonary capillary wedge pressure is suggestive of hypovolemia *(Stoelting: Basics of Anesthesia, ed 3, pp 211-213).*

968. **(E)** Mitral stenosis is the sole valvular lesion in approximately 25% of patients with rheumatic heart disease. In general, women are affected more frequently than men. Patients usually experience a latency period of approximately 2 to 4 decades between the initial bout with rheumatic fever and the onset of symptoms. In mitral stenosis, the area of the mitral valve orifice is markedly reduced, which impairs left ventricular filling. Left atrial volume and pressure, pulmonary venous pressure, and pulmonary capillary wedge pressure are also elevated with severe stenosis. If stenosis is significant, transudation of fluid into the pulmonary interstitial space can occur, which reduces pulmonary compliance and increases the work of breathing. The goals in the anesthetic management of these patients should be to prevent rapid ventricular heart rates, minimize increases in central blood volume and pulmonary artery pressure, and avoid marked decreases in systemic vascular resistance. These patients may be more susceptible than normal individuals to the ventilatory depressant effects of sedative drugs, such as diazepam and narcotics. Marked increases in central blood volume caused by overtransfusion or the Trendelenburg position can precipitate right-sided heart failure. Because the ability to vary cardiac stroke volume is very limited, a decrease in systemic vascular resistance must be compensated for by an increase in heart rate, which may cause cardiac decompensation by reducing diastolic filling time. Factors which increase pulmonary vascular resistance, such as hypercarbia, hypoxia, acidosis, or lung hyperinflation, should be avoided. There is no evidence to suggest that the use of N_2O increases the incidence of cardiac decompensation when used for general anesthesia in these patients *(Stoelting: Basics of Anesthesia, ed 3, pp 254 & 255)*.

969. **(A)** Hemodynamically unstable cardiac dysrhythmias can result in hypoperfusion and metabolic acidosis. If metabolic acidosis is confirmed on arterial blood gases, IV sodium bicarbonate should be administered. Adverse effects associated with administration of sodium bicarbonate are well documented and include severe plasma hyperosmolality, paradoxic CSF acidosis, hypernatremia, and hypercarbia, particularly in patients who are not adequately ventilated *(Miller: Anesthesia, ed 4, p 2551)*.

970. **(B)** Hypercyanotic attacks occur in approximately 35% of children with Tetralogy of Fallot. These attacks usually occur without provocation but can be associated with episodes of excitement, such as crying or exercise. The mechanism for these attacks is not known; it is believed, however, that hypercyanotic attacks occur as a result of spasm of the infundibular cardiac muscle or a decrease in systemic vascular resistance; both will exacerbate the right-to-left intracardiac shunt. Phenylephrine, an α-adrenergic receptor agonist, is the drug of choice for treatment of hypercyanotic attacks, presumably because phenylephrine increases systemic vascular resistance, which reduces the intracardiac right-to-left shunt and improves arterial oxygenation. Propranolol is also effective presumably because it reduces spasm of the infundibular cardiac muscle *(Stoelting: Anesthesia and Co-existing Disease, ed 3, p 43)*.

971. **(A)** Hetastarch is a high molecular weight hydroxyethyl starch which belongs to a group of colloids which structurally resemble glycogen. Hetastarch is most frequently used to expand the intravascular volume in patients who are hypovolemic. Administration of hetastarch is associated with several complications including transient elevations in serum amylase, anaphylactoid reactions, and coagulopathy. The effect of hetastarch on hemostasis is dose related and thought to occur as a result of decreased procoagulants and quantitative and qualitative decrease in platelet function *(Rogers: Principles and Practice of Anesthesiology, p 933)*.

972. **(D)**   Aortic stenosis usually occurs from progressive calcification and stenosis of a congenitally abnormal (usually bicuspid) valve. When aortic stenosis occurs in association with rheumatic fever, the mitral valve is usually also affected. The most frequent clinical symptoms associated with aortic stenosis include angina, which can occur in the absence of coronary artery disease, dyspnea on exertion, and syncope. When any of these symptoms is present, life expectancy is less than 5 years. In aortic stenosis, the left ventricle must eject blood through a markedly stenotic aortic valve orifice. This results in a compensatory concentric increase in the thickness of the left-ventricular wall (with minimal change in left ventricular chamber size). With severe and chronic disease, the left ventricle chamber becomes dilated, and myocardial contractility diminishes. Hemodynamically significant disease is defined by the presence of a valvular pressure gradient greater than 50 mm Hg. Left-ventricular filling is highly dependent on atrial contractions, because of decreased left ventricular compliance. Loss of normal atrial contractions during a junctional rhythm or atrial fibrillation may produce a significant decrease in stroke volume, cardiac output, and blood pressure. An increase in heart rate reduces diastolic filling time resulting in a decrease in stroke volume and cardiac output *(Stoelting: Basics of Anesthesia, ed 3, pp 257 & 258)*.

973. **(C)**   Some form of congenital heart defect occurs in approximately 0.8% of life births. The most common congenital heart defect is a ventricular septal defect which results in a left-to-right intracardiac shunt. The result of such shunting is an increase in pulmonary blood flow, which over time leads to pulmonary hypertension, right ventricular hypertrophy, and in advanced cases, congestive heart failure. Patients with small ventricular septal defects (i.e., a pulmonary-to-systemic blood flow ratios less than 1.5:1) are typically asymptomatic. The anesthetic management of patients with ventricular septal defects is similar to that in patients with atrial septal defects. The overall goal in these patients is to maintain pulmonary blood flow so that controlled ventilation of the lungs is well tolerated. Generally speaking, drugs or events that increase arterial blood pressure and/or systemic vascular resistance should be avoided, since this would increase the magnitude of the left-to-right shunt. Conversely, a decrease in these parameters will tend to decrease the magnitude of the shunt. Hyperventilation of the lungs will cause an acute respiratory alkalosis resulting in a decrease in pulmonary vascular resistance and subsequently, an increase in the left-to-right shunt *(Stoelting: Basics of Anesthesia, ed 3, p 259)*.

974. **(A)**   Curare may increase the magnitude of the right-to-left intracardiac shunt by two mechanisms: arteriolar vasodilation secondary to the release of histamine from mast cells and sympathetic ganglionic blockade. Positive airway pressure also increases right-to-left shunting by increasing pulmonary vascular resistance. Ketamine increases systemic vascular resistance and is, therefore, a useful drug for induction and maintenance of general anesthesia in these patients *(Stoelting: Basics of Anesthesia, ed 3, pp 260 & 261)*.

975. **(C)**   The treatment and anesthetic management of patients with hypertrophic cardiomyopathy should be directed toward reducing the obstruction to left ventricular outflow. In general, left ventricular outflow obstruction is reduced by decreasing myocardial contractility and heart rate, and by increasing systemic vascular resistance. The anesthetic management of these patients should begin in the preoperative period which should focus on reducing anxiety, which increases heart rate. Administration of anticholinergics such as atropine is questionable since it may cause tachycardia *(Stoelting: Anesthesia and Co-existing Disease, ed 3, pp 99-102)*.

976. (A) There have been several large cooperative studies initiated in the 1970s to define the benefits of surgical treatment of coronary artery disease as compared with medical treatment. Additionally, these studies have provided useful information regarding the risk factors for postoperative morbidity and mortality. The variables identified by these studies to be predictive of mortality include female sex, age (mortality increases with age), preoperative congestive heart failure, left main coronary stenosis or left main coronary equivalent, unstable angina, failed angioplasty, and the need for reoperation. It is thought that smaller vessels and a higher incidence of diabetes may account for the higher mortality in females compared with men *(Thomas: Manual of Cardiac Anesthesia, ed 2, pp 277-278)*.

977. (E) Autoregulation is the intrinsic ability of a vascular system to adjust its resistance to maintain blood flow constant over a wide range of mean arterial pressures. Arterial systems which are autoregulated include the cerebral, renal, coronary, hepatic arterial, and intestinal systems, and muscle circulation *(Miller: Basics of Anesthesia, ed 3, pp 290, 301, & 333; Barash: Clinical Anesthesia, ed 2, p 1003)*.

978. (D) The internal jugular veins can be cannulated to provide intravenous access for fluid and pharmacologic therapy, to gain access to the central circulation for hemodynamic monitoring, and for administration of hypertonic solutions. Cannulation of the right internal jugular vein is preferred over the left internal jugular vein because 1) the dome of the right lung and pleura is lower than the left lung, 2) there is a straight line to the right atrium, and 3) the large thoracic duct located near the left internal jugular vein is not endangered. The usual reason for cannulation of the left internal jugular vein is the inability to cannulate the right internal jugular vein *(McIntyre: Textbook of Advanced Cardiac Life Support, ed 2, chapter 6, p 9)*.

979. (A) Prevention of perioperative myocardial ischemia is an important goal in the anesthetic management of patients with coronary artery disease. Abrupt discontinuation of oral nitrates, ß-blocking agents, and calcium channel entry blocking medications must be avoided. Continuing ß-blocking agents and calcium channel entry blocking medication has been shown to reduce the incidence and severity of tachydysrhythmias, reduce coronary artery vasospasm, and hypertension. Calcium entry blockers do not decrease MAC; however, they may potentiate the effects of muscle relaxants *(Miller: Anesthesia, ed 4, pp 25 & 1767)*.

980. (A) Prolonged QT interval syndromes predispose patients to ventricular dysrhythmias, some of which may be fatal. Acquired prolonged QT interval syndromes can occur in association with electrolyte disturbances, such as reduced concentrations of potassium, calcium, or magnesium. These electrolyte disturbances should be included in the differential diagnosis of intractable ventricular tachycardia or ventricular fibrillation. Hypernatremia is not a cause of prolonged QT interval syndromes *(Stoelting: Basics of Anesthesia, ed 3, pp 235-237; Barash: Clinical Anesthesia, ed 2, p 801; Kaplan: Cardiac Anesthesia, ed 3, p 178)*.

981. **(D)** One important goal in the anesthetic management of patients with Wolff-Parkinson-White syndrome is to avoid events and drugs which increase the activity of the sympathetic nervous system, since this will accelerate conduction of cardiac impulses from the atria via the Kent fibers (accessory pathway) to the ventricles and predispose the patient to tachydysrhythmias. For this reason, drugs such as anticholinergics, ketamine, and pancuronium, which increase sympathetic nervous system tone, should be used cautiously, if at all. General anesthesia can usually be induced safely with thiopental, benzodiazepines, or etomidate. Tracheal intubation should be performed only after the depth of anesthesia is sufficient to adequately blunt the sympathetic response to direct laryngoscopy. Vecuronium is recommended to facilitate tracheal intubation and to provide skeletal muscle paralysis during surgery, because it has minimal effects on the cardiovascular system *(Stoelting: Basics of Anesthesia, ed 3, pp 262 & 263).*

982. **(A)** Both ketamine and pancuronium have sympathomimetic properties that can cause tachycardia and hypertension. In patients with aortic stenosis, left ventricular emptying during systole and myocardial perfusion during diastole are reduced by tachycardia. Likewise, in patients with mitral stenosis, left atrial emptying into the left ventricle during diastole, and subsequently left ventricular end-diastolic volume (i.e., preload) and cardiac output are reduced by tachycardia. For these reasons, anesthetic agents and adjuvants, or events that can cause tachycardia should be avoided in patients with aortic or mitral stenosis. In patients with mitral valve prolapse, the degree of prolapse into the left atrium is increased when left-ventricular end-diastolic volume is reduced. Therefore, any anesthetic agent or event which reduces left-ventricular end-diastolic volume, such as hypovolemia (i.e., decreased preload), afterload reduction, or increased myocardial contractility, will reduce left ventricular end-diastolic volume and augment prolapse of the mitral valve leaflet. This can cause cardiac dysrhythmias and augment mitral regurgitation, which can reduce cardiac output and cause hypotension in these patients *(Stoelting: Basics of Anesthesia, ed 3, pp 254, 255, & 258).*

983. **(A)** Patients with congenital prolonged QT interval syndromes are treated with ß-adrenergic receptor antagonists or left stellate ganglion block. Other drugs that can be used include verapamil, phenytoin, primidone, or bretylium. Anesthetic management of these patients should include 1) avoidance of event or drugs that increase sympathetic nervous system activity and 2) immediate availability of equipment needed to treat life-threatening cardiac dysrhythmias *(Stoelting: Basics of Anesthesia, ed 3, p 263; Stoelting: Anesthesia and Co-existing Disease, ed 3, pp 76-77).*

984. **(A)** The approximate distances from the most frequently used insertion sites to the right atrium are shown in the table below *(Barash: Clinical Anesthesia, ed 1, p 574).*

Distances From Insertion Sites to the Right Atrium

Insertion site		Distance to Right Atrium (cm)
Internal jugular vein	Right	20
	Left	25
Antecubital vein	Right	50
	Left	55
Femoral vein		40
Subclavian vein		10

985. **(C)** The $S\overline{v}O_2$ reflects the overall ability of cardiac output to adequately meet metabolic needs, and is thus a comprehensive measure of cardiac performance. There are several factors that can influence $S\overline{v}O_2$. These factors are easily understood by rearranging the Fick equation as follows:

$$S\overline{v}O_2 = SaO_2 - \frac{\dot{V}O_2}{CO \cdot O_2 \ content}.$$

See explanation to question 106 for complete definition of O_2 content. Thus, $S\overline{v}O_2$ can be reduced by a decrease in SaO_2, CO, and [Hgb], and an increase in $\dot{V}O_2$. These factors must be accounted for when interpreting $S\overline{v}O_2$ measurements *(Miller: Anesthesia, ed 4, pp 1192 & 1193)*.

986. **(D)** The indicator dye dilution technique can be used to measure cardiac output or for the diagnosis if intracardiac shunts. The indicator dye dilution curve shown in the figure of the question is that of a normal heart. The concentration of the indicator dye (i.e., photometric absorbance) is measured as a function of time. Note that following injection of the indicator dye, there is a large concentration peak, followed by a smaller recirculation peak. The recirculation peak typically occurs approximately 10 to 20 seconds following the large concentration peak. The indicator dye dilution curve shown in figure A was obtained from a patient with a small left-to-right intracardiac shunt. Note that the recirculation peak occurs earlier than normal. In patients with right-to-left intracardiac shunts (Figure B), the indicator dye dilution curve is characterized by an early small initial peak followed by a larger recirculation peak *(Miller: Anesthesia, ed 4, pp 1186 & 1187)*.

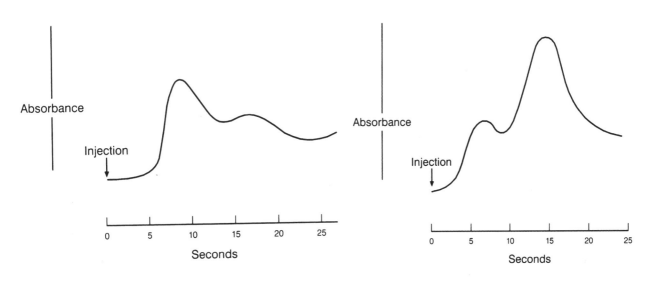

Figure A   **Figure B**

987. **(E)** Primary "idiopathic" pulmonary hypertension is pulmonary hypertension caused by an undetermined etiology. The characteristic features of primary pulmonary hypertension are hypoxia, as well as increased PVR, pulmonary artery pressure, and right ventricular pressure, and in severe cases, right ventricular failure and death. The mainstay of medical therapy for patients with primary pulmonary hypertension is prophylactic anticoagulation (to reduce the likelihood of pulmonary embolism) and vasodilator therapy. The primary objective of vasodilator therapy in these patients is to reduce PVR (afterload) and, concomitantly, right ventricular work. This would reduce pulmonary artery pressures and improve right ventricular failure, cardiac output, and pulmonary gas exchange. Vasodilation can be achieved with α-adrenergic receptor antagonists, such as tolazoline, phentolamine, and prazosin, ß-adrenergic receptor agonists, such as isoproterenol and terbutaline, and direct-acting vasodilators, such as hydralazine, nitroprusside, and nitroglycerin. Other pharmacologic agents that have proven useful in reducing pulmonary vascular resistance include prostaglandins (prostacyclin and prostaglandin E_1) and cyclo-oxygenase inhibitors, such as indomethacin *(Kaplan: Cardiac Anesthesia, ed 3, pp 839 & 840)*.

988. **(A)** Intraventricular conduction disturbances are classified into left bundle-branch block, right bundle-branch block, or hemiblock. Each of these conduction disturbances can occur alone or in any combination. Left bundle-branch block is the most serious of these conduction disturbances since it is always associated with significant cardiac disease. Right bundle-branch block is usually of no clinical significance or may occur in association with chronic lung disease or atrial septal defects. Right bundle-branch block associated with a hemiblock of the left intraventricular conduction system may be serious. Right bundle-branch block with left posterior hemiblock can progress to complete heart block. In contrast, right bundle-branch block with left anterior hemiblock progresses to complete heart block only 10% of the time *(Miller: Anesthesia, ed 4, pp 1245-1248)*.

989. **(D)** There are two basic types of oxygenators commonly used for cardiopulmonary bypass, i.e. bubble oxygenators and membrane oxygenators. In general, bubble oxygenators are easier to use and less expensive and less complex than are membrane oxygenators. In addition, bubble oxygenators require a lower priming volume than do membrane oxygenators. However, the turbulence created by gas bubbling in blood causes hemolysis of erythrocytes. This disadvantage is most significant with prolonged cardiopulmonary bypass (i.e., >90-100 minutes). Membrane oxygenators are preferable when prolonged cardiopulmonary bypass is anticipated *(Miller: Anesthesia, ed 4, p 1791)*.

990. **(C)** There are many factors that affect pacemaker thresholds. Some raise the pacemaker threshold, i.e., make it more difficult to pace while others decrease the pacemaker threshold, i.e., make it easier to pace. Some changes are easily understood on the basis of physiology. For example, the effect of acute electrolyte changes on the membrane potential can be calculated using the modified Nernst equation. Other changes can be explained on the basis of myopotentials. For example, non-rate responsive generators may interpret myopotentials coming from muscle mass in the vicinity of the heart as electrical cardiac activity and inhibit pacing. Such myopotentials could theoretically be caused by a dose of succinylcholine or shivering postoperatively. Stress is associated with a decrease in the pacemaker threshold while sleep and rest are associated with an increase. Hypoxia causes an increase in the pacemaker threshold whereas hypocarbia causes a decrease. Toxic doses of procainamide may cause an increase in pacemaker threshold *(Thomas: Manual of Cardiac Anesthesia, ed 2, p 383)*.

Factors Affecting Pacemaker Thresholds

Drug or Event	Pacemaker Threshold Changes
Rest and sleep	↑
Stress	↓
Glucose	↑
HCO_3^-	NC
P_aO_2	↓ with ↑ P_aO_2
	↑ with ↓ P_aO_2
P_aCO_2	↓ with ↓ P_aO_2
	↑ with ↑ P_aCO_2
K^+	↓ with ↑ serum K (see text)
	↑ with ↓ serum K (see text)
Na^+	↑ with 3% NaCl infusion
Sympathomimetics	
Ephedrine 25 mg q 6 hr	↓
Isoproterenol low-dose	↓
Isoproterenol high-dose	↑
ß-Blockers	↑, no effect is sleep or rest
Procainamide	↑ if toxic dose
Quinidine	? probably like procainamide
Digoxin	↓ acutely ?, but clinically NC
Glucocorticoid	↓
Mineralocorticoid	↑

Abbreviations and symbols: ↑ = increase (more difficult to pace); ↓ = decrease (easier to pace); NC = no change

991. **(A)** The scenario described in this question is consistent with occlusion of the right coronary artery and right ventricular ischemia. The area of myocardium supplied by the right coronary artery include right atrium, right ventricle, the interatrial septum, sinoatrial node, and atrioventricular node. Consequently, occlusion of the right coronary artery can also result in a first-, second-, or third-degree heart block. If type 2 second-degree heart block or third-degree heart block occurs, a temporary transvenous pacemaker should be placed *(Stoelting: Pharmacology and Physiology in Anesthetic Practice, ed 2, p 710).*

992. **(D)** The table below summarizes the hemodynamic goals in the anesthetic management of the five most common valvular heart lesions *(Thomas: Manual of Cardiac Anesthesia, ed 2, p 89).*

Hemodynamic Goals*

	Aortic Stenosis	Mitral Stenosis**	Aortic Regurgitation	Mitral Insufficiency[†]	Tricuspid Insufficiency[‡]
Preload	↑	↑	↑	↑	-
Afterload	-/↑	-	-/↓	-/↓	-/?↓
Contractility	-	-	-	-/?↑	-/↑
Rate	Avoid extremes	↓	-/↑	-/↑	-
Rhythm	Maintain sinus	Usually AF	-	-	-
MVO_2	Potential problem	-	-	Potential problem if CAD present	-

Abbreviations: AF, atrial fibrillation; MVO_2, myocardial oxygen demand; CAD, coronary artery disease.

*With coexisting lesions, hemodynamic goals are based on the most severe lesion but often represent a "compromise" if goals are contradictory.

**Be alert for right ventricular dysfunction; control of pressure-volume relationship becomes very important.

[†]If coronary artery disease is present, the goals of a slow, small, well-perfused heart may predominate.

[‡]Usually a secondary lesion. Control of pressure-volume relationship and improving contractility may be beneficial.

993. **(E)** Calculation of cardiac output by the thermodilution technique employs the Stuart-Hamilton equation which is defined as follows:

$$Q = V_i(T_b - T_i)K/(dT_b/dt)$$

where Q is the cardiac output, V_i is the injectable volume, T_b and T_i are the body and injectable temperatures respectively, and dT_b divided by dt is the change in body temperature with time. Any condition that reduces the measured change in body temperature with time (i.e., which reflects greater dilution) is erroneously recorded as an increased cardiac output *(Thomas: Manual of Cardiac Anesthesia, ed 2, p 38).*

994. **(D)** All of the drugs listed in this question have positive inotropic properties. However, dopamine is the only drug listed that increases myocardial contractility by activating ß receptors *(Thomas: Manual of Cardiac Anesthesia, ed 2, p 326).*

995. **(B)** 996. **(A)** 997. **(E)** Cardiac pacemaker and muscle cells maintain transmembrane concentration gradients for sodium, potassium, calcium, and magnesium via energy-dependent, active transport pumps. The resting cell membrane potential depends on the maintenance of the sodium and potassium concentration gradients across the cell membrane. The intracellular threshold potential depends on the maintenance of calcium and magnesium gradients across the cell membrane. Alterations in any of these gradients can alter the electrophysiology of excitable cardiac cells, which can be detected on the ECG. With hypokalemia, the PR interval and QT interval are prolonged, the ST segment is depressed, the T wave is flat, and a U wave may be present. With hyperkalemia, the PR interval is markedly prolonged (or absent), the QRS complex is broadened, the ST segment is elevated, and the T waves are peaked. Hypercalcemia may be associated with ECG changes such as prolonged PR interval, widened QRS complex, and short QT interval. Hypocalcemia and hypomagnesemia will prolong the QT interval *(Barash: Clinical Anesthesia, ed 2, p 1162; Stoelting: Anesthesia and Co-existing Disease, ed 3, pp 321 & 332).*

REFERENCES

American Academy of Pediatrics and American Heart Association s Textbook, *Neonatal Resuscitation,* 1994.

American Society of Anesthesiologist Committee on Transfusion Medicine: *Questions and Answers About Transfusion,* ed 2, Park Ridge, American Society of Anesthesiologists, 1993.

Atrach HK: Maternal Mortality in the United States, 1979-1986, *Obstet Gynecol* 76:1055-1060, 1990.

Barash PG, Cullen BF, and Stoelting RK (eds): *Clinical Anesthesia,* ed 2, Philadelphia, J.B. Lippincott Company, 1992.

Barash PG, Cullen BF, and Stoelting RK (eds): *Clinical Anesthesia,* Philadelphia, J.B. Lippincott Company, 1989.

Berry FA (ed): *Anesthetic Management of Difficult and Routine Pediatric Patients,* ed 2, New York, Churchill Livingstone, 1990.

Brown DL (ed): *Atlas of Regional Anesthesia, Philadelphia,* W.B. Saunders Company, 1992.

Brunner JMR, Leonard PF (eds): *Electricity, Safety, and the Patient,* Chicago, Year Book Medical Publishers, Inc., 1989.

Chantigian RC: Antepartum Hemorrhage (Chapter 15) in Datta S, Ostheimer GW (eds): *Common Problems in Obstetric Anesthesia,* Chicago, Year Book Medical Publishers, Inc., pp 236-244, 1987.

Chestnut DH (ed): *Obstetric Anesthesia,* St. Louis, Mosby–Year Book, 1994.

Cemente CD (ed): *Anatomy: A Regional Atlas of the Human Body,* ed 3, Baltimore, Urban & Schwarzenberg, 1987.

Cottrell JE, Smith DS (eds): *Anesthesia and Neurosurgery,* ed 3, St. Louis, Mosby–Year Book, 1994.

Cousins MJ and Bridenbough PO (eds): *Neural Blockade in Clinical Anesthesia and Management of Pain,* ed 2, Philadelphia, J.B. Lippincott Company, 1988.

Cummins RD (ed): *Textbook of Advanced Cardiac Life Support,* ed 2, Dallas, American Heart Association, 1990.

Cummins RD (ed): *Textbook of Advanced Cardiac Life Support,* ed 1, Dallas, American Heart Association, 1994.

Davison JK, Eckhardt WF III, and Perese DA (eds): *Clinical Anesthesia Procedures of the Massachusetts General Hospital,* ed 4, Boston, Little, Brown and Company, 1993.

Eger EI: *Anesthetic Update and Action,* Baltimore, Williams & Wilkins, 1974.

Ehrenwerth J, Eisenkraft JB (eds): *Anesthesia Equipment: Principles and Applications,* St. Louis, Mosby–Year Book, 1993.

Eisenkraft JB: Potential for barotrauma or hypoventilation with the Drager AV-E ventilator, *J Clin Anesth,* 1:452-456, 1989.

Faust RJ: *Anesthesiology Review,* ed 2, New York, Churhill Livingstone, 1994.

Firestone LL, Lebowitz PW, and Cook CE (eds): *Clinical Anesthesia Procedures of the Massachusetts General Hospital,* ed 3, Boston, Little, Brown and Company, 1988.

Frigoletto JD and Umansky I: Erythroblastosis fetalis: Identificaiton, management and prevention, *Clin Perinatol,* 6: 321-331, 1979.

Gravenstein: *Manual of Complications During Anesthesia,* Philadclphia, J.B. Lippincott Company, 1991.

Gregory GA (ed): *Pediatric Anesthesia,* ed 3, New York, Churchill Livingstone, 1994.

Guyton AC (ed): *Textbook of Medical Physiology,* ed 7, Philadelphia, W.B. Saunders Co., 1986.

Kaplan JA (ed): *Cardic Anesthesia,* ed 3, New York, Grune & Stratton, Inc., 1993.

Kaplan JA (ed): *Cardic Anesthesia,* ed 2, New York, Grune & Stratton, Inc., 1993.

Michenfelder JD (ed): *Anesthesia and the Brain,* New York, Churchill Livingstone, 1988.

Miller RD (ed): *Anesthesia,* ed 4, New York, Churchill Livingstone, Inc., 1994.

Miller RD (ed): *Anesthesia,* ed 3, New York, Churchill Livingstone, Inc., 1990.

Miller RD (ed): *Anesthesia,* ed 2, New York, Churchill Livingstone, Inc., 1986.

Morgan GE, Mikhail MS (ed): *Clinical Anesthesiology,* Norwalk, Appleton & Lange, 1992.

Motoyama EK and Davis PJ (eds): *Smith's Anesthesia for Infants and Children,* ed 2, St. Louis, C.V. Mosby Company, 1990.

Raj PP: *Practical Management of Pain,* ed 2, St. Louis, Mosby–Year Book, 1992.

Rogers: *Principles and Practice of Anesthesiology,* St. Louis, Mosby–Year Book, 1993.

Scheller MS, Jones BR, and Benumof JL: The influence of fresh gas flow and inspiratory-expiratory ratio on tital volume and arterial CO2 tension in mechanically ventilated surgical patients, *J Cardiothoracic Anesth* 3:564-567, 1989.

Shnider SM, Levinson G (eds): *Anesthesia for Obstetrics,* ed 3, Baltimore, Williams & Wilkins, 1993.

Snell RS and Katz J (eds). *Clinical Anatomy for Anesthesiologists,* ed 1, San Mateo, Appleton and Lange, 1988.

Stoelting RK, Dierdorf SF, and McCammon RL (eds): *Anesthesia and Co-existing Disease,* ed 3, New York, Churchill Livingstone, Inc., 1993.

Stoelting RK, Dierdorf SF, and McCammon RL (eds): *Anesthesia and Co-existing Disease,* ed 2, New York, Churchill Livingstone, Inc., 1988.

Stoelting RK and Miller RD (eds): *Basics of Anesthesia,* ed 3, New York, Churchill Livingstone, Inc., 1994.

Stoelting RK and Miller RD (eds): *Basics of Anesthesia,* ed 2, New York, Churchill Livingstone, Inc., 1989.

Stoelting RK (ed): *Pharmacology an Pysiology in Anesthetic Practice,* ed 2, Philadelphia, J.B. Lippincott, 1991.

Thomas SJ (ed): *Manual of Cardiac Anesthesia,* ed 2, New York, Chruchill Livingstone, Inc., 1993.

Wass CT: Improving Neurology Outcome Following Cardiac Arrest, *Anesthesiology Clinics of North America,* 13:869-903, 1995.

Wedel DJ (ed): *Othopedic Anesthesia,* New York, Churchill Livingstone, 1993.

West JB (ed): *Respiratory Physiology-The Essentials,* ed 5, Baltimore, Williams & Wilkins, 1995.

West JB (ed): *Respiratory Physiology-The Essentials,* ed 4, Baltimore, Williams & Wilkins, 1990.

West JB (ed): *Respiratory Physiology-The Essentials,* ed 3, Baltimore, Williams & Wilkins, 1985.

Wood M, Wood AJJ (eds): *Drugs and Anesthesia: Pharmacology for Anesthesiologists,* ed 2, Baltimore, Williams & Wilkins, pp 240-241, 1990.

Index

A

a/A ratio (*see* Arterial-to-alveolar ratio)

Abdominal cramping, digitalis overdose and, 74, 100

Abdominal viscera, pain description in, 313, 333

Abducens nerve, retrobulbar block and, 307, 329

Acetazolamide, CSF production inhibition and, 73, 99

Acetylcholine, neurotransmitter effects, 343, 362

Acid-base disturbances, 43, 57

Acquired immunodeficiency syndrome, transfusion-associated, 149

Addison's disease, metabolic abnormalities and, 180, 207

Adenine-glucose-mannitol-sodium chloride, 155

Adrenal suppression, propofol and, 87, 115

β-Adrenergic receptor agonists, bronchial asthma and, 108

β-Adrenergic receptor blockade, labetalol and, 87, 116

α-Adrenergic receptor blockade, labetalol and, 87, 116

Adult respiratory distress syndrome, sepsis and, 156, 186

Adults, anesthetic requirements, 122, 133

Afterload reduction, 345, 364

Aging
conduction velocity in peripheral nerves, 180, 208
FEV_1 levels and, elderly compared to younger people, 43
increasing closing capacity and, 49, 63
P_aO_2 levels and, elderly compared to younger people, 43

postoperative pulmonary complications and, 172, 200

progressive kyphosis, 57

pulmonary gas exchange and, 57

scoliosis and, 57

serum albumin and, 180, 208

ventilatory response to hypercarbia and, elderly compared to younger people, 43

ventilatory volumes/capacities and, 57

vital capacity levels and, elderly compared to younger people, 43

Air embolism, 15, 34

Air flow, in obstructed tracheal, 1

Airborne bacteria, O_2 concentrations and, 10, 29

Air-oxygen dilution systems, Venturi principle mechanisms and, 6, 24

Airway anatomy, infants compared to adults, 223, 237

Airway laser surgery, igniting materials and, 16, 34

Airway obstruction, upper (*see* Upper airway obstruction)

Airway resistance, short-term abstinence from cigarette smoking and, 182, 208

Albumin
half-time in plasma, 142, 150
neonatal resuscitation and, 255, 270

Alcohol abuse, postoperative pain and, 78, 105

Aldomet (*see* α-Methyldopa)

Alkaline phosphatase, plasma concentration, biliary obstruction and, 159, 189

Allodynia, reflex sympathetic dystrophy and, 306, 328

Altitude, high
CO_2 absorber functioning and, 18, 36
gas flow and, 14, 33

Alveolar concentration of anesthetic gases, 123, 134

Alveolar concentration, minimum, 87, 116, 172, 200
decrease during pregnancy, 251, 266
decreased, during pregnancy, 255, 271
factors lowering, 127, 137
for halothane, 218, 233
hyperkalemia and, 88, 117
hypernatremia and, 88, 117
hyperthyroidism and, 88, 117
increase for volatile anesthetics, 174, 201
lidocaine and, 88, 117
lithium and, 88, 117
oil:gas partition coefficient and, 162, 192
physiologic and pharmacology factors, 201
volatile anesthetics and, 121, 132

Alveolar membrane, thickness, 48, 62

Alveolar ventilation *see* Alveolar ventilation
distribution in lungs, 45, 59
F_A/F_I ratio and, 122, 133

Alveolar washout, halothane versus enflurane, 125, 135

Alveolus, radius of, 2

Alzheimer's disease, scopolamine administration and, 162, 192

Ambulation, deep-vein thrombosis prevention after lung biopsy and, 157, 187

Amide-type local anesthetics, plasma clearance, 320, 339

Aminophylline, bronchial asthma and, 81, 108

Amiodarone, hypothyroidism and hyperthyroidism and, 346, 365

Amniotic fluid embolism diagnosing, 250, 266